The Return of the White Plague

The Return of the White Plague

Global Poverty and the 'New' Tuberculosis

Edited by

MATTHEW GANDY

and

ALIMUDDIN ZUMLA

VERSO

London • New York

First published by Verso 2003
© in the collection Verso 2003
© in individual contributions the contributors 2003
All rights reserved

1 3 5 7 9 10 8 6 4 2

Verso
UK: 6 Meard Street, London W1F 0EG
USA: 180 Varick Street, New York, NY 10014–4606
www.versobooks.com

Verso is the imprint of New Left Books

ISBN 1–85984–669–6

British Library Cataloguing in Publication Data
The return of the white plague : global poverty and the
'new' tuberculosis
1. Tuberculosis   2. Poverty
I. Gandy, Matthew   II. Zumla, Alimuddin
614.5'42

ISBN 1859846696

Library of Congress Cataloging-in-Publication Data
A catalog record for this book is available from the Library of Congress

Typeset in 10.2 on 13.6 Sabon by
SetSystems Ltd, Saffron Walden, Essex
Printed in the UK by Bath Press

Contents

Prologue: The Return of Old Diseases and the Appearance
of New Ones   1
    Richard Lewontin and Richard Levins

Introduction   7
    Matthew Gandy and Alimuddin Zumla

PART I   History and Context

1 Life without Germs: Contested Episodes in the History of
Tuberculosis   15
    Matthew Gandy

2 Immigration, Race and Geographies of Difference in the
Tuberculosis Pandemic   39
    Nicholas B. King

3 Gender and Tuberculosis: A Conceptual Framework for
Identifying Gender Inequalities   55
    Anna Thorson and Vinod K. Diwan

4 War and Disease: Some Perspectives on the Spatial and
Temporal Occurrence of Tuberculosis in Wartime   70
    Matthew Smallman-Raynor and Andrew D. Cliff

PART II   The 'New' Tuberculosis

5 The Present Global Burden of Tuberculosis   95
    Léopold Blanc and Mukund Uplekar

6   Tuberculosis and HIV Infection in Sub-Saharan Africa   112
    *Anthony D. Harries, Nicola J. Hargreaves and
    Alimuddin Zumla*

7   The Recent Tuberculosis Epidemic in New York City:
    Warning from the De-Developing World   125
    Deborah Wallace and Rodrick Wallace

8   Private Wealth and Public Squalor: The Resurgence of
    Tuberculosis in London   147
    Alistair Story and Ken Citron

9   The Social Impact of Multi-drug-resistant Tuberculosis:
    Haiti and Peru   163
    Paul Farmer and David Walton

10 *The House of the Dead* Revisited: Prisons, Tuberculosis
    and Public Health in the Former Soviet Bloc   178
    Vivien Stern

PART III   Advocacy and Action

11 Rethinking the Social Context of Illness: Interdisciplinary
    Approaches to Tuberculosis Control   195
    Christian Lienhardt, Jessica Ogden and Oumou Sow

12 Reflections on the Role of Science in Tuberculosis Control   207
    T. Mark Doherty, Martin E. Munk and Peter Andersen

13 Global Poverty and Tuberculosis: Implications for Ethics
    and Human Rights   222
    Solomon R. Benatar

    Epilogue: Politics, Science and the 'New' Tuberculosis   237
    Alimuddin Zumla and Matthew Gandy

    Notes   243

    About the Contributors   303

    Resource List   309

    Acknowledgements   312

    Index   313

PROLOGUE

The Return of Old Diseases and the Appearance of New Ones

Richard Lewontin and Richard Levins

In the 1950s, the common-sense view of public health leaders was that infectious disease had been defeated in principle and was on the way out as an important cause of sickness and mortality. Medical students were told to avoid specializing in infectious disease because it was a dying field. The Epidemiology Department at the Harvard School of Public Health specialized in cancer and heart disease.

The public health leaders were wrong. In 1961, the seventh pandemic of cholera hit Indonesia; in 1970, it reached Africa, and in the 1990s, South America. After retreating for a few years, malaria came back with a vengeance. In 1976, Legionnaire's disease appeared at a convention of the American Legion in Philadelphia. Lyme disease spread in the northeast of the USA. Cryptosporidiosis affected 400,000 people in Milwaukee. Toxic shock syndrome, chronic fatigue syndrome, Lassa fever, Ebola, Venezuela haemorrhagic fever, Bolivian haemorrhagic fever, Crimean–Congo haemorrhagic fever, Argentine haemorrhagic fever, hanta virus and, of course, AIDS, have confronted us with new diseases. And tuberculosis has increased to become the leading cause of death in many parts of the world. The doctrine of the epidemiological transition was dreadfully wrong. Infectious disease is a major public health problem everywhere.

Why were public health leaders caught so completely by surprise?

Part of the answer is that science is often wrong because we study the unknown by making believe it is like the known. Often it is, making science possible, but sometimes it is not, making science even more necessary, and surprise inevitable. Physicists in the late 1930s were lamenting the end of atomic physics. All the fundamental particles were already known – the electron, the neutron, the proton had been measured. What more could there be? Then came the neutrinos, positrons, mesons, antimatter, quarks, strings. And each time, the end was declared.

But the answer to our question demands something more than the obvious fact that science will often be wrong. Before we can explain why public health professionals were caught by surprise, we have to ask what made the idea of the epidemiological transition seem so plausible to the theorists and practitioners of health in the first place.

There were three main arguments. First, infectious disease had been declining as a cause of death in Europe and North America for nearly 150 years since the causes of mortality were first systematically recorded. Smallpox was almost gone, TB was decreasing, malaria had been driven out of Europe and the United States, polio had become a rarity, the childhood scourges of diphtheria and whooping cough were on their way out. Women were no longer dying of tetanus after giving birth. Just look ahead: the other diseases would go the same way. Second, we had ever better 'weapons' in the 'war' against disease: better laboratory tests to detect them, drugs, antibiotics and vaccines. Technology was advancing, while the germs had to rely on their only ways of responding, by mutations. Of course we were winning. Third, the whole world was developing. Soon all countries would be affluent enough to use the advanced technologies and acquire a modern health portrait.

Each of these arguments was loosely plausible, and each of them was wrong. The problem is that although they seem to be historical arguments, they completely lack an understanding of historical contingency, or of the way in which historical changes alter the conditions of future change.

First, public health professionals had too short a time horizon. If instead of counting only the last century or two they had looked at a longer period of human history they would have seen a different picture. The first confirmed eruption of plague, the Black Death, hit Europe in the time of the Emperor Justinian when the Roman Empire was in decline. The second spread in fourteenth-century Europe during the crisis of feudalism. What the relation of economic and political events was to these outbreaks is unclear, but when the historical record is more complete the causal paths are easier to follow. The great plague of northern Italy at the beginning of the seventeenth century was directly consequent on the famine and widespread movement of armies during the dynastic wars of the period. And the most devastating epidemiological event we know of accompanied the European conquest of the Americas, when a combination of disease, overwork, hunger and massacre reduced the native American population by as much as 90 per cent. The Industrial Revolution brought the dreadful diseases of the new cities that Engels wrote about in relation to Manchester.

So instead of the claim that infectious disease is in irreversible decline, we have to assert that every major change in society, population, use of the land, climate, nutrition or migration is also a public health event with its own pattern of diseases.

Waves of European conquest spread plague, smallpox and TB. Deforestation exposes us to mosquito-borne, tick-borne or rodent-carried diseases. Giant hydroelectric projects and their accompanying irrigation canals spread the snails that carry liver flukes and allow mosquitoes to breed. Monocultures of grains are mouse food, and if the owls and jaguars and snakes that eat mice are exterminated, the mouse populations erupt with their own reservoirs of diseases. New environments such as the warm, chlorinated circulating water in hotels allow Legionnaire's bacteria to multiply. It is a widespread germ, usually rare because it is a poor competitor, but it tolerates heat better than most, and can invade the larger but still microscopic protozoa to avoid chlorine. Finally, modern fine-spray showers provide the bacteria with droplets that can reach the furthest corners of our lungs.

Public health was narrow in another way: it looked only at people. But if veterinarians and plant pathologists had been consulted, new diseases would frequently have been seen in other organisms. African swine fever, mad cow disease in England, the distemper-type viruses in North Sea and Baltic mammals, the tristeza disease of citrus, the golden mosaic of beans, the leaf-yellowing syndrome of sugar cane, tomato gemini virus and the variety of diseases killing off urban trees would have made it obvious that the eradication of some diseases would not prevent the emergence of others.

The third way public health was too narrow was in its theory, in paying no real attention to evolution or the ecology of species inter-actions. Theorists of public health did not realize that parasitism is a universal aspect of evolving life. Parasites usually cannot do too well in the free soil or water and so they adapt to the special habitats of the inside of another organism. They escape competition (almost) but have to cope with the partly contradictory demands of that new environ-ment: where to get a good meal, how to avoid the body's defences, and how to find an exit and get to somebody else. The subsequent evolution of parasites responds to the internal environment, to the external conditions of transmission, and to whatever we do to cure or prevent the disease. Large populations of crops, animals or people are new opportunities for bacteria and viruses and fungi, and they keep trying.

A deep problem has been a failure to appreciate the evolutionary change that occurs in disease organisms as a direct consequence of the attempts to deal with them. In the optimistic climate of the 1950s and 1960s and beyond, public health theorists did not really consider how the bugs would react to medical practice, even though drug resistance had been reported since the late 1940s and pest managers already knew of many cases of pesticide resistance. The faith in 'magic bullet' approaches to disease control and the widespread use of military metaphors ('weapons in the war on . . .', 'attack', 'defence', 'come in for the kill . . .') made it harder to acknowledge that nature too is active, and that our treatments necessarily evoke some responses.

Finally, the expectation that 'development' would lead to worldwide prosperity and major increases in the resources applied to health improvement is a myth of classical development theory. During the Cold War, challenges to the World Bank/IMF approach to develop-ment were marginalized as communist. But in the actual world of dominance by already formed rich economies, the poor nations obvi-ously could not close the gap with the rich, and even when their total economies grew this did not mean that the mass of people prospered or that more resources were devoted to social need.

More deeply, social processes of poverty and oppression and the actual conditions of world trade were not the stuff of the 'real' science that deals with microbes and molecules. So, a cholera outbreak is seen by 'real' scientists only as the coming of cholera bacteria to lots of people. But cholera lives among the plankton along the coasts when it isn't in people. The plankton blooms when the seas get warm and when run-off from sewage and from agricultural fertilizers feeds the algae. World trade is carried in freighters that use seawater as ballast which they discharge before coming into port, along with the beasts that live in that ballast water. Small crustaceans eat the algae, fish eat the crustaceans and cholera bacteria meet the eaters of fish. If the public health system of a nation has already been gutted by structural adjustment of the economy, then the full explanation of the epidemic is, jointly, *Vibrio cholerae* and the World Bank.

So, at one level of explanation, the failure of public health theory identifies mistaken ideas and too narrow a vision. But these in turn require further explanation. The doctors who looked only at the past 150 years were educated people. Many studied the classics. They knew that history did not begin in nineteenth-century Europe. But earlier times somehow did not matter to them when they thought about health. The rapid development of capitalism had led to ideas about the unique novelty of our own time, immortalized by Henry Ford as 'history is bunk'. The doctors shared American (and, though less extreme, European) pragmatism, an impatience with theory (in this case evolution and ecology). Therefore they did not see the commonality of plants and people as species among species. Ministries of health do not talk to ministries of agriculture. Agriculture schools are rural and state-supported, their students often drawn from farming communities. Medical schools are urban and usually private, and their students come from the urban middle class. These two groups of students neither fraternize nor read the same journals. The pragmatism of both groups is reinforced by the sense of urgency to meet an immediate human need.

The development of a coherent epidemiology is thwarted by the false dichotomies that permeate the thinking of both communities: the either/ors of biological/social, physical/psychological, chance/determinism, heredity/environment, infectious/chronic and others.

One more level of explanation helps to understand the intellectual barriers that led to the epidemiological surprise. The narrowness and pragmatism of public health theory are characteristic of the dominant ways of thought under capitalism, where the individualism of economic man is a model for the autonomy and isolation of all phenomena, and where a knowledge industry turns scientific ideas into marketable commodities – precisely the magic bullets that the pharmaceutical industry sells people. The long-term history of capitalist experience encourages those ideas that are reinforced by the organizational structure and economics of the knowledge industry, thus creating the special patterns of insight and ignorance that characterize each field and make inevitable its own particular surprises.

Introduction

Matthew Gandy and Alimuddin Zumla

> The flushed appearance of many of the passers-by in the streets of London indicates to what an extent the polluted atmosphere of the capital, particularly in the workers' quarters, fosters the prevalence of consumption.
>
> Friedrich Engels, 1845[1]

> The problem of tuberculosis control is, of course, dominated by economic considerations.
>
> René and Jean Dubos, 1952[2]

> Tuberculosis was a major world health problem 50 years ago, and it is an even greater problem today.
>
> Gordon L. Snider, 1997[3]

The resurgence of disease is one of the most telling indictments of the failure of global political and economic institutions to improve the lives of ordinary people. A public health crisis has become one of the markers of a new world order alongside the growth of poverty, environmental degradation and community breakdown. In the wake of the terrorist attacks of 2001 much media attention has been devoted to the threat of biological terrorism, yet the spread of infectious diseases such as HIV/AIDS, malaria and tuberculosis presents a much more real danger to the lives of the world's poor. But what lies behind this public health catastrophe? Why does infectious disease now threaten to undermine all efforts to improve the lives of millions of people?

In the early 1970s there were still more than twenty nations with new annual case rates for tuberculosis of over 150 per 100,000 people. High-profile public health successes such as the eradication of smallpox in 1977 masked the degree to which this decade marked a watershed in global efforts to contain disease. Since 1973 over thirty new infectious diseases have been recognized including HIV, Ebola and cryptosporidiosis. Furthermore, diseases that were once considered in decline or under control such as cholera, malaria and TB have made startling comebacks, marking a fundamental reversal in many of the twentieth-century global advances in public health.[4]

The dramatic increase in the global prevalence of TB since the 1980s has brought about a stark reversal in the public health optimism of earlier decades. A disease that according to many commentators was destined for complete eradication in the 1970s has rapidly become the centre of a global public health crisis. The 'new' TB is in fact derived from a combination of different developments such as collapsing health care services, shifting patterns of poverty and inequality, the spread of HIV, and the emergence of virulent drug-resistant strains. Further, the geography of the TB pandemic defies simple categorizations: the borough of Newham in east London, for example, now has a higher rate of TB than India.

In a Western context the disease has gained political prominence through a series of high-profile outbreaks which have challenged public health complacency. In New York City during the early 1990s, for example, the deadly appearance of multi-drug-resistant TB in hospitals and prisons focused national attention on a problem that was quietly drifting out of control. And in the spring of 2001 the British TB crisis was suddenly exposed to national media attention by the discovery of a virulent strain of TB in an inner-city school in Leicester.[5]

In South Asia, sub-Saharan Africa, Latin America and elsewhere, the rapid spread of HIV threatens to precipitate a further explosion in new TB cases as bodily resistance to the disease is lowered for many millions of people. The return of TB has shattered the public health complacency that developed in the wake of the antibiotic revolution of the 1940s and 1950s. The combined effects of HIV and TB are already having catastrophic social and economic consequences in sub-Saharan Africa, yet no coherent political response has yet emerged at a regional or an international level. And the spread of virulent strains of drug-resistant TB threatens to overwhelm global efforts to secure improvements in public health.

TB is a disease caused by a small rod-shaped bacterium *Mycobacterium tuberculosis*. The commonest means of infection is through the inhalation of bacteria into the lungs. Only a small number of TB bacilli need to be inhaled for a person to become infected, yet not all infected people will go on to develop the disease. On arrival in the lungs these small numbers of bacteria are attacked by defensive cells known as alveolar macrophages which ingest and attempt to destroy the bacteria. If the macrophages succeed in this task then the infection has been successfully prevented from progressing any further. If, however, the macrophage cell cannot destroy the bacteria then they will begin to multiply and overwhelm the defensive cell. As infection progresses to the second stage the bacteria begin to infect other, immature macrophage cells. The body's immune system responds by sending additional defensive macrophage cells from the blood stream which multiply and attempt to restrict the further advance of infection. During this so-called symbiotic phase the numbers of bacteria and macrophages grow rapidly and they form a cluster within the infected tissue. At stage three of the infection the body initiates what is known as a delayed-type hypersensitivity reaction in order to kill the infected cluster of macrophage cells. The toxic chemicals emitted by the bacteria induce the human body to produce characteristic swellings or lesions. In some cases these lesions may be hidden within the lungs, or in other cases large glandular swellings may appear on the neck, armpits or groin. The human immune system reacts to the presence of clusters of TB bacteria by surrounding the pathogens with a thick waxy coat in order to prevent the spread of the disease. During stage four of the disease, newly arriving macrophages may surround the lesion and destroy any escaping bacteria so that the infection is successfully contained. These lesions serve to block off infected tissue from the rest of the body and may succeed in preventing the further advance of the disease. Over time these lesions may become encapsulated or calcified, and these 'walled-off' clusters of bacteria can lie dormant for years but may be activated if the person's immune system is damaged or weakened. The stress of war or forced migration, for example, or the debilitating effects of HIV on the body's immune system, can all play a role in the reactivation of dormant infection within the body. The breakdown of these lesions leaves a cavity and discharges infective material via the blood and lymph system to other parts of the body. This fifth and much the most dangerous stage of the disease involves the release of many millions of bacteria and may overwhelm the body's defensive mechanisms. This is also the moment at which the infection becomes highly contagious through the proliferation of bacteria in the lungs which can then be easily spread to other people through everyday activities such as coughing, sneezing, talking and spitting.[6]

The historical impact of TB mortality is indicated by the litany of well-known poets, writers and musicians who suffered from the disease. These include, amongst others, the Brontë sisters, Anton Chekhov, Frédéric Chopin, Fyodor Dostoevsky, Ralph Waldo Emerson, Johann Wolfgang von Goethe, Heinrich Heine, D. H. Lawrence, Immanuel Kant, John Keats, Katherine Mansfield, George Orwell, Jean-Jacques Rousseau, John Ruskin and Robert Louis Stevenson. 'There is no limit to human suffering,' Katherine Mansfield wrote. 'When one thinks: "Now I have touched the bottom of the sea – now I can go no deeper," one goes deeper.'[7] And John Keats, a century earlier: 'There is blood in my mouth . . . bring me a candle and let me see this blood . . . I cannot be deceived in the colour. That drop of blood is my death warrant.'[8] One of the most vivid literary descriptions of all is provided by Charles Dickens:

> There is a dread disease which so prepares its victims, as it were, for death; which so refines it of its grosser aspect, and throws around familiar looks, unearthly indications of the coming change – a dread disease, in which the struggle between soul and body is so gradual, quiet, and solemn, and the result so sure, that day by day, and grain by grain, the mortal part wastes and withers away, so that the spirit grows light and sanguine with its lightening load, and, feeling immortality at hand, deems it but a new term of mortal life – a disease in which death takes the glow and hue of life, and life the gaunt and grisly form of death.[9]

In its commonest form TB is marked by a gradual destruction of the lungs leading, if untreated, to increasing incapacity and death. In addition to breathlessness and coughing the symptoms may include fever, malaise, weight loss, anaemia, the disruption of metabolic functions and psychological disturbances. Before the spread of HIV some 85 per cent of reported cases of TB were limited to infection of the lungs with the remaining cases involving the infection of other parts of the body. In addition to pulmonary TB the disease may affect the brain, the bones, the skin, the lymph nodes, the genitals or any part of the body as the bacteria eat away at human tissue. People whose bones have become infected may experience a deterioration in skeletal strength and the twisting or deformation of the spine. Infection of the brain may result in tubercular meningitis, whereas glandular swellings associated with TB have been historically referred to as 'scrofula'. With the spread of HIV infection the incidence of non-pulmonary TB has become more widespread which has further complicated the recognition and treatment of the disease and its interaction with other factors such as poverty, malnutrition and access to adequate medical care. Since about one third of the world's adult population are already infected with TB the potential consequences of the interaction of TB with HIV infection, poverty and other factors are immediately apparent. Yet there has been insufficient dialogue between different branches of scientific expertise, which has led to an intellectual hiatus between the small-scale focus of bio-medical interventions and disease epidemiology's focus on the wider structural factors.[10]

The centrepiece of recent global efforts to control TB has been the directly observed therapy, short-course (DOTS) programme initiated by the World Health Organization in the early 1990s. The core of the DOTS strategy is to ensure universal access to properly trained medical staff and a regular supply of drugs which are free at the point of delivery. Though the DOTS programme has certainly made an impact on the problem it can provide only part of the solution to a multi-faceted public health crisis that is driven by an array of different social, economic and political factors.[11] The role of the World Health Organization and other international agencies is crucial to the success of global efforts to eradicate infectious disease, yet their scientific remit and political constraints place them largely outside the crucial arenas of political and economic decision making that will determine the long-term outcome of this humanitarian crisis.

This book provides a survey of current thought on the spread and control of TB. It is international in scope and aims to foster dialogue between a range of different disciplines. All the contributors share the view that the current situation is serious, that current public health strategies are insufficient to meet the scale of the challenge, and that the prevalence of TB remains inextricably linked to wider factors such as poverty and social exclusion. Yet this apparent consensus masks a series of important tensions between the chapters over themes such as the potential role of new drugs and vaccines, the role of gender differences in the experience of illness, the relative significance of TB resistance in accounting for the changing dynamics of disease epidemiology, and the effectiveness of recent global efforts to control the disease under various programmes directed by the World Health Organization and other international agencies.

The book is divided into three parts. In Part I we review historical and conceptual dimensions to the impact of TB on human societies. The roles and significance of race, gender and class are examined to trace the social and political context for the control of TB. The complexity of TB epidemiology is illustrated through historical themes such as the effects of war, the development of institutional responses to disease and rival explanations for the decline of TB since the middle decades of the nineteenth century. In Part II we address the contemporary TB pandemic. Critical dimensions to the current crisis such as the impact of HIV infection and the spread of drug-resistant TB strains are examined. We trace the advance of the disease not only through the developing world but also in the affluent global cities of London and New York. In Part III we present a critical forum of views from medical and health care professionals to highlight the connections between our understanding of TB and the implications for health policy.

PART I

History and Context

1

Life without Germs:
Contested Episodes in the History
of Tuberculosis

Matthew Gandy

The understanding and control of tuberculosis is one of the most significant chapters in the history of humankind. In a detailed chronology of the disease from classical times until the twentieth century the Italian historian Arturo Castiglioni remarked on 'the marvelous progress from demonism to bacteriology'.[1] For Castiglioni, writing in 1933, the science of bacteriology marked a decisive advance in the progressive development of Western civilization. The decline of TB was a marker on a path towards a better future in which rational knowledge would prevail over the ignorance, superstition and neglect of the past. Yet Castiglioni's faith in the centrality of science to the eradication of disease masks the full complexity of the epidemiology of TB. The rapid decline of the disease from the middle decades of the nineteenth century, before the disease was fully understood, and its more recent resurgence point to an array of social, economic and political developments beyond the confines of the laboratory.

Few other diseases have caused human suffering on the scale of TB. The classical medical scholar Hippocrates (460–370 BCE) considered 'phthisis', or pulmonary TB as it is now known, to be the 'greatest and most terrible disease'.[2] A combination of historical and archaeological evidence shows that TB was widespread in early Hindu, Greek and Roman societies, and gradually spread for over 2,000 years.[3] By the early nineteenth century the 'White Plague' had become the principal cause of death in much of Europe and North America and it is estimated that the prevalence of TB infection neared 100 per cent in rapidly growing cities such as London and Paris.[4]

The history of TB is complicated, however, by the diversity of manifestations of the disease and the absence of definitive data before the introduction of mass screening in the late nineteenth century using the bacterial culture tuberculin and X-ray photography.[5] In 1726, for instance, the English physician Richard Blackmore was unable to clearly distinguish 'scrophulous tumours' from other 'Morbifick viscous coagulations'. 'So immense is the variety of Knots and Tumours to which all Parts of the Body, External and Internal, are obnoxious,' Blackmore wrote, 'that to reduce them to their proper Classes and assign the Limitations and essential Boundaries that discriminate and divide them, seems impracticable.'[6] Other manifestions of the disease in addition to 'scrofula' (glandular TB) include infections of the spine (widely referred to as 'gibbus' or 'Pott's disease'), infections of the skin (known as 'lupus') and infections of the brain. The disease can affect almost any part of the body and produce a variety of symptoms, which have often caused it to be confused with bronchitis, typhoid or a variety of other illnesses.[7] Indeed, the powerful stigma surrounding the diagnosis of TB, and its long-standing hereditarian associations, has fostered a degree of confusion and uncertainty concerning many medical records in the pre-bacteriological era before the advent of compulsory notification and the widespread adoption of other modern public health measures.

For much of medical history, TB proved not only difficult to classify but also mysterious in its apparently indiscriminate prevalence. During the nineteenth century we find a variety of different explanations for TB. In addition to hereditary and 'constitutional' causes, for example, the English physician Sir James Clark, writing in 1837, lists 'improper diet, impure air, deficient exercise, excessive labour, imperfect clothing, want of cleanliness, abuse of spiritous liquors, mental causes and contagion'. Clark despaired at the 'total inefficacy of all means hitherto adopted for diminishing the frequency or reducing the mortality of this class of diseases'.[8] The American physician William Beach, writing in 1840, dismissed the notion that TB might be contagious and chose to emphasize 'hereditary disposition' marked by features such as 'prominent shoulders' or a 'narrow chest'. Like many of his contemporaries Beach suggested travel as the only alternative for patients who had not responded to 'proper medicine'. 'It is well known,' Beach wrote, 'that warm climates have considerable influence in removing tubercles from the Lung, by the genial and uniform temperature imparted, hence the

Brazils, and West India climate, have sometimes benefited, when other means have failed'.[9]

The diversity of nineteenth-century perspectives on the disease belied the fact that medical science could offer no satisfactory explanation or cure. In 1868, for example, the founder of modern cellular pathology, Rudolf Virchov, considered TB to be a kind of tumour and fiercely rejected the newly emerging contagion theories developed by the French surgeon Jean-Antoine Villemin.[10] Villemin had succeeded in infecting animals with TB under laboratory conditions and presented a direct challenge to the prevailing 'hereditarian' consensus in northern Europe. In fact, modern theories of contagion can be traced to the Veronese physician Gerolamo Fracastoro (1483–1553) who warned against the 'seeds of contagion' lingering in the rooms and belongings of phthsis sufferers.[11] Fracastoro's views proved influential in Italy but failed to make much impact in northern Europe where hereditary and 'constitutional' explanations prevailed. Theories of contagion held implications for the responsibilities of municipal government which conflicted with the narrowly perceived self-interest of political and economic elites. In eighteenth-century Italy, for example, legislative measures to ensure the disinfection of infected homes in Lucca, Florence, Naples and Venice were short-lived in the face of opposition on the grounds of cost.[12]

In the last two decades of the nineteenth century the contagion theories developed by Fracastoro and Villemin were radically advanced by the emerging science of bacteriology which could now identify the role of microbial pathogens in the spread of disease. The discovery of the TB bacterium by the Prussian bacteriologist Robert Koch in 1882 marked a decisive shift in the balance of the epidemiological debate: Koch declared that in the 'battle with this horrible plague . . . we are no longer dealing with an indefinable Something, but with a definite parasite whose vital processes are, for the most part, known, and which can be studied further'.[13] Yet even after Koch's discovery of the TB bacterium, alternative theories of hereditary or 'constitutional' transmission persisted for many years. And Koch was himself the subject of fierce criticism for disputing the significance of bovine TB in transmitting the disease to humans through infected milk.[14] In fact the history of TB was marked from the outset by rival bodies of medical thought rooted in alternative explanations for the transmission of the disease. The gradual acceptance of various 'germ theories' undermined

the moralistic discourses of nineteenth-century medicine and strength-
ened the political salience of the public health movement. Yet by the
middle decades of the twentieth century the recognition that TB was a
social disease rooted in poverty and poor housing became gradually
obscured by an emphasis on the success of new forms of biomedical
intervention. The discovery of relatively cheap and individualized
courses of antibiotic treatment such as streptomycin and isoniazid
succeeded in virtually eliminating the disease from more affluent societies but also served to shift attention away from the structural factors
that had contributed towards the spread of the disease in the past.

This chapter continues with an exploration of the intersections
between Romanticism, anti-urban sentiment and the development of
the sanatoria movement in the pre-bacteriological era. My starting
point is the nineteenth century, which marks a transition between the
aestheticization of tubercular mortality and an emerging recognition of
the contagious nature of the disease. I turn next to the debate surrounding the McKeown thesis and rival explanations for the widespread
decline of TB in the second half of the nineteenth century. My focus
then moves to the twentieth century in order to evaluate explanations
for persistent regional and social disparities in the incidence of TB.
Evolving interpretations of the relations between race, class and disease
reveal how hereditarian views became reconfigured within a racialized
topography of illness. I conclude with an examination of the global
resurgence of TB since the early 1980s, and suggest that the success of
TB eradication programmes during the 1950s and 1960s in the developed world served to deflect attention from the global scale and
political complexity of the problem. The return of TB has undermined
this earlier wave of scientific optimism and fostered a renewed recognition of the connection between disease and poverty.

Romanticism, anti-urbanism and the sanatoria movement

During the modern era, TB became widely perceived as 'a disease of
humid and dank cities'.[15] Ever-greater numbers of people were
crowded into dilapidated and makeshift housing in the rapidly growing
cities of Europe and North America, and those who could find work
were widely subjected to dusty, confined or physically exhausting
working conditions in the textile, metalworking and other industries

which contributed towards a greater susceptibility of infection.[16] Yet the absence of any clear understanding of the epidemiology of the disease led to a generalized indictment of urban life rather than any systematic analysis of the changing living and working conditions that placed many people at much greater risk than hitherto of contracting respiratory diseases. As the literary critic Susan Sontag observes:

> When travel to a better climate was invented as a treatment for TB in the early nineteenth century, the most contradictory destinations were proposed. The south, mountains, deserts, islands – their very diversity suggests what they have in common: the rejection of the city.[17]

The association between TB and urban living conditions fed into long-standing medical discourses surrounding climate and pulmonary TB. From Hippocrates onwards many physicians had recommended changes in climate to alleviate the symptoms of consumption as a form of 'physiological therapy'.[18] Consequently, wealthier sufferers sought to leave cities in search of warm and dry climates where they might alleviate their symptoms.[19] Hereditarian and 'constitutional' conceptions of TB had allowed dual cultures of disease to emerge: for the poor TB was a disaster, yet for the rich the illness was transformed into an intense personal experience.[20] The nineteenth-century internalization of TB as, for wealthy sufferers, a disease of the self rests on an interplay between Romantic anti-urbanism and pre-bacteriological epidemiology. Romantic depictions of pulmonary TB contributed towards the aestheticization of death and at the same time emphasized the unique individual sensitivities of the tubercular self in a grotesque parody of the enhanced social and cultural subjectivity of the Enlightenment. The literary Romantic movement, which was especially influential between 1760 and 1830, sought to transform the moral stigma of the TB death into a profound experience of individual sensitivity 'which dissolved the gross body, etherealized the personality, expanded consciousness'.[21] The disappearance or 'consuming' of the body became a metaphor for spiritual transcendence, in contrast to the widespread revulsion associated with pulmonary TB by earlier scholars and physicians.[22] The 'consumptive' lover dying as a consequence of rejection is a recurring cultural trope in Romantic literature which served to trivialize the suffering associated with the disease.[23] The actual death from TB of leading figures within the Romantic movement such as the poets Novalis (1801), Ernst Schulze (1817) and John Keats (1821) intensified the association between artistic genius and consumption, thereby separating the experience of illness (and creativity) from any wider social context. TB became associated with a heightened state of creativity in the shortened lives of poets and artists (a creativity believed by contemporaries to be caused by the intoxicating effects of the illness) yet widespread opiate addiction among wealthy sufferers is a more plausible explanation for this 'mental effervescence'.[24]

The search for a climatic cure fostered the development of specialized institutions devoted to the treatment of TB. The first of these sanatoria were private health institutions, catering for the wealthier classes, which originated in Germany in the late 1850s and early 1860s. The commercial success of Hermann Brehmer and other pioneers of this new treatment soon attracted international attention. The construction of sanatoria across Europe and North America formed part of a wider reaction against the insalubrity of modern cities and was closely allied with the back-to-nature movements that emerged in nineteenth-century Europe and North America with their emphasis on forests, mountains and open-air pursuits. A second phase of development occured in the early twentieth century with the widespread construction of public sanatoria in Europe, North America and elsewhere, as the state played a much more active role in the eradication of TB.[25] The sanatoria evolved into elaborate institutions where patients, of whom an increasing number were working class, undertook a combination of rest and exercise aimed at eliminating infection and building up bodily defences. Though sanatoria had originally emerged as a kind of 'safe haven' from the urban and industrial chaos of the nineteenth century they gradually became an extension of urban modernity itself through their adoption of the modernist principles of 'hygienist' urban design.[26] Esoteric treatments such as heliotherapy (sunbathing) formed part of a wider aim to reconnect mind, body and nature in a new mode of modern living.[27] With the rapid growth of the sanatoria movement the promotion of rigorous treatment regimes replaced the original emphasis on specific locations such as islands and mountains. The spread of institutionalized treatment 'swept the pine trees from the path' and challenged the therapeutic role of climate.[28]

Reports of patient improvement lent a perceived scientific rationale to the burgeoning sanatoria movement but such claims remained controversial. 'These albums of cured cases,' the physician Pierre

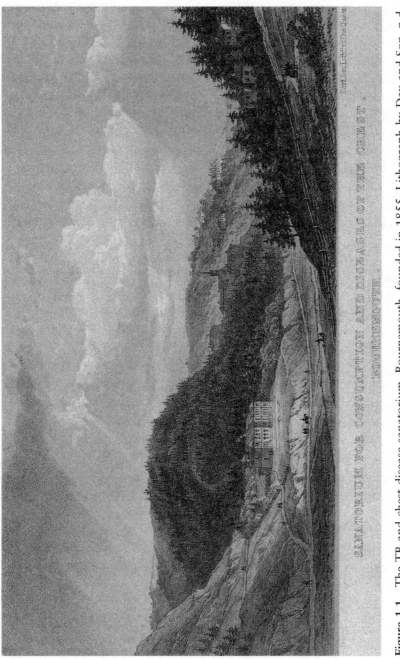

SANATORIUM FOR CONSUMPTION AND DISEASES OF THE CHEST,
BOURNEMOUTH.

Day & Son, Lith.rs to The Queen

Figure 1.1 The TB and chest disease sanatorium, Bournemouth, founded in 1855. Lithograph by Day and Son, n.d. Source: Wellcome Library for the History and Understanding of Medicine, London.

Hulliger mocked, 'have no scientific value: they are advertising results.'[29] By the 1930s a wide-ranging critique of sanatoria began to emerge based on their limited impact on the wider health problem, the unreliability of their medical records and the absence of any effective aftercare. Most critically, the provision of expensive and ineffective sanatoria treatment diverted attention and, more important, resources away from the more radical prescriptions that might have had any real impact on the disease.[30]

The second phase of the sanatoria movement grew out of the radical disjuncture in the experience of TB in nineteenth-century Europe and North America. Nineteenth-century conceptions of TB reworked existing disease metaphors within a specific historical and cultural context derived from the Romantic reaction to rapid urbanization. Yet by the late nineteenth century the 'perverted sentimentalism' of the past had been replaced by a renewed sense of fear and disgust.[31] No longer a 'romantic affliction', the disease was now unambiguously perceived by middle-class commentators as a menacing and disgusting stigma of poverty. In 1912, for example, the British physician de Carle Woodcock described TB as 'in truth a coarse, common disease, bred in foul breath, in dirt, in squalor. . . . The beautiful and the rich receive it from the unbeautiful poor. . . . The scrofula which deforms the already coarsened features of the stunted slum dweller is tubercle.'[32]

The development of the modern sanatorium reflected a shift in prevailing conceptions of TB from a constitutional affliction to be countered with a 'change of air' towards a contagionist emphasis on the eradication of disease through a programme of institutional segregation and intervention. Yet even when bacteriological insights into the disease began to be accepted in mainstream medical opinion, the idea that the disease was associated with specific categories of people continued to suffuse scientific and political debate.[33] The fatalistic spectre of 'tubercular urbanism' would blight the lives of the urban poor for many decades after the first tentative steps towards public health reform. And in much of the developing world the impact of TB was yet to be fully experienced.

Social reform, the McKeown thesis and the epidemiological transition

Evidence from Europe and North America suggests that TB was in widespread decline from the middle decades of the nineteenth century onwards, before the introduction of any systematic attempts to prevent its spread (see Figure 1.2). This significant time lapse between the recorded decline of TB and coordinated control efforts is one of the most contentious themes in the history of disease: it forms the basis of the historian Thomas McKeown's influential view that TB and other infectious diseases declined as a by-product of wider social and economic advances rather than as a result of any specific medical interventions.[34] The core of the so-called 'McKeown thesis' is a rejection of the role of physicians, scientists and hospital administrators in the decline in morbidity and mortality – the so-called epidemiological

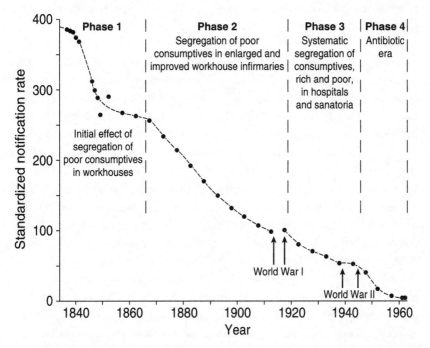

Figure 1.2 The historical decline in TB, 1840 to 1960. Source: Data derived from various sources including Thomas McKeown, *The Modern Rise of Population*, London: Edward Arnold 1976.

transition – that occurred during the second half of the nineteenth century:

> The history of TB illustrates, perhaps better than that of any other infection, a general point about the contribution of therapy. Effective clinical intervention came late in the history of the disease, and over the whole period of its decline the effect was small in relation to that of other influences.[35]

The principal flaw with McKeown's argument, however, is that the decline in TB mortality is difficult to attribute simply to improved nutrition or higher standards of living. Whilst McKeown is right to be sceptical about some of the claims of physicians, scientists and the 'heroic' genre of medical history, he overlooks the significance of wider public health reforms. Alternative perspectives on the history of disease have emphasized the critical importance of institutional and legislative change fostered by the political salience of the public health movement.[36] An emphasis on public health advocacy reveals the significance of specific measures aimed against TB such as effective patient segregation, housing improvements and the control of bovine TB.[37] The historian Leonard Wilson, for example, contests the McKeown thesis by emphasizing the role of segregation for infective TB patients. He points to the growing role of workhouse infirmaries, hospitals and other institutions during the nineteenth century using evidence from Britain, Prussia and the USA. From the late 1840s onwards, for instance, before the infectivity of the disease was understood, British workhouses admitted ever greater numbers of consumptive patients: the issue then, in the pre-bacteriological era, is not the effectiveness of treatment but the impact of containment on rates of infection.[38] Yet Wilson's emphasis on segregation does not fully explain why a higher proportion of those infected with TB, the majority of the population at the time, did not go on to develop the full symptoms of the disease. It is this complex relationship between infection, resistance and illness that fuels rival interpretations of the epidemiological transition in nineteenth-century Europe and North America.[39] The 'nutritionists', who adhere to the McKeown thesis, emphasize general improvements in resistance, whereas the 'contagionists' point to reduced sources of infection.

The uneven social and geographical incidence of the disease also works against any generalized mode of explanation. In France, for

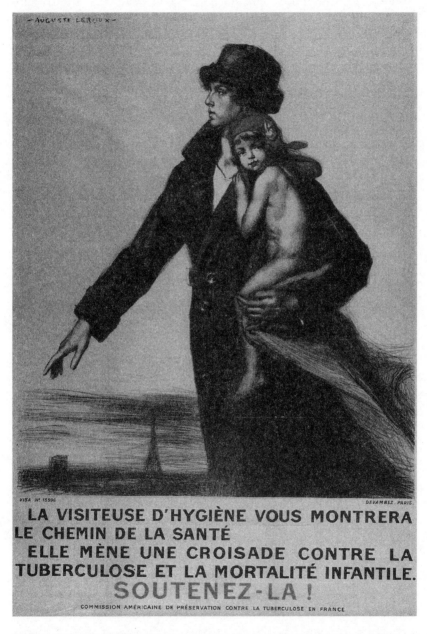

Figure 1.3 A health visitor promoting a campaign against TB and infant mortality. Colour process print by Auguste Leroux, 1918. Source: Wellcome Library for the History and Understanding of Medicine, London.

instance, high mortality rates for TB, almost double those of Britain and Germany, persisted well into the twentieth century. 'France has a death rate from TB that is especially unfavourable,' observed Robert Koch in 1910; '. . . there can be no question of a general, regular, uniform decrease in mortality from consumption'.[40] Koch's analysis of the prevalence of TB in early-twentieth-century European cities showed that it was far higher in Paris than in Hamburg, Copenhagen or London. The historian Allan Mitchell has amplified these observations by showing that these regional and national differences are not explained by stark variations in general welfare and nutrition; instead, he attributes them to the failure of the French authorities to implement the kind of local sanitary measures and national health reforms that were being pursued in Britain and Germany. As Mitchell notes of early-twentieth-century France, 'The construction of inexpensive public housing (*habitations à bon marché*), still left in private hands, had scarcely begun to alleviate wretched conditions in the "dark spots" (*îlots noirs*) of French cities'.[41] In an interesting defence of the Mc-Keown thesis, however, the historian David Barnes refutes the accuracy of available mortality data for late-nineteenth-century France. Barnes uses local rather than national data to question the argument made by Mitchell and others that levels of TB in France continued to increase at a time of falling rates in Britain and Germany. Barnes also suggests that French workers had a lower standard of living compared with Britain and Germany which may have limited their resistance to infection and hence led to the observed disparities in TB mortality. He emphasizes the role of workplace reform rather than municipal public health measures in order to provide a wider historical interpretation of the political dynamics of mortality decline in nineteenth-century Europe.[42] Thus the French case is especially interesting for the historiography of TB because it offers contradictory interpretations of the relationship between disease epidemiology and different aspects of social reform.

It appears that the McKeown thesis can be interpreted in two radically different ways. On the one hand the emphasis on general social and economic improvements behind the epidemiological transition can be perceived as a pretext to dismiss the role of medical science in large-scale improvements in human health. Robert Koch, for example, was quick to point out that the decline in TB since the middle of the nineteenth century could not be attributed to improved methods of treatment.[43] On the other hand the scepticism towards the role of the medical sciences can be interpreted as an argument for structural reform in preference to a reliance on clinical intervention.[44] Here again, the observations of Koch are germane to contemporary debate. Koch contended that two critical factors explained the sharp variations in the incidence of the disease: the construction of hospital facilities and improvements in housing. Hospital facilities played a crucial role in segregating infective patients from the general population, and better housing reduced levels of overcrowding and infection within the home. Using the most detailed data available Koch was able to show that the relative increase in rates of infection in early-twentieth-century Norway, for instance, could be attributed to inadequate hospital provision. He also suggested that regional variations in the disease across northern Europe could be influenced by differences in housing design such as the use of cramped sleeping rooms or *Butzen*. Similar observations have been made in Britain where general improvements in TB mortality during the first half of the twentieth century mask stark regional disparities driven at least in part by differences in housing design. The overcrowded tenements of Glasgow, for example, saw rates of TB peak in 1949 despite forty years of attempts to control the disease.[45]

The generalized decline in TB since the middle decades of the nineteenth century – which began first in Britain, Germany and Belgium and occurred at a later stage in France, Ireland, Norway and elsewhere – cannot, then, be attributed to only one factor. If we add the possibility that widening resistance to infection may also have played a role then the picture becomes even more complicated.[46] The tension in the historical literature between 'nutritionist' and 'contagionist' perspectives has obscured the relationship between public health interventions and broader social and political developments. Legislative advances in fields such as workplace safety and housing provision must be viewed within the context of more general patterns of social and economic improvement.

Furthermore, the bacteriological insights from the 1880s onwards did begin to contribute towards a more focused and coordinated set of public health policies. The comprehensive efforts to fight TB in New York City in the 1890s, for example, were praised by Robert Koch for their efficiency, scientific rationale and willingness to challenge private interests in the pursuit of wider goals.[47] The city's new diagnostic research laboratory was 'a superb technical innovation, a medico-scientific and political counterpart to the Brooklyn Bridge', and unlike any other facility yet constructed.[48] Similarly, the city's introduction of compulsory notification for the disease in 1897 marked a radical extension in the power of municipal government to override the objections of individual physicians and patients in the interest of public health.[49] Yet the nineteenth-century public health movement displayed a profound ambivalence towards the structural determinants of ill health since the purification of urban space it proposed was a process which sought simultaneously to transform both the social and the environmental characteristics of cities. Concern with housing design, sanitation and workplace safety was coupled with an emphasis on the morality and living habits of the working classes in the new industrial cities.

Class, race and death in the twentieth century

The production of more accurate data on morbidity and mortality in the last decades of the nineteenth century began to reveal the disproportionate concentration of TB among specific social groups. The relationship between TB, race and social class became more evident not only because of the changing politics of public health but also because the partial retreat of the disease had highlighted its higher prevalence among the poor, non-whites and other marginalized groups.[50] A parallel discourse of differential susceptibility to TB began to develop alongside the sanitarian emphasis on improved hygiene. Instead of new bacteriological insights dispelling the earlier hereditarian emphasis of the nineteenth century, the 'constitutional' dimensions to disease epidemiology became reformulated in terms of different degrees of racial resistance to TB.

The recognition of differential mortality by race provoked a complex array of arguments which sought to use prevailing cultural and biological conceptions of human difference as a means to explain widening inequalities in human health. In the British colonies, for example, a theory of 'virgin soil' populations emerged which attributed high rates of TB mortality among non-whites to the lack of 'tubercularization' or disease resistance amongst people who had not yet undergone the full effects of industrialization and urbanization. The influential pathologist Lyle Cummins posited that Europeans owed their higher survival rates to long-standing low-level exposure to the disease coupled with the spread of new hygienic living practices which prevented the illness from taking root in all but the most weakened or intemperate individuals. In contrast, non-European peoples were characterized by Cummins as biologically inferior and culturally backward which rendered them susceptible to TB as a 'disease of civilization'. The high rates of TB experienced in Africa, India and elsewhere in the colonial world were widely seen as an inevitable and necessary marker on the path to a Westernized society which had achieved a more stable relationship between the human immune system and the virulence of the TB bacillus.[51] Yet at the heart of this 'tubercularization' debate lay a profound confusion over whether the observed racial differences in mortality could be attributed to a Lamarckian process of acquired immunity or to a longer-term history of Darwinian evolution. Arguments about the relative significance of inherited or acquired immunological characteristics were supplemented by the proposal of a cultural hierarchy of disease resistance ranging from the 'childlike' susceptibility of colonized peoples to the supposedly hardier responses of urbanized European societies.

In the United States the control of TB amplified middle-class antipathy towards the 'lower classes' and heightened anxieties over immigration and racial mixing. Surveys carried out in the early twentieth century revealed that the rate of TB mortality was three times higher for black Americans than for white Americans.[52] These general figures mask even greater differences in many of the larger towns and cities. In Charleston, South Carolina, for example, the rate of TB mortality for blacks in 1900 was seven times higher than for whites. How were these disparities to be explained? A variant of the 'tubercularization' thesis suggested that former slaves had been protected from the disease through their 'healthy' outdoor life on Southern plantations. The implication was that high rates of TB among African-Americans were an unfortunate yet inevitable consequence of their emancipation.[53] Yet the social conditions under which most African-Americans lived could not be discounted altogether as a cause of their higher mortality. In 1920, for example, George E. Bushnell, a colonel in the US Medical Corps and director of the National Tuberculosis Association, combined a version of the tubercularization thesis with a recognition of the impact of poverty on ill health. 'Because of his color the negro is barred from much productive industry,' Bushnell wrote. 'As he therefore cannot compete with the whites in earning capacity, he is relegated to the worst habitations in the most insalubrious locations and to arduous or poorly paid toil everywhere.' But instead of calling for government action to improve living conditions, Bushnell chose instead to insist on improvements in the behaviour of poor blacks, the majority of whom he characterized as 'extraordinarily untrained, improvident and reckless; so that there must be taken into account not only poverty but a poverty which is tenfold worse because of the failure to make proper use of the scanty means at hand'.[54] A new concern with what the historian Marion Torchia describes as the 'Negro health problem' emerged which combined a mix of nineteenth-century moralism and white self-interest in order to avoid the possibility of infection by black maids, servants and other workers in daily contact with affluent middle-class homes.[55] As the historian Jessica Robbins notes of the shifting politics of TB in the United States:

> The acceptance of the germ theory had given TB a new and threat-ening social dimension. The tuberculous patient was not only an individual sufferer but also a potential source of infection and danger to others. The overwhelming majority of these patients were among the working-class poor. The prescription for health, physicians believed, was fresh air, good food, and plenty of rest – all of which were beyond the means of the urban poor. Professionals and reform-ers engaged in a protracted debate over what, if anything, should be done about this social problem.[56]

To acknowledge fully the structural causes of TB threatened to open up a much wider progressive agenda for social reform. For conservative health commentators it was essential, therefore, to persist with individ-ualized modes of explanation which emphasized putative connections between 'immoral living habits' and susceptibility to infection. In Canada, for example, the chief medical officer, Peter Bryce, described TB as one of a group of social diseases along with alcoholism, syphilis and feeble-mindedness: 'We find them so often intermingled,' Bryce wrote, 'that it seems quite impossible to determine which disease is the determinant or dominant one.'[57] The idea of differential degrees of immunity provided a scientific veneer for official indifference towards much higher levels of TB among poor and marginalized sections of society. Evolutionary conceptions of TB implied that control of the disease would occur through a long-term immunological transition rather than through any kind of medical intervention.[58] At root, however, anxieties over class, race and disease flowed from fears that these stigmatized groups would act as reservoirs for the contagion of wider society. Hereditarian views persisted in the post-bacteriological era as part of an emerging discourse of disease and national identity which would find its most virulent expressions under European fascism. Jews, for example, were denounced in Nazi Germany as 'a racial TB among nations'.[59] Thus even in the context of the widespread retreat of the disease across Europe and North America, TB retained a powerful metaphorical resonance for racial and ethnic hatred.

Improvements in diagnosis after the discovery of the TB bacillus in 1882 were not matched by major advances in treatment for many decades. Koch's claim, for example, to have discovered a cure for TB in 1890 through the production of the bacterial culture tuberculin was discredited. Although the incidence of TB declined during the twentieth century those who contracted the disease still suffered a high mortality rate. And even when improved treatments became available, the most vulnerable sections of society – principally the urban poor – were often unable to gain access to adequate medical care.[60] In the post-bacteriological era there were repeated innoculation experiments aimed at furthering scientific understanding of bacterial immunity. In 1914, for example, the American physician Guy Hinsdale predicted that 'future generations will be provided with a practical and efficient method of destroying this insatiate monster'. It would be some years, however, before the efforts of Trudeau, Gilliand, de Schweinitz and others would lead towards any definitive advance in the development of an effective vaccine. The most critical advance in TB inoculation was achieved by the French scientists Albert Calmette and Camille Guérin who began testing a bovine-derived vaccine in 1922. Initially the Bacille Calmette-Guérin (BCG) vaccine was only widely adopted in France and other countries – such as Spain and Canada – with strong cultural ties to French science.[61] In the USA, by contrast, the rejection of the BCG vaccine reflected a long-standing antipathy towards universal health interventions which might strengthen the role of the state in the advancement of public health (despite the pioneering early efforts of some municipal authorities). American scientists feared that the introduction of BCG would subvert the self-improvement ethos of the New Deal and at the same time draw attention to the persistence of the disease in spite of the twentieth-century rhetoric of scientific success.[62] In essence, the varied national responses to the

BCG vaccine reflected different conceptions of the relationship between health care and social policy, a tension which was temporarily obscured by advances in the antibiotic treatment of TB sufferers from the 1940s onwards.[63]

In 1944 the treatment for TB was transformed with the first use of the antibiotic streptomycin by Selman Waksman to cure infected patients. This was followed in 1951 by the use of another powerful antibiotic, isoniazid. Taken together, these new drugs revolutionized the treatment of TB and contributed towards a sharp decline in the environmental emphasis of the past. Unlike the BCG vaccine which aimed to prevent the progression from infection to illness, the widespread use of antibiotic drugs from the early 1950s onwards sought to cure patients who had already become ill. Within thirty years the rate of TB mortality in the developed world had fallen by more than 90 per cent. The discovery of streptomycin instituted a new phase in the control of TB which would increasingly emphasize issues of patient compliance over any wider discussion of the social and economic dimensions to disease epidemiology. The very success of the antibiotic revolution in health care served to disengage clinical medicine from the wider public health agendas of the past. The historical construction of the term 'non-compliance' reveals how bio-medical perceptions of patient deviance emphasized that particular groups are 'difficult' or 'recalcitrant' in terms of cooperating with medical authorities. Thus the issue of uneven access to adequate treatment in the antibiotic era became widely framed in terms of individual deficiencies or anti-rational belief systems rather than any acknowledgment of the social context in which the disease might be spread.[64] In apartheid South Africa, for example, persistent racial disparities in rates of infection were routinely dismissed on the grounds of cultural difference and a preference for traditional medicine. Yet a wealth of evidence from South Africa showed how poor housing and working conditions, combined with inequalities in access to medical care, had contributed towards widening health disparities in the twentieth century.[65] At a global scale, the antibiotic revolution of the 1940s and 1950s was highly uneven in its social and geographical impact, leaving much of the world's population languishing under high rates of infection with only haphazard access to treatment. Most critically, however, the early success of antibiotic drugs served to mask the continuing prevalence of TB infection. The 'magic bullet' of drug therapy diverted attention from the social and economic conditions in which the TB bacillus could continue to thrive.

Global poverty and the 'new' TB

The antibiotic revolution of the 1940s and 1950s led a range of leading public health campaigners, scientists and physicians confidently to predict the eradication of TB by the year 2000.[66] By the early 1980s TB appeared to be largely a disease of historical interest in the West, a consensus that indicated a dangerous complacency in the face of the continuing high prevalence of the disease in many developing countries. As recently as 1987, for example, the *Oxford Textbook of Medicine* predicted the virtual eradication of TB in 'most technically advanced countries' before the year 2050.[67] Yet those who considered TB in a global context were far less optimistic. In 1964, for instance, the executive director of the International Union against Tuberculosis, John Holm, issued this warning:

> For about half of the world's population no organized efforts are made to control tuberculosis, and this is the half where the problem is most serious. For the other half, efforts to control tuberculosis are conducted in a haphazard manner. Only a small fraction of the world's population is covered by well-organized programs in which the most modern means to control tuberculosis are systematically employed.[68]

The turning point in global efforts to control TB can be traced to the United States in the mid-1980s where a sudden increase in cases was observed in urban areas: between 1985 and 1992 there was a rise in TB cases of over 20 per cent.[69] Cities such as New York faced a rapid and unexpected spread of TB which quickly escalated into a public health emergency. This surge in reported cases can be attributed to increases in poverty and homelessness during the 1980s combined with the effects of HIV infection and the spread of drug-resistant TB strains. The emerging public health crisis facing deprived inner-city neighbourhoods represented a microcosm of the changing global incidence of the disease. It soon became apparent that the problems facing inner-city America were surfacing on a global scale in response to the combined effects of drug resistance, HIV and poverty.

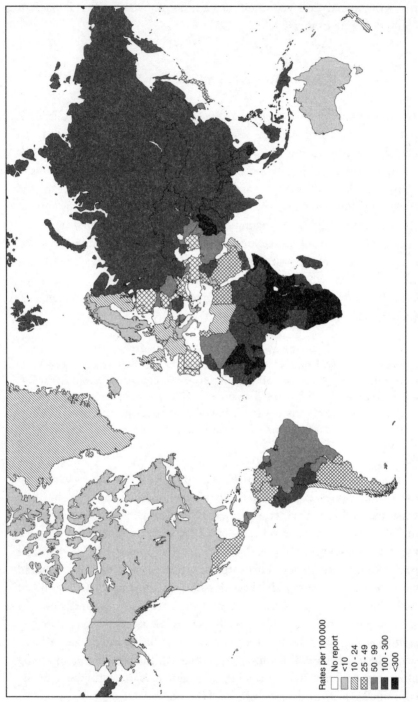

Figure 1.4 The global incidence of TB in 2001. Source: World Health Organization.

Rates per 100000

No report
<10
10 - 24
25 - 49
50 - 99
100 - 300
<300

The development of drug resistance is thought to be responsible for around 10 per cent of new TB cases worldwide.[70] The problem of drug resistance was encountered soon after the discovery of streptomycin and other anti-TB drugs and led to the gradual emergence of multi-drug treatment programmes. Factors involved in the emergence of drug-resistance include the poor supervision of therapy, the use of badly prepared combination preparations, inconsistent prescribing practices, erratic drug supplies, and unregulated over-the-counter sales of drugs.[71] The most commonly encountered resistance is to a single drug, usually streptomycin or isoniazid, and most TB bacteria with such resistance respond adequately to a multi-drug treatment programme. The emergence of resistance to rifampicin is much more serious, however, as this is the most powerful anti-TB drug, with the ability to sterilize lesions by destroying near-dormant 'persister' bacilli. Furthermore, most rifampicin-resistant strains are also resistant to isoniazid; by convention, TB due to strains resistant to these two agents, with or without additional resistances, is said to be multi-drug-resistant. The use of standard short-course treatment becomes not only ineffectual but may even be positively harmful as resistance to other drugs such as pyrazinamide and ethambutol also develops as part of the so-called 'amplifier effect'.[72] In Russia and other states of the former Soviet Union, mutant forms of TB, variously referred to as multi-drug-resistant TB (MDR-TB), have been rapidly spreading in response to chronic overcrowding in the prison system and severe cutbacks in primary health care. The problems and costs of managing each case of MDR-TB are enormous. Successful therapy requires prolonged courses of less effective, more expensive and more toxic drugs, under long-term supervision.[73] The incidence of MDR-TB in New York City has been reduced by such a strategy, although at very great cost: the cost of the management of a single case can exceed US$250,000.[74] In the case of New York, the spread of MDR-TB was facilitated by reductions in public health expenditure during the 1980s, but the city ended up having to spend ten times more than it saved in order to bring TB under control.[75]

A second factor behind the resurgence of TB is the AIDS pandemic. This is estimated to contribute around 10 per cent of TB cases worldwide. In Africa, however, HIV is responsible for at least 20 per cent of TB cases.[76] Given that one third of the world's population carry quiescent TB infection the effects of immune system damage can be expected to have devastating consequences: the most recent data suggest that in parts of sub-Saharan Africa, for example, more than one third of the adult population are now infected with HIV. Infection by HIV is currently the most important predisposing factor for the development of overt TB in those infected by TB before or after becoming HIV positive and by the late 1990s there were estimates of at least 11 million co-infected persons.[77] The increasing recognition of links between TB and HIV among patients has had the adverse effect of adding to the stigma of TB symptoms and has hindered cooperation between patients, health care workers and local communities.[78] The return of TB has also exposed tensions between different conceptions of medicine and individual liberty: in the USA, for example, the threat of MDR TB and co-infection with HIV has led to calls for punitive public health strategies based on mandatory screening and treatment, case notification to public agencies, aggressive contact tracing and the use of quarantine. Such measures, reminiscent of early-twentieth-century approaches to public health, are in conflict with contemporary conceptions of individual liberty.[79]

A third dimension to the 'new' TB is the effects of global social and economic change. Mass movements of people in response to war, increased economic insecurity, community breakdown and other factors have been involved in the spread of TB and other infectious diseases associated with overcrowding, makeshift housing and poor sanitation.[80] In addition to short-term disruption we must consider the longer-term social and economic shifts that have emerged since the early 1970s. There is now increasing evidence that growing poverty, infrastructural decay and declining health services have facilitated the spread of TB, diphtheria, sleeping sickness and other preventable diseases.[81] In the case of Vietnam, for instance, recent research has shown how the scaling down of established public health care systems during the 1990s has resulted in increased costs, more erratic drug availability and sinking morale among low-paid community health workers at the forefront of health care provision.[82] A substantial body of evidence suggests that TB has a disproportionate impact on the economically poor: 95 per cent of all TB cases and 98 per cent of TB deaths occur in the developing world where problems of ill health contribute towards cycles of economic hardship in the context of high unemployment and weak social security and health care provision. Similarly, the spread of TB and other preventable diseases in the so-called de-developing enclaves of urban America and the poverty-stricken cities of the former Soviet Union can only be fully understood with reference to the dynamics of global political and economic change since the Second World War.[83] Changing patterns of economic and social investment have contributed towards a new geography of wealth and poverty with significant implications for the epidemiology of disease. With the advent of more diffuse patterns of urbanization and the greater mobility of capital investment it has become far easier for public health crises to be effectively ignored where they present no generalized threat to the overall well-being of an increasingly globalized economic system.

In 1948 the newly created World Health Organization defined health as 'a state of complete physical, mental and social well-being, not merely the absence of disease and infirmity'.[84] This definition rests on an explicit recognition of the connections between health care and wider ethical and political ideals, yet recent advances in bio-medicine have served to obscure any meaningful connection between health and social justice. The last thirty years has seen a shift from collective forms of health care to an increasing emphasis on health as an individualized dimension to personal development. The historical synergy between health reform and social justice has been displaced by an increasing emphasis on the individual patient (or consumer) rather than the wider social and political context for disease. The profit-driven restructuring of global health care has led to widening health inequalities as the world's poor find themselves unable to benefit from the latest techno-logical and pharmaceutical advances. In comparison with other major health afflictions, TB remains relatively neglected: the funding of TB control worldwide, for example, continues to be very low in compari-son with other infectious diseases: just $8 of external aid is spent for each patient death compared with $137 for malaria, $925 for AIDs and over $38,000 for leprosy.[85] Of the 1,240 new drugs that were licensed between 1975 and 1996, only thirteen dealt with the world's killer diseases that primarily afflict people from tropical and poor countries. In 1998, for example, the World Health Organization failed to persuade pharmaceutical leaders to collaborate over the develop-ment of a combined drug for TB to make public health campaigns simpler and more cost-effective because the potential profit margins were too low.[86]

The problems of poverty and community breakdown have had a

devastating effect on global public health and threaten to overwhelm the prospects for greater social cohesion and economic development. Whilst new technological advances may play a useful role in the treatment of TB the eventual eradication of the disease will rest on wider structural changes in modern societies. Most sufferers from TB have limited political and economic power and their plight remains of only marginal significance in global affairs. Yet the corrosive effect of ill health on social development threatens to expose the specious logic behind a new world order in which much of humanity is condemned to poverty and serfdom. If there is one lesson to be learned from the diseased cities of nineteenth-century Europe and North America, it is that the contemporary global public health crisis will be solved not by medical intervention but by political transformation.

2

Immigration, Race and Geographies of Difference in the Tuberculosis Pandemic

Nicholas B. King

For nearly five months, anyone of Tibetan origin who has come to the Peace Bridge just north of Buffalo, N.Y., has been immediately segregated from others trying to cross into Canada, forced to don a bright yellow surgical mask and wait outside the Canadian immigration office, no matter the weather.... The Tibetans are eventually taken, usually by taxi with a driver who also wears a mask, to a doctor in Niagara Falls, who gives them a chest X-ray. Only when the doctor pronounces them TB-free can the Tibetans proceed. Even then, Canadian agents at the border have sometimes greeted the bewildered immigrants in biohazard jumpsuits.[1]

Italy next weekend enters the Schengen Agreement in favour of the free movement of people within most of Europe's borders, raising the spectre of a surge of illegal, diseased and violent Third World immigrants.... To survive in hiding, many illegal immigrants turn to crime, or live in unhealthy conditions. Doctors say such conditions help contagious diseases such as tuberculosis, which immigrants may have already contracted elsewhere, to manifest themselves after their arrival.[2]

Some state agencies expressed fears that the opening of the checkpoints would encourage the influx of Karen and Burmese immigrants into Thailand and these aliens might

bring with them contagious diseases such as tuberculosis,
elephantiasis, syphilis, malaria and leprosy.[3]

In the years since 1993, when the World Health Organization (WHO)
declared tuberculosis a 'global health emergency', numerous observers
have argued that any response to this disease must be international in
scope, and requires the collaborative effort of both developed and
developing nations.[4] However, as the above quotations illustrate, the
resurgence of TB has also been met with a renewed concern over the
borders that separate people, particularly those borders associated with
the nation-state. This concern is supported by overwhelming evidence
of significant disparities in TB morbidity and mortality according to
race, ethnicity and place of birth. In a number of countries, higher case
rates of TB and mortality among immigrants and racial and ethnic
minorities have presented public health officials with a dilemma: how
do they address significant disparities in health while maintaining
policies and practices that are equitable, just and non-discriminatory?

Using insights from history, social science and public health, this
chapter examines the role that health disparities and national borders
play in international responses to the TB pandemic.[5] In the past, both
the association of disease with immigrants, and the recognition of
racial and ethnic health disparities have been accompanied by the
stigmatization of socially marginalized populations. The widespread
discrimination that has accompanied the recent HIV/AIDS pandemic
reminds us that these pernicious social responses are still a very real
danger.

There is also the danger that uncritical interpretations of statistics
on health disparities will oversimplify what is in fact an extraordinarily
complex disease. The disproportionate burden of TB on certain populations is seldom the result of a single obvious cause. Moreover, while
statistics often appear incontrovertible, the appropriate interpretation
of and response to them is not. Any social or public health policy that
seeks to address these health disparities must take into account the fact
that both the production of official statistics and the subjective interpretation of them take place within national and social contexts laden
with debates over racial, ethnic and national difference.[6]

Disease, borders and difference

Scientists and public health officials have responded to differential TB morbidity and mortality rates in several ways. One strategy has been to assume that health disparities are caused by essential differences between people – that is, that TB disproportionately affects certain populations because they are intrinsically different in some way. Under this essentialist view, biological, physiological, genetic or cultural differences cause certain people to be more or less susceptible to TB infection, activation or mortality. As a consequence, if TB morbidity or mortality is higher among certain racial or ethnic groups, it is because those groups are essentially different in some way.

Essentialist explanations for health disparities have often been expressed as origin narratives. A group of people disproportionately affected by a disease is identified as the *cause* or the *source* of that disease, and is seen as a threat to the public's health. In this way, a particular disease is identified as somehow coming from outside – whether that 'outside' refers to a foreign country, or simply to a group of people who in some way are seen as outside the 'general population'. For example, during the early 1980s the recognition that Haitians seemed to suffer disproportionately high rates of HIV/AIDS led many Americans to identify Haiti as the historical 'source' of this disease. This identification was later proved to be wholly erroneous.[7]

Essentialism has also often been expressed in geographical terms. The association of infectious disease with outsiders, especially during periods of the expansion of international migration and commerce, has a long history. The derogatory epithets most commonly directed against immigrants have perennially been 'dirty' and 'diseased'. Since the early sixteenth century, syphilis has alternatively been known as 'morbus gallicus' (the French pox) in Italy, 'le mal de Naples' (the disease of Naples) in France, 'the Polish disease' in Russia, 'the Russian disease' in Siberia, 'the Portuguese disease' in India and Japan, 'the Castilian disease' in Portugal, and 'the British disease' in Tahiti.[8] During the successive waves of immigration to the USA in the late nineteenth and early twentieth centuries, Americans frequently blamed immigrants for the spread of various infectious diseases. In the most famous instance of nativist anxieties determining public health policy, the Irish immigrant Mary Mallon – popularly known as Typhoid Mary

– was incarcerated for twenty-five years on a small island near New York City.[9] More recently, having first identified Haiti as the geographical origin of the HIV/AIDS epidemic, Americans subsequently relocated its origin to Africa. Conversely, the Soviet Union, Japan and Germany blamed the USA for the origin and spread of the disease.[10]

In the last decade of the twentieth century, concerns over the porousness of national borders in a globalizing era framed US and European responses to new and emerging infections. The intensification of international travel and commerce has led to increasing anxiety among affluent residents of the industrialized West, who are increasingly fearful that they are under siege by infectious diseases hitherto thought to be confined to developing nations.[11] This is perhaps best illustrated by US media coverage of a 1994 outbreak of the Ebola virus in Zaire (now Democratic Republic of Congo), which made clear the renewed fear that foreigners might be vectors of a deadly disease: 'We want to know whether Ebola is headed *our* way. Could it reach critical mass in a Third World capital, then engulf the globe? And what if Ebola somehow mutated into an airborne form? Could coughs and sneezes become the agents of mass death?'[12]

TB has also long been associated with racial and ethnic difference.[13] At the turn of the last century, American nativists called TB 'the Jewish disease', despite contemporary evidence that demonstrated lower rates of TB among Jewish immigrants than among native-born Americans. American Southerners believed that African-Americans suffered from a peculiar form of 'negro consumption', and eugenicists, blaming Italian, Jewish and Irish immigrants for importing TB into the USA, argued for selective breeding and strict immigration restrictions.[14] Essential racial, ethnic and cultural differences were also constant reference points for European colonials' explanations of health disparities in Africa and South Asia during the nineteenth and early twentieth centuries.[15]

Essentialism has often proved attractive for a number of reasons. First, it has allowed observers to reduce a complex problem, involving a number of different causal factors, to a clear and distinct problem with a single cause. This reductionism has been practically useful in numerous arenas: in epidemiology, it has facilitated the gathering of basic statistics on the distribution of the disease over time and across space; in public health, it has enabled the provision of efficient, specific and cost-effective targeted interventions in an era in which funding for TB has been severely constrained; and in the political arena it has facilitated the implementation of policies designed to prevent the spread of the disease. Reductionism has also been politically attractive in a negative sense, allowing pre-existing racist or nativist sentiments to be clothed in the garb of objectivity and scientific authority, and leading to victim-blaming and stigmatization of socially marginalized groups as disease-ridden.[16]

Essentialism has also been attractive because it explains phenomena in terms of 'natural' characteristics that are observable and immutable. Again, this has a practical utility, as it encourages scientific study of the biological or physiological roots of a problem. However, it has also been used as a justification for failing to address the problems of socially marginalized populations. If certain social groups suffer from higher rates of disease because of essential physical differences, then social policy is (under this argument) powerless to address health disparities. This style of thinking is illustrated by a comment by Montana Lieutenant Governor Dennis Rehberg, who bluntly noted in 1994, 'The problem with AIDS is: you got it, you die. So why are we spending money on the issue?'[17]

Essentialism is by no means the only framework available to those who wish to understand and respond to the contemporary TB pandemic. Many public health researchers have adopted 'anti-essentialist' methods of explaining health disparities, emphasizing the contingent and multi-factoral causes of TB morbidity and mortality. Rather than focusing on the tuberculosis bacillus as the single cause of TB, the anti-essentialist viewpoint argues that multiple factors – including poverty, nutrition, homelessness, residential crowding, drug and alcohol use, institutionalization (in hospitals, shelters, and detention facilities such as prisons and refugee camps), and access to health care – contribute to both the spread of infection and the incidence of active cases. These factors are neither natural nor immutable. Rather, they are contingent upon more general social conditions which display immense historical and geographic variability. For these reasons, TB has often been referred to as a 'social disease', or 'poverty's penalty'.[19]

The distinction between essentialist and anti-essentialist theories of disease causation is important because it shapes the ways in which public health officials respond to health disparities. If TB is the result of a number of contingent causes, then disparities according to race, ethnicity or place of birth may be more closely associated with the present social or economic conditions of a group than with some essential biological or cultural difference. And if this is true, then an appropriate response would not focus on determining or preserving essential differences between racial, ethnic or national groups, but instead would target contingent social and economic conditions.[20] An anti-essentialist understanding of health disparities, rather than assuming that pre-existing categories such as race, ethnicity and nationality necessarily predetermine health disparities, would enquire into the ways in which contingent factors – such as social and economic justice – are mapped onto differences in morbidity and mortality.

Immigration: a cause of the spread of TB

It has become commonplace in a number of nations to identify immigration as a 'cause' of the rising incidence of TB. This observation is supported by substantial epidemiological evidence that, in the developed world at least, TB appears to be imported from elsewhere. As summarized in Table 2.1, studies conducted throughout the 1990s attributed a large proportion of cases in North America, Western Europe and Australia to the foreign-born. In some areas, the observed rates of TB among immigrants have been astonishing. In Western Australia, for example, immigrants accounted for 88 per cent of cases, while in the Netherlands incidence rates of TB in the Somalian community were 1,000 per 100,000 person-years – 200 times the Dutch national rate.[21]

Changes in TB case rates among immigrants have received the most attention in the USA. Between 1986 and 1994, the foreign-born accounted for 25.8 per cent of the total reported cases of TB, and their case rate was more than four times that of people born in the USA. They also have been identified as the most significant contributor to the overall increase in cases in the USA. Between 1985 and 1992, the foreign-born accounted for 60 per cent of the total increase in reported cases, with five border states (New York, New Jersey, Florida, Texas and California) accounting for a full 92 per cent of the increase. Over the next three years, cases in the foreign-born increased 10.6 per cent, while those in the US-born decreased 24 per cent. By 2000, the foreign-born accounted for 40 per cent of cases in the USA, upwards of 50 per cent in many European countries, and 80 per cent in Australia.[22] Recently, immigrants have also been identified as the source of increasing rates of drug-resistant TB worldwide.

Table 2.1 Percentage of TB cases attributed to the foreign-born, by country.

Country/Region	Percentage of reported cases of TB attributed to the foreign-born	Date of report
Australia	73	1992
Western Region	88	1997
Canada	57.8	1995
Southern Alberta	70.6	early 1990s
Montreal	77.3	early 1990s
Denmark	38	1991
Israel	57*	1999
Italy	22.8	1999
Netherlands	56	1997
New Zealand	66	1997
Sweden	41	1991
Switzerland	51	1991
USA	36.1	1996
California	66.2	1995
Los Angeles	62	1993
New Jersey	37	1995

* Cases of MDR-TB only

Sources: Australia: Mario C. Raviglione *et al.*, 'Global Epidemiology of tuberculosis: Morbidity and Mortality of a Worldwide Epidemic', *Journal of the American Medical Association*, vol. 273:3 (18 January 1995): 220–26. Canada: E. Anne Fanning, 'Globalization of Tuberculosis', CMAJ, vol. 158:5 (10 March 1998): 611. Denmark, Sweden and Switzerland: Raviglione *et al.* Israel: J. Sosna, *et al.*, 'Drug-resistant Pulmonary Tuberculosis in Israel, A Society of Immigrants: 1985–1994', *International Journal of Tuberculosis and Lung Disease*, vol. 3 (August 1999): 689–94. Italy: L. R. Codecasa *et al.*, 'Tuberculosis Among Immigrants from the Developing Countries in the Province of Milan, 1993–1996', *International Journal of Tuberculosis and Lung Disease*, vol. 3 (July 1999): 589–95. Netherlands: R. Bwire, 'Tuberculosis Screening Among Immigrants in The Netherlands: What is Its Contribution to Public Health?' *Netherlands Journal of Medicine*, vol. 56 (2000): 63–71. New Zealand: Adrian Harrison, 'Tuberculosis in Immigrants and Visitors', *New Zealand Medical Journal*, vol. 112 (24 September 1999): 363–5. USA: S. Jody Heymann *et al.*, 'The Need for Global Action Against Multidrug-Resistant Tuberculosis', *Journal of the American Medical Association*, vol. 281:22 (9 June 1999): 2138–40; Raviglione *et al.*; Kathryn DeRiemer, 'Tuberculosis Among Immigrants and Refugees', *Archives of Internal Medicine*, vol. 158 (13 April 1998): 753–60; Zhiyuan Liu, 'Distinct Trends in Tuberculosis Morbidity Among Foreign-Born and US-Born Persons in New Jersey, 1986 Through 1995', *American Journal of Public Health*, vol. 88 (July 1998): 1064–7.

After reviewing the sobering epidemiological evidence of disparities in health according to place of birth, many observers have concluded that increased immigration is a significant cause of the rising incidence of TB in the developed world. This has led public health officials to recommend a range of responses, from better policing of national borders and tighter controls on legal and especially illegal immigration, to better screening and treatment of the people crossing those borders.[23] However, framing the problem of international TB control in these terms raises a number of difficult issues with regard to epidemiology, public health and social policy.

National borders and the politics of blame

The identification of immigration as a cause of increased TB case rates focuses attention on the bodies of people crossing international borders. This focus is rhetorically useful, in that it alerts the often-complacent lawmakers and citizenry of the industrialized West to the importance of investing in international TB prevention and control. On a more practical level, governmental institutions are already in place to process and monitor the movement of bodies across national borders, providing a convenient location for data collection and preventive public health measures.

Yet the close association of immigrants and disease also raises the ugly spectre of racist and nativist hatred and the scapegoating of immigrants for social problems.[24] While it may be convenient to regard such beliefs as relics of the past, the 1980s and 1990s saw a marked resurgence of nativist and anti-immigrant sentiment in the industrialized nations of Western Europe and the USA, precisely the countries that consider themselves to be under siege by TB carried in from outside. A 1994 *Journal of the American Medical Association* report claiming that the foreign-born were responsible for 60 per cent of the recent increase in TB in the USA attracted the interest of anti-immigration groups such as the Federation for American Immigration Reform, which invoked the threat of tubercular immigrants as a justification for cracking down on legal and illegal immigration. In the same year, voters in the state of California passed Proposition 187, a statute that prohibited publicly funded facilities from providing non-emergency medical care to illegal immigrants.[25] In addition, it required such facilities to verify the immigration status of prospective patients, and to notify the Immigration and Naturalization Service and the Attorney General of California if they suspected that a patient was an illegal alien, thus effectively transforming physicians into border police. Though eventually ruled unconstitutional in a federal court, this proposition inspired the introduction of several federal bills aimed at eliminating social services for illegal immigrants. As numerous observers noted at the time, the immigration and welfare reform policies of the 1990s discouraged immigrants from seeking care out of fear of the immigration authorities and, in some extreme cases, these policies denied care to potentially infectious individuals.[26]

It is also important to note that 'immigrant' is an extremely ambiguous term.[27] Two contrasting definitions of this word uneasily coexist. On the one hand, the term seems to denote a contingent property, pertaining to the recent movement of bodies in space: an 'immigrant' is someone who crosses a national border, often with the purpose of eventually residing in the destination country. However, most of the institutions of the nation-state (such as the Immigration and Naturalization Service in the USA) do not treat all such border crossings similarly, as international travellers and workers are exempt from the screening that 'immigrants' must undergo. Not all bodies that cross national borders are immigrant bodies.

On the other hand, in the social and political arenas, 'immigrant' is often used less as a description of the contingent movement of bodies through geopolitical space, and rather more as a description of (or proxy for) essential racial or ethnic characteristics. Much of the anti-immigrant sentiment in the USA and Western Europe is a reaction to the presence of racial or ethnic minorities rather than to the movement of bodies in space.[28]

The difficulty is that there is considerable slippage between these two definitions of 'immigrant'. The social and medical response to the prevalence of TB among 'immigrants' cannot be disentangled from the symbolic definition of the nation-state and its citizenry; likewise, the legitimate observation that certain social groups might have a higher incidence of TB than others can too easily be transformed into fear and stigmatization of 'diseased and violent Third World immigrants'.[29]

Immigration and epidemiological knowledge

Blaming immigration for the recent rise in TB cases also obscures significant complexities in the dynamics of transmission of TB between individuals and populations. Since TB can remain latent for many years, careful distinctions must be made between TB cases that are the result of recent transmission (e.g., 'secondary cases'), and cases that are the result of reactivation of old infections. Using molecular epidemiological techniques, recent studies have demonstrated that most TB cases among immigrants to the USA are the result of reactivation of latent infections.[30] The activation of latent infections in recent immigrants is likely to be due to the peculiar stresses that they face during migration. Many are forced to move because of economic deprivation, natural disasters, political instability and wars in their home country.[31] During migration and upon arrival in their destination country, they are subject to a number of factors that contribute to the reactivation of TB infections. These include the stress of relocation, concurrent illness and poor overall health, poor nutrition, cramped living conditions in institutions such as refugee camps, hospitals, prisons and holding facilities, lack of access to adequate health care, and socioeconomic marginalization in the form of inadequate housing, low income and poor working conditions.

It is thus inaccurate to say that immigrants transport TB from one country to another. Most immigrants do not *transport* active cases of TB, but rather *develop* active cases within the first few years after their arrival.[32] The higher rate of TB among immigrants thus owes as much to the hardships they face during and shortly after migration, as it does to their country of origin. Focusing too closely on immigrants as vectors of disease conceals the causal roles played by inadequate health care and social and economic injustice in their destination country.

A number of recent studies also call into question the assumption that immigrants are a significant source of new infections in their destination countries. Studies of the transmission of TB in San Francisco found that, in eight of nine 'clusters' of TB cases (89 per cent), the direction of transmission was from US-born to Mexican-born individuals, not the reverse; the US-born, though accounting for only 27 per cent of the total cases, accounted for 51 per cent of the secondary cases.[23] Another study indicated that only 2 of 115 secondary cases in the US-born could be directly attributed to foreign-born sources, and a similar study in the UK found no evidence of cross-infection between immigrants from South Asia and the rest of the population.[34] The low incidence of transmission between foreign-born and native-born populations illustrates the danger of assuming that 'immigrants' – even those from high-prevalence countries – are responsible for transmission of TB to native-born populations. The fear of the 'threat' that immigrants present is not only politically alarming but also epidemiologically unsound. In addition, it indicates that social, geographic and economic borders between people *within* countries may be far more significant than the political borders *between* countries.

Finally, blaming 'immigration' for the increased incidence of TB vastly oversimplifies an extraordinarily complex problem regarding the causes of TB incidence and transmission. Focusing too closely on the role of individual carriers of the tubercle bacillus diverts attention from the more complicated socioeconomic and structural problems that contribute to the spread of TB. It is, for example, much simpler to identify Russians as potential carriers and screen them upon entry into the USA, than it is to interrogate the role of the recent 'shock therapy'-driven transition to a market economy in the explosion of TB in that country.[35] It is a time-consuming but easily intelligible task to divide the world geographically into 'low-incidence' and 'high-incidence' nations, identify people who cross the borders between these areas, and either prevent them from crossing these borders, or, more humanely, treat them once they do. It is a much less intelligible task to identify the complicated transnational factors of political economy responsible for the increased incidence in TB among socially and economically marginalized populations worldwide.

Health disparities and racial difference

As with immigration, there is considerable epidemiological evidence establishing a link between race, ethnicity and TB. Since the early 1970s, researchers have noted clear and alarming racial and ethnic disparities in infection rates, morbidity and mortality from TB.

Over the course of the twentieth century in the USA, mortality from TB declined more slowly in minority groups than the nation as a whole, even following the mid-century chemotherapeutic revolution. The resurgence of TB in the 1970s and 1980s also affected racial and ethnic minorities disproportionately. Between 1985 and 1992, TB cases in the nation as a whole increased 20 per cent. However, there was a profound differential distribution according to race: during this period, TB cases increased 27 per cent among blacks, 75 per cent among Hispanics and 46 per cent among Asian/Pacific Islanders, but decreased 10 per cent among non-Hispanic whites, and 23 per cent among American Indians.[36] In 1993 in the UK, although they accounted for only about 5 per cent of the population, non-whites accounted for 56 per cent of the cases of TB (up from 16.4 per cent of cases in 1965).[37] We should also note that race and ethnicity do not necessarily map clearly onto nationality – indeed, some studies indicate that race is more important than place of birth as a risk factor for TB in the USA.[38]

While the evidence for racial and ethnic disparities in health is clear, the explanation for such disparities is not. To begin with, the categories of 'race' and 'ethnicity' have for some time been the objects of substantial controversy. For much of human history, these categories have been assumed to be essential forms of human difference – that is, rooted in fundamentally physical or biological characteristics, such as skin colour, blood type or genetic makeup. More recently, scientists and other scholars have argued that in fact these categories are 'social constructions' – that is, that race and ethnicity are social or cultural categories, and do not directly correspond to measurable physiological, biological or genetic differences.[39]

The impact of this reformulation of racial and ethnic categories on the understanding of health disparities is profound. On the one hand, if such differences are essential in nature, then one could reasonably assume that health disparities arise out of biological differences. Indeed, a number of scientists have speculated that genetic differences may be responsible for disparities in TB incidence between blacks and whites, though at this time no definite linkage between race, genetics and health disparities has been proved.[40] If, on the other hand, racial and ethnic differences are social constructions, then many health disparities cannot necessarily be explained by reference to physiology, biology or genetics.[41]

What then might account for the significant, measured racial and ethnic disparities in TB incidence and mortality? Two interconnected possibilities are likely: first, that disparities according to race and ethnicity are in fact the result of another variable, such as income level or access to health care; second, that despite their questionable physical or biological foundations, perceptions of racial and ethnic difference still have significant social consequences.

TB has long been recognized as a disease that targets the socially and economically marginalized, especially those who are poor, homeless, or confined to crowded institutions such as jails, prisons and shelters. In many countries, those categorized as racial or ethnic minorities are disproportionately represented among these groups – thus engendering a vicious cycle of stigmatization and social and economic marginalization. For example, in the USA, although they made up only one tenth of the total population, African-Americans have accounted for 38 per cent of the homeless – and in some urban areas this percentage has approached 80 per cent.[42] African-Americans have also been disproportionately more likely to be incarcerated in jails or prisons, to use intravenous drugs, and to be severely economically marginalized.[43] One contemporary study found that adjusting for six indicators of socioeconomic status (crowding, income, poverty level, public assistance, unemployment and education) accounted for roughly half of the racial disparity in TB case rates among native-born Americans.[44] Another study of TB rates in urban areas found that death rates of whites and blacks living in poor sections of a given city were generally almost three times – and in some cases as much as six times – the rate of those living in affluent areas. In a number of cities TB mortality rates among poor whites were significantly higher than among non-whites.[45]

It is difficult to disentangle fully the relationship between socioeconomic status and racial difference. However, it is clear that observed racial or ethnic disparities in health often obscure underlying disparities according to socioeconomic status, place of residence (for example, in areas with high rates of poverty, or with a high amount of residential crowding), and institutionalization rates. Disparities in health that may at first seem to arise from essential racial or ethnic differences are often in fact the result of contingent socioeconomic differences.[46] In addition, whether or not essential racial or ethnic differences exist, the perception that they do has important consequences. Recent epidemiological work indicates that racism and racial discrimination play a significant role in health inequalities, and contribute to higher rates of physical and mental health problems among racial minorities.[47] Social and economic discrimination against racial and ethnic minorities often leads to higher rates of homelessness, incarceration, and lack of access to health care and social services, all of which are important risk factors for TB.[48]

For these reasons, researchers and policymakers must take great care in identifying the causes of, and the appropriate responses to, observed racial or ethnic differences in TB case rates. Even if scientists and social scientists are able to articulate the complex relationship between health, race and political economy in a fair and just manner, the historical record indicates that it can easily be oversimplified on the social and political level. Historical scholarship also alerts us to the role that racial discrimination can play in medical research and practice. Physicians and scientists, like other members of a society, often consciously or unconsciously exhibit the racial biases and essentializing tendencies prevalent in that society. In its most extreme forms, this has contributed to racist and unethical practices such as eugenics and the Tuskeegee Syphilis Study.[49] The likelihood that contemporary TB control efforts will replicate these ethical lapses is remote. However, it is worth noting that, in the past, the humanitarian motivations of public health workers have not always been enough to ensure that pernicious measures – such as forcible detention of 'unruly' populations of alcoholics and vagrants – will not be used to achieve the laudable ends of TB control.[50]

Rethinking geographies of difference

> Such cases [of transnational TB] remind us that much of the current literature conflates administrative boundaries with those of biological salience. Although turbulence may be introduced at national borders, they have proven ineffective in stopping the expansion of MDR-TB outbreaks. So too have prison walls and city limits.[51]

For those concerned about the global TB epidemic, thinking in terms of borders and difference is often immensely constructive. Epidemiologists ask how and why this disease affects some people more than others, and why some borders are more effective than others at containing its spread. Using the knowledge gained from epidemiological research on disease and difference, public health officials design specific interventions targeted at those populations most at risk of developing TB. When compared to less specific programmes, targeted interventions are typically more efficient, cost-effective and successful at curing the sick and preventing the spread of the disease.

However, focusing on borders and difference brings risks as well as rewards. The historical record indicates that essentialist understandings of difference have played a role in the institution of some of the more pernicious nationalist and racist social policies during human history, and for this reason they should be deployed cautiously. An uncritical reliance upon essentialist understandings of difference risks introducing elements of stigmatization and racism into social policies and public health practices. Even the most scrupulously objective scientific study of health disparities can be misused in the public sphere. It is tempting to believe that scientific advances, such as the discovery of a new vaccine or a 'miracle drug', will eventually render the subjectivism of politics and social policy irrelevant. However, with the threat of drug-resistant TB increasing, it would be folly to wait for that time.

In addition, focusing on borders and difference may also ultimately obscure as much as it reveals about the incidence and transmission of infectious disease. In the future, successful global TB control will have to rely upon a fundamental reworking of these categories in epidemiology and public health. For example, researchers and public health officials would do well to think in *transnational* as well as *international* terms. This means focusing less on the transgression of borders by individuals, and more on the formation of transnational connections between spaces and populations once thought to be disconnected or insulated from one another. The notion that TB is transmitted from 'high-incidence' to 'low-incidence' countries may have less utility than a recognition that particular neighbourhoods in different cities are connected through transnational social networks that transcend national borders.[52]

Finally, future responses to TB will have to be built not upon an essentialized geography of national, racial or ethnic differences, but rather upon a transnational geography of contingent differences in levels of poverty, social justice, nutrition, employment and access to health care and adequate housing. The most salient observation for TB control in the future may be that TB, rather than being 'transported' across national borders, is activated in disparate locations by similar social conditions. A genuinely global response to the resurgent TB pandemic does not simply mean that the affluent residents of the West should address the disease in other countries, either out of humanitarian concern or national self-interest. It means that we must fundamentally rethink the geographies of difference that influence the incidence and transmission of TB worldwide.

3

Gender and Tuberculosis: A Conceptual Framework for Identifying Gender Inequalities

Anna Thorson and Vinod K. Diwan

Gender of itself is not the cause of morbidity and mortality in tuberculosis, but it is a powerful indicator of disadvantage, a marker of the many factors that influence health and the utilisation of health services.

I. Smith[1]

Few scientific studies have been published on gender aspects of tuberculosis, even though TB kills more women than any other infectious disease, including malaria and AIDS, and available data show that more women die from TB than from all causes of maternal deaths put together.[2]

The concept of gender was introduced by the American anthropologist Gayle Rubin in 1975 in order to distinguish the predetermined biological characteristics of the sexes from the socio-cultural factors that create 'maleness' or 'femaleness' as well as the power relations between men and women.[3] The use of the term 'gender' instead of 'sex' served a purpose by taking a standpoint that opposed the essentialist view on femaleness and maleness as created by biological sex, and thus being predetermined and unchangeable. The fast development thereafter in feminist and gender research has given the concept of 'gender' new and wider definitions. The dichotomy of the division into biological sex and social sex (gender) and the conception of predetermination have been criticized by recent post-structuralist thinkers, who have suggested that sex should be viewed not as predetermined, but instead as gendered in itself.[4] This abstract concept would indicate that there is a possibility of multiple genders, and that categorizing men and women into two defined groups with some kind of common characteristics is actually impossible. Women belonging to groups other than the white, Western middle-class groups that have dominated feminist theory have also raised points of criticism. Strategies of a universal feminism have been considered problematic and likely to be oversimplifying due to the wide variety of complex realities that women all over the world experience.[5]

We choose here to define gender as including not only the biological differences between men and women but also the wide variety of behaviours, expectations and roles attributed by social structures to men and to women.[6] The use of gender in this way emphasizes the problems in distinguishing the respective influences of what are traditionally viewed as 'biological factors' and 'social factors'. An example is the issue of height. Mean height among both women and men has increased in high-income countries. The reason for this is believed to be social development with better nutrition. Thus social factors create changes in biology. Another example is the current trends of body weight in modern society. Many women diet, which may affect not only their own bodies but, through lack of nutrients in the pregnant woman, also the development of the unborn child.

Gender relations are power relations in which women and men are subject to a hierarchical ordering which leads to inequities in health and well-being. These relations are often of special significance to women, since female subordination is present in most societies, leading to inequality and discrimination also in health. Gender relations are closely linked to other structural factors such as ethnicity, race and social class, which must be taken into account when carrying out a gender analysis of health. All women and men do not live under the same conditions, but other structural factors interact with gender to create conditions of health or ill health, in which women most often are the disadvantaged.[7]

Ill health in the family is also most often a greater burden on women than on men, because of the female's role as a carer. Still, men too suffer from specific risks of ill health related to their gender role, such as, for example, an increased risk of accidents at work. Paradoxically women in most countries live longer then men, whereas in most contexts they report more morbidity. Whether the female longevity in these countries is a result of genetic disposition or a consequence of a combination of social, environmental and genetic factors is not well explored. It can be concluded, however, that the acknowledgement of gender as a determinant of health shows clearly the need for diagnostic and treatment approaches that take gender into account.

Research within the field of gender and health has been developing in Western countries but has mainly been limited to diseases common in these parts of the world. In low- and middle-income countries women's health issues have until recently been restricted to conditions related to reproductive functions. The view of women as important primarily for their reproductive role has been supported by a focus on reproductive health in many aid and development programmes directed at low-income countries.

Infectious diseases are still the most common cause of death in the world today. However, research and control strategies for infectious diseases have traditionally been focused on biomedical theories of disease causation. Reductionism and a narrow approach have been key features of the medical disciplines working with these strategies. Not until recently has an interest been taken in the social context of the diseases. Considering that it is estimated that women make up 70 per cent of the world's poor,[8] the interaction between gender and poverty needs to be recognized in health research and policy making.

Gender-related inequities in infectious diseases have thus previously been a neglected research area but are now becoming recognized as factors of importance for the understanding of communicable diseases.[9] Information on how gender transforms into differential impacts of disease is still limited, but gender differences in infectious diseases in poor countries have been studied in some settings. The different activities that men and women undertake lead to different exposures to infectious microbes. Household chores such as collecting water may put women of reproductive age at a higher risk of acquiring an infection such as schistosomiasis than men of the same age.[10] Social stigma associated with infectious diseases is also a factor of great importance to access to health care and health-seeking behaviour. Because of the gender inequities existing in many societies, where women have less access to power both in the family and in societal spheres and where women are more dependent on marriage and traditional family structure, women are considered more vulnerable to social stigma than men. Filariasis and leprosy are diseases whose effect on physical appearance are likely to have particularly adverse consequences for women. Being diagnosed with leprosy may in some societies severely reduce a women's chances of marriage or affect her position in the household. Women have been found to hide their leprosy symptoms more than men, and several studies have shown fear of stigmatization to be an important barrier to seeking timely treatment.[11] It has also been reported from a quantitative study on leprosy in India that more women were diagnosed with leprosy in general surveys and contact surveys, while fewer were detected by passive case finding (that is, where case detection requires an active initiative from the patient rather than the health care provider) such as referral, voluntary reporting and school surveys[12]. Similar gender-related differences between active and passive case finding have been shown to exist for other infectious diseases. A study in Thailand showed that six times more men than women attended malaria clinics even though the prevalence of malaria, based on population screenings, is the same for both sexes.[13] In Colombia when cases of leishmaniasis were investigated through active case finding, the disease was found to be equally frequent among both men and women, although the disease had earlier been considered twice as common in men.[14]

TB kills about one million women per year and it is estimated that almost one billion women and girls are infected with TB.[15] In women aged fifteen to forty-four in poor countries TB is the third most important cause of morbidity and mortality combined. Yet very little is known about how gender differences may create gender inequalities in relation to TB control programmes.[16] The pathology of *Mycobacterium tuberculosis* is complicated and a stepwise process takes place in the development of infection, disease and outcome of treatment. Gender is an important determinant of the outcome of each step of the process. The conceptual framework shown in Figure 3.1 provides a basis for gender analysis of the different stages of TB.[17]

Is TB infection really higher among men?

A recent review of past epidemiological studies suggests that age- and sex-based differences in TB infection exist. An analysis of tuberculin surveys around the world during 1948–51 showed that the prevalence of TB infection was equal between males and females during childhood, and that between ten and sixteen years of age male prevalence began

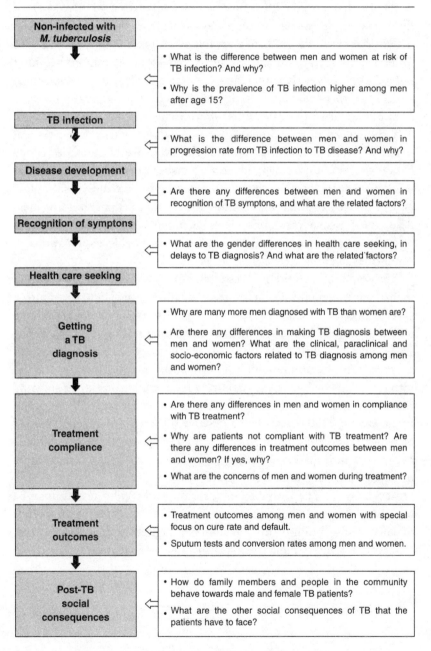

Figure 3.1 Framework for a gender analysis of TB.

to exceed that of female. Similar results on the prevalence of TB infection are reported from studies in Africa, India and South Korea.[18] A theory that is often presented as an explanation of the observed difference in prevalence is that men in general have a wider social network that would lead to a greater exposure to the bacteria. This difference in social contacts is considered to be of importance after puberty, following the differentiation into gender roles that in most societies starts at that age. On the other hand *Mycobacterium tuberculosis* is known to be transmitted more easily indoors than outdoors, and the infection rate increases exponentially with the time spent together with an infectious individual. These are features describing better the traditional female gender tasks (spending time indoors working with household chores, taking care of sick individuals, close and prolonged contact with family and relatives) than those of men. Also, the possible variations in social habits of men and women in different cultural contexts seem too large to enable explanations of similarities in global prevalence patterns.

The common method of investigating the prevalence of TB infection is through tuberculin testing, that is, measuring the skin reaction to a specific injected substance. However, the observed differences between men and women in the results after tuberculin testing need not necessarily indicate a difference in prevalence of infection, but could instead be explained by immunological differences in the response to TB infection. This hypothesis is supported by a study from Japan showing that more male than female TB patients – that is, people who had progressed to TB disease – had a positive tuberculin reaction.[19] A study of senior schoolchildren in Kuwait who were given the tuberculin test, found that boys had a delayed-type hypersensitivity reaction to more mycobacterial sensitins than girls as well as larger scars after BCG revaccination.[20] These studies indicate that tuberculin testing may be less sensitive in women and thus the published figures on the prevalence of and/or susceptibility to infection may suffer from a gender bias. Research to address these theories has so far been scarce.[21]

Do women have a higher rate of progression from infection to disease?

A higher rate of progression from infection to disease among reproductive-age women has been described in several studies. In a longitudinal study conducted in Bangalore, India,[22] where subjects were actively screened for TB, females had up to a 130 per cent higher risk than men of progressing from TB infection to disease between the ages of ten and forty-four years. In Puerto Rico, tuberculin-positive individuals were followed for on average 18.7 years, and the progression to active TB (all forms) was 17 per cent higher among women; the male rate was higher only in the 1 to 6 years age group.[23] Similar results have been shown in a study from Alaska, and in several studies from high-income settings.[24] An argument against these findings has been that women are more likely to use health services during their reproductive years, and thus are more likely to be diagnosed with TB at this time in life. This argument does not explain the findings in the Bangalore study where active case finding was used, and it also seems simplistic to generalize about the health-seeking behaviour of women in these different contexts.

Different causes have been suggested to explain why women of reproductive age would have a higher progression from infection to active TB. One of the most common theories has been that the stresses of pregnancy would affect the immune response and thus allow the onset of disease. However, scientific studies have produced contradictory and inconclusive results on the relation between TB and pregnancy.[25] The hormonal and physiological changes in females during the post-partum period have also been discussed as a risk factor to progression to disease, but this relation has not been shown in scientific studies. A case control study comparing the incidence of pregnancy or childbirth over the previous six months between TB and non-TB patients showed no difference in frequency of reproductive events between the women with TB and those without TB.[26] In summary it may be stated that despite a relatively large number of studies carried out addressing this aspect of TB, the relation between pregnancy and progression to active TB disease is not clear.[27] It is also noteworthy that despite the inconclusiveness of the research, it remains one of the few fields where an interest in how TB affects women has been explored. The strong focus on TB and pregnancy, compared to the lack of interest in other aspects of the impact of TB in women, shows how research relating to gender issues has been reduced to an interest in effects on female reproduction. This focus emphasizes the societal view of women as of primary importance for their function as childbearers and carers. The spheres of women's lives that do not include reproduction have been of marginal interest to the research world.

Gender difference in symptoms recognition and health care seeking

Strategies for TB control worldwide are based on passive case detection, that is, as already noted, a situation where the active initiative for case detection comes from the patient rather than from the health care provider. Therefore the patient's perceived symptoms and recognition of ill health are crucial for case detection. TB is clinically a complicated disease where low-grade symptoms may be present for a long time, imitating a common cold or general tiredness. This feature makes patients' recognition of symptoms a complicated and diverse procedure. How case detection among patients with TB-suggestive symptoms relates to gender has not been fully explored.

In a population-based study from rural Vietnam, it was found that among men and women with TB-suggestive symptoms (prolonged cough), women did not start to seek health care action later than men, but there was a gender difference in the type of health care sought.[28] Women in this study more often sought the low-qualified health care providers, and women also delayed longer in seeking hospital care. These findings are similar to data from qualitative studies in Vietnam where men with TB were said to neglect their symptoms until a late stage of the disease, and then to seek hospital care directly, without any attempt at self-medication or any visit to private practitioners.[29] Women with TB, on the other hand, were described as first practising self-medication, or visiting a private practitioner, before seeking any public health care.

The recognition of symptoms and health-seeking behaviour need to be regarded not only in relation to physical experience of ill health, but also as consequences of fear of serious or stigmatizing diseases that may influence healthcare-seeking behaviour. The association of stigma with TB is widespread. In Northern European countries where TB was a high-incidence disease in the middle of the twentieth century, TB was strongly linked to social stigma. Examples from art and literature of descriptions of TB victims belonging to socially marginalized groups are numerous.[30] Qualitative studies from Vietnam have shown that the general knowledge of TB among men and women without TB is fairly good. Still, women are more concerned than men about the social stigma of the disease and its adverse consequences for their lives, whereas men's concerns are related more often to the economic consequences.[31] Unmarried women are especially vulnerable socially since a diagnosis of TB is likely to reduce the chances of marriage.[32] The relation between stigma and gender, and how these factors interact to create disadvantages for women in some contexts, has not been an issue when strategies for control have been developed.

Global TB control strategies focus primarily on pulmonary, contagious TB. However, TB has many different forms and clinical manifestations. In a large study on extra-pulmonary TB (TB outside the lungs) it was found that more women than men were diagnosed with extra-pulmonary forms of TB.[33] In separate studies on TB in organs other than the lungs, women were found to get these diagnoses at least as often as men.[34] Since global and national TB control strategies focus on the prevention of pulmonary, contagious TB, the diffuse, 'atypical' symptoms of extra-pulmonary TB are less often recognized by patients and healthcare providers.

Diagnosis and gender

About one third of all reported new TB cases are women, and two thirds men.[35] It is not known whether this is a genuine difference in incidence, the result of an under-reporting of female cases or a combination of both. Historically, in countries with a high prevalence of TB in the beginning and middle of the twentieth century, notification of TB showed a different pattern. In Denmark (1939–41), Norway (1937), and England and Wales (1952–54), notification rates were similar for both sexes below age 15 but higher among women until their mid-twenties or early thirties. After age 40, notification rates for men were higher in most of these countries.[36] In low-income countries with about the same notification rates of TB today as in Europe in the middle of the twentieth century, a reversed pattern is seen with higher notification rates among younger men. However, a study carried out in eastern Nepal in the early 1980s that compared active case detection with passive case detection showed interesting results. When using active case finding, 46 per cent of the detected cases were females; however, of the group who had to refer themselves to health care, only 28 per cent were females.[37] These findings are consistent with the previously described undernotification of other infectious diseases and give support to the hypothesis of an under-reporting of female TB cases.

A study of prevalence data in comparison with notification data was recently carried out with the aim of defining gender differences in access to health care.[38] Age- and sex-specific TB prevalence rates of smear-positive TB – representing active case finding – were obtained from TB prevalence surveys reported to the World Health Organization or published in the literature and were compared to sex-specific notification rates from the same fourteen countries in 1996. A patient detection ratio was calculated. The female/male ratio of notification rates was below 1 and decreased with increasing age in almost all countries. The female/male prevalence ratios were less than 0.5 in surveys in the Southeast Asia and Western Pacific Region, and approximately 1 in Africa. The main conclusions from the study were that male–female differences in detection rates are due not to differential access to health care, but instead to differences in the actual incidence of TB. Still, methodological weaknesses mean that it is impossible to get conclusive evidence from this study. The African prevalence studies used were carried out many years before the notification rates used and the possibility of estimating prevalence may be dependent on the length of sputum positivity among men and women. Further population-based prevalence studies are needed before an undernotification of female cases due to gender differences in access to health care can be ruled out in all settings.

TB, together with some other diseases including syphilis and systemic lupus erythematosus, belongs to a group of diseases that are known within the medical world as 'great pretenders'. The labelling is intended as a reminder of the multiple different ways in which these diseases may present themselves. Considering the complicated immunological response to the TB bacillus and the different forms of TB that exist it is easy to understand the logic of the expression. Still there are some key symptoms of TB that are of importance to case detection of contagious, pulmonary TB. These are cough with sputum production or haemoptysis (expectoration of blood), persisting for more than three weeks. The WHO recommends that TB diagnostics are carried out in all patients who present with these symptoms in a high-prevalent TB setting. In low-income settings where resources are scarce, case detection relies mainly on the physicians' ability to recognize patients with these symptoms. In a study of sputum smear-positive pulmonary TB patients in Vietnam it was shown that women were diagnosed on average two weeks later than men, due to a delay in diagnosis at TB units.[39] This finding suggests a failure to recognize women as potential TB patients. In another study, factors that could influence diagnostic interventions were examined. It was found that among male and female patients with sputum smear-positive pulmonary TB, men significantly more often presented blood or sputum expectorates together with cough at the time of diagnosis.[40] If these symptoms, which worldwide programmes tell doctors are typical of TB, are less common in women with pulmonary TB, the possibilities for diagnosing a female patient with pulmonary TB, compared to a male patient, are reduced. Examples of how gender blindness may generate misconceptions about typical symptoms exist from internal medicine and specifically the case of acute myocardial infarction (heart attack). 'Typical symptoms' turn out to be male symptoms, which proved to be less effective for identifying females at risk.[41] Similarly the Vietnamese study on symptoms points at the danger of using male TB symptoms as normative for both men and women. Even though TB is one of the main causes of morbidity and mortality globally, methods for diagnosing it are still poor. New molecular genetic methods are expensive, and require highly equipped laboratories. Detection strategies in low-income countries still rely on sputum smear microscopy for case detection. The production of a sputum sample may be culturally sensitive in some settings and especially so for women, since women in some cultures, like Pakistan and Bangladesh, are not allowed to spit. Moreover, biological differences between male and female TB, such as the locations of pulmonary lesions, have been shown to exist. These differences also are likely to have an effect on the sensitivity of sputum testing for men and women. Interactions between cultural restrictions against producing sputum samples and the lower likelihood of women's sputum containing mycobacteria may thus have an impact on the actual number of female cases diagnosed with sputum smear-positive TB. Therefore the reported notification rates of TB may in some contexts not reflect the actual TB incidence, but instead a gender-biased estimate.

Treatment compliance and gender

Compliance or adherence to treatment is an extremely important issue of TB control, not only for the success of curing the disease in the individual patient, but also from a public health perspective. Low compliance means risks of continuing transmission of the disease and, in the case of incorrect drug intake, the possible development of drug resistance. Currently the TB control strategy dubbed directly observed therapy, short-course (DOTS), recommended by the World Health Organization, is being widely implemented. The strategy includes five components supposed to increase the efficacy and treatment success of the TB control programme. One important component is the concept of direct observed therapy (DOT) itself, requiring that health care personnel (or specially allocated staff) should literally observe the taking of the medicine, in order to ensure compliance with treatment. During the initial treatment phase the DOTS model requires either daily visits by the patient to TB dispensaries or clinics, or home visits by the health care personnel. These demands may be difficult to cope with for both men and women, and especially so for women in low-income countries, who lack resources in terms of time, money and power. Moreover, the need for a regular contact with the TB unit or health centre may have stigmatizing effects since the TB diagnosis will be evident to other people in the community. In qualitative studies, stigma has been shown to be of special importance to women,[42] and it may create reluctance to get involved with the TB programme. A randomized controlled trial carried out in South Africa showed that among men and women with TB, self-supervised treatment was more successful than the directly observed therapy. The link between treatment success and self-supervised treatment was especially strong for the female patients.[43] Clearly, more knowledge is needed about how the DOTS strategy affects women and men specifically. The 'one size fits all' approach to its implementation may create situations where female TB patients are disadvantaged. Moreover, a recent review focusing on the effectiveness of the whole DOT concept declares that 'the WHO's focus on DOT as central to improved adherence has not been helpful'.[44] More research into other methods to enhance compliance such as customized information programmes and family involvement, for example, should be carried out, and new programmes should be implemented according to the specific needs of women and men in different cultural environments.

In fact, little research has been carried out on relations between gender and treatment compliance. A recent survey presents qualitative studies on gender and compliance carried out in Vietnam.[45] When asked specifically about compliance, women were said to be more compliant in general. Men were thought to drop out of treatment before it was finished because they had to return to work and fullfill their role as 'the pillar of the household'. The quality of the encounter between doctor and patient also seems of importance for compliance. When interaction between doctor and patient was limited, dropping-out from treatment occurred. The sex of the physician also influenced the quality of the encounter. Several male doctors reported limited interaction with female patients because of poor communication, and described their encounters with female patients as 'difficult'.[46]

To ensure compliance to treatment there has to be a mutual responsibility shared by the patient and the TB doctors/programme. The goal should thus be to have open, transparent and well-informed communication between the TB programme providers and the patient. It is evident that this goal is difficult to achieve if the doctors perceive the patients as difficult and hard to communicate with.

A study from Bangalore, India, examined the case fatality rate (deaths due to TB compared to the population with TB) and found it to be 27–41 per cent higher for females aged 5–24 whereas male and female case fatality rates were similar after the age of 25.[47] These findings are in line with results from a survey carried out in China in 1990 in which women were found to have higher TB mortality rates from birth through to the age of 29. After age 29, men had higher mortality rates.[48] A similar pattern with a higher female vulnerability is suggested in a cross-sectional study conducted in Bolivia during 1993–96, in which variables predicting death from TB were identified. Female sex was found to be one of the risk factors associated with dying from TB among the hospitalized patients included in the study.[49]

Poor nutritional status is well known to be associated with an impaired immune defence,[50] and there is strong evidence suggesting a link between poor nutritional status and the severity of TB disease.[51] The power structure in many low-income countries often transforms into inequalities in food allocation, which means that young women may be especially vulnerable to TB and thus have an increased risk of a fatal outcome. The higher mortality rates could also be explained by the higher rate of progression from infection to disease among women of reproductive ages.

Social consequences – rejection and isolation of women

The traditional medical view of infectious diseases would postulate that once the disease is diagnosed, treatment is started and the eradication of the mycobacteria is in progress, the patient should also be on the road to a happy cure. However, in qualitative studies of TB patients many social consequences of TB were reported. In studies from Vietnam, initially strong negative reactions to TB were described. Thereafter patients' fears of a deadly disease and of enacted stigma were to some extent replaced by interest in more practical matters such as the cost, the distance to the TB unit and how to protect the family from becoming sick. The economic burden on the family was believed to be largest when the husband got TB, since in Vietnam the man is the major generator of income to the family. The social consequences of TB could be said to reflect the general power structure of the society. In the Vietnamese studies it was found that the reactions of family members were strongly influenced by the status of the person being diagnosed with TB. Men were in general mostly well treated and supported, whereas women could be left without support and even be rejected by the family. TB was also mentioned as a reason for divorce among couples, especially those who already had marital problems. The worry about divorce was believed to be more important to female TB patients since women were described as being the weaker party in marriage. It was also said that for an unmarried young woman, getting TB could be disastrous since she would have difficulty in finding a husband.[52]

Isolation within the community was mentioned as one of the consequences that seemed to be specific for female TB patients. Women patients described how they felt isolated by relatives and neighbours and how people no longer visited them or wanted to spend time with them. Men did not express fear of isolation in this way. The reason may be either that women with TB are more isolated than men, or that the impact of isolation is perceived more strongly by women. Apart from the studies mentioned above, the issue of the social consequences of TB has not been subject to much research. More knowledge is needed since post-TB social consequences are likely to be related to healthcare-seeking behaviour, compliance with treatment and probably also to symptom recognition and general case detection.

A gender-sensitive organization of TB control is essential when establishing TB control programmes aimed at reaching the whole population, yet this issue has been systematically neglected. It is to be hoped that increased awareness of gender inequalities in health will lead to increased research resources and efforts to understand inequities in health care. Very little is known about how the currently recommended models of control and treatment of TB affect women and men in different contexts. A gender analysis of TB is crucial to the future fight against the White Plague.

4

War and Disease: Some Perspectives on the Spatial and Temporal Occurrence of Tuberculosis in Wartime

Matthew Smallman-Raynor and Andrew D. Cliff

> Of all the diseases that flourish in the festering communities left in the wake of a modern war, tuberculosis is the most widespread and the most tenacious; its effects will continue to be felt for many years after other wartime epidemics have ceased.[1]

The social, physical and environmental circumstances of war are conducive to the rapid propagation of all manner of infectious diseases.[2] With war comes the heightened mixing of both military and civil populations, thereby increasing the likelihood of the transmission of infectious disease. The combatants may be drawn from a variety of epidemiological backgrounds, they may be assembled and deployed in disease environments to which they are not acclimatized, and they may carry infections to which the inhabitants of war zones have little or no acquired immunity. For all involved, resistance to infection may be compromised by mental and physical stress, trauma, nutritional deprivation and the deleterious consequences of rapid exposure to multiple disease agents. Insanitary conditions, enforced population concentration and overcrowding, the destruction of health infrastructure, the interruption or cessation of disease control programmes, and the collapse of the conventional rules of social behaviour further compound the epidemiological unhealthiness of war.

That infectious diseases exacted a heavy human toll in many past wars – frequently outstripping battle and violent injury as the leading causes of death in both military and civil populations – is evidenced for a sample of nineteenth- and twentieth-century conflicts in Table 4.1. During the Austro-Prussian War of 1866, for example, the 43,000 battle-related deaths in the belligerent armies are to be set against the 280,000 soldiers and civilians left for dead by the cholera epidemic that spread as a consequence of the war. Likewise, the Franco-Prussian War (1870–71) sparked concurrent epidemics of smallpox, typhoid and typhus fevers that claimed the lives of some 300,000 French and German nationals while, perhaps more famously, upwards of 25 million are believed to have perished in the global pandemic of Spanish influenza that spread with demobilization in the wake of the First World War (1914–18).[3]

Yet, as Table 4.1 also shows, the early years of the twentieth century mark something of a watershed in the epidemiological history of war. Due in part to developments in the firepower of belligerent states and in part to improvements in military hygiene and disease control, the Russo-Japanese War (1904–05) and the First World War signalled the start of an enduring trend in which more soldiers died in battle than in military lazarets.[4] At the same time, the great war pestilences that had racked the military and civil populations of earlier centuries – cholera, dysentery, plague, smallpox, typhoid, typhus and yellow fever – were joined, and in some cases supplanted, by such conditions as cerebrospinal meningitis, respiratory tract infections, sexually transmitted infections and tuberculosis as the most potent disease threats of war.[5] Indeed, such were the developments that, in 1947, Marc Daniels could proclaim TB 'the major health disaster of the Second World War'.[6]

As part of an ongoing project concerned with the spatial and temporal dynamics of war epidemics,[7] this chapter draws on a sample of late nineteenth- and twentieth-century conflicts to illustrate how the socioeconomic dislocation of war may affect patterns of TB activity at different spatial levels. Our consideration begins with a brief overview of the factors that may contribute to a wartime increase in TB activity, and the problems inherent in the data available to analyse that activity. Few strategies of modern warfare have proved as epidemiologically divisive as population reconcentration and, in the next section, we examine how the environmental conditions engendered by such a strategy were to fuel the spread of TB – amongst a host of infectious diseases – in one city (Havana, Cuba) during a nineteenth-century war (the Cuban Insurrection of 1895–98). Turning to the twentieth century and the two world wars, a geographical consideration of the epidemic

Table 4.1 Deaths in military and civil populations for sample wars of the nineteenth and twentieth centuries.

Force	Military Deaths Battle[a]	Disease	Country	Civil Deaths All causes	Diseases
Napoleonic Wars: Spanish War (1808–14)					
France	100,000	300,000			
Britain	10,716	24,053			
Russo-Polish War (1829–30)					
			Poland	326,000	?
Crimean War (1853–56)					
France	20,240	75,375			
Britain	4,602	17,580			
Russia	35,671	37,454			
American Civil War (1861–65)					
Union	93,443	186,216			
French Expedition to Mexico (1862–67)					
France	1,729	4,925			
Austro-Prussian War (1866)					
Austria	38,183	18,952	Austria	?	165,292[b]
Prussia	4,450	6,427	Prussia	?	114,776[b]
Franco-Prussian War (1870–71)					
France	138,871	25,077[c]	France	?	89,954[b]
Germany	28,276	14,825	Germany	?	176,977[b]
Russo-Turkish War (1877–78)					
Russia	34,742	81,166			
Austrian Expedition to Bosnia and Herzegovina (1878)					
Austria	1,205	2,099			
Cuban Insurrection and Spanish–American War (1895–98)					
Cuba	5,180	3,437	Cuba	218,000	?
Spain	9,143	53,440			
USA[d]	698	5,509			
Philippine-American War (1899–1902)					
Philippines	20,000	?	Philippines	?	200,000[b]
Boer War (1899–1902)					
Britain	7,534	14,382	S Africa	19,600[e]	?

Table 4.1 (*Continued*)

Military			Civil		
	Deaths			Deaths	
Force	Battle[a]	Disease	Country	All causes	Diseases
Russo-Japanese War (1904–05)					
Japan	58,900	27,200			
Russia	34,000	9,300			
First World War (1914–18)					
All forces	8,000,000	3,115,000	Global	10,080,000[f]	25,000,000[g]
France	1,385,000	500,000	France	140,128[h]	?
Germany	2,000,000	400,000	Germany	692,000[h]	?
Britain	934,000	250,000	Gt Britain	281,038[h]	?
Civil War, Soviet Russia (1917–22)					
Red Army	308,517[i]	283, 079[i]			
Second World War (1939–45)					
All forces	16,933,000[i]	2,363,500[i]?	Global	34,325,000	?
(Second) Vietnam War (1965–75)					
USA	45,941	10,000[i]	Vietnam	2,058,000	?

[a] Includes battle wounds. [b] Cholera deaths only. [c] Smallpox deaths only. [d] March 1898 – June 1899. [e] Death in Transvaal concentration camps to March 1902. [f] Excludes deaths from Spanish influenza. [g] Estimated influenza deaths, 1918–19. [h] Estimated excess deaths. [i] Deaths for 1918–20 only, including prisoners of war. [j] Includes all non-combat deaths.

Source: based principally on information in: Friedrich Prinzing, *Epidemics Resulting from Wars*, Oxford: Clarendon Press, 1916; Samuel Dumas and K. O. Vedel-Petersen, *Losses of Life Caused by War*, Oxford: Clarendon Press, 1923.

ascendancy of TB in the European theatre is followed by an examination of the spatial parameters that underpinned one prominent epidemiological feature of wartime Britain: the rise of pulmonary TB among young adult women in the First World War. To underscore the enduring nature of the association between war and TB, the chapter concludes with a brief review of disease activity in high- and low-intensity conflicts during the latter half of the twentieth century.

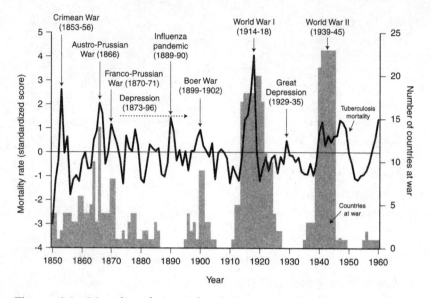

Figure 4.1 Mortality from pulmonary TB in England and Wales, 1850–1960. The annual series of TB mortality, plotted as a line trace, has been detrended and is expressed in standard Normal score form. For reference, the number of European countries at war in each year is plotted as a bar chart. Source of data: Registrar-General of England and Wales, *Annual Reports*, London: HMSO.

TB as a war pestilence

The signature of war can be deciphered in many past records of TB activity. By way of illustration, Figure 4.1 shows that wartime peaks in the series of TB mortality for England and Wales reflect not only conflicts in which Britain held a military stake (the Crimean War, the Boer War and the two world wars), but also the overspill from continental European wars in which Britain maintained a non-belligerent status (the Austro-Prussian War and the Franco-Prussian War).[8]

Specific factors that may contribute to a wartime increase in TB activity, and which could account for past mortality fluctuations of the type depicted in Figure 4.1, are well known and include a broad range of primary environmental influences on the transmission of, and host resistance to, the tubercle bacillus.[9] The crowding of both military and civil populations – arising from the destruction of housing infrastructure, billeting and close-quarter accommodation in such facilities as military assembly and training camps, concentration and prison camps, refugee camps, hospitals and air raid shelters – provides conditions ripe for the aerosol transmission of the tubercle bacillus. Protein–calorie malnutrition, resulting from the disruption of agricultural production and the shredding of food supply lines, food rationing and distribution controls, is aetiologically linked to a reduction in human resistance to pre-existing or new tubercular infection; additionally, as part of a general war effort, increased employment in munitions production and/or certain other 'dusty' industries may serve as a further stimulant to latent pulmonary infection. The physical exertion and mental stress that typically accompany a war may also weaken resistance to infection, while the adverse consequences of disruption of TB control programmes, including the military requisitioning of dedicated hospital facilities and sanatoria, are illustrated by the experience of some European countries during the First World War.[10]

As for any infectious disease, however, the analysis of TB occurrence in wartime is confronted by an insidious problem in epidemiological studies: the quality of the data available for examination. The destruction of public health infrastructure, the redeployment, transfer or elimination of health resources and personnel, the collapse of communications systems, the lack of diagnostic capabilities, censorship, propaganda, and the intentional falsification of information all conspire to limit the availability and reliability of TB statistics in wartime. While these problems are compounded by difficulties surrounding the recognition, clinical distinction and classification of tubercular diseases in earlier centuries,[11] the testimony of medical staff attached to the United Nations Relief and Rehabilitation Administration (UNRRA), operating in Europe in the immediate aftermath of the Second World War, provides some insight into the limitations of TB statistics in a modern theatre of war:

> When we went into the liberated countries, in our innocence we asked for figures to show the TB death-rates during the war years. . . . In some countries, public health records were lost or destroyed; in a couple of Polish cities, wartime records were preserved only through the grim tenacity of a few doctors who could foresee their use . . . the unreliability of many statistics was apparent when one examined their source. . . . In examining pre-war figures we were convinced that the desire to please a dictator who took a benevolent interest in

TB may well have made rather steeper a decline in the death-rates. Figures of incidence were quoted . . . but it was soon apparent that they could be of no value.[12]

According to the same source, the mortality records for Yugoslavia 'everywhere were destroyed', no records were available for Greece while, for the Nazi concentration and extermination camps, information regarding the occurrence of TB was largely dependent on post-war autopsies conducted on the dead of such places as Belsen and Dachau.[13] But the experience of occupied Europe in the Second World War provides just one example and, in the latter half of the twentieth century, high- and low-intensity conflicts in Vietnam, Cambodia, Lebanon, Nicaragua and the former Yugoslavia, among many other countries, have been associated with acute or chronic disruption of surveillance for TB and other infectious diseases.

Insurrection, population reconcentration and disease: Havana, Cuba (1895–98)

Although detailed accounts of TB activity in conflicts prior to the First World War are generally lacking, a novel archival source in epidemiological studies – the sanitary dispatches prepared by officers of the US Marine Hospital Service and reprinted in the US *Public Health Reports* – provides a window on the epidemic occurrence of TB, alongside a series of other infectious diseases (including enteric fever, smallpox and yellow fever), in one nineteenth-century conflict: the Cuban insurrection against Spain (February 1895 to August 1898).[15] Details of the data source, the insurrection and its association with the Spanish-American War (April to August 1898) are given elsewhere,[16] but, as Table 4.1 indicates, the hostilities plunged the Caribbean island of Cuba into four years of disease turmoil. Of the estimated 290,000 Spanish and Cuban soldiers and civilians who perished during the war and its immediate aftermath, some 275,000 (95 per cent) are believed to have succumbed to disease and the deprivations of war rather than to battle. While yellow fever devastated the largely unacclimatized contingent of 200,000 Spanish troops deployed to combat the Cuban *insurrectos*, it was the Spanish military response to insurrectionary activity that was to have the gravest epidemiological ramifications for the island. In a draconian attempt to quash rural support for the Cuban Revolutionary Army, the Spanish authorities issued an order for the reconcentration of the rural population of Cuba on 17 February 1896. Under this order, rural civilians were directed to relocate to towns and cities; travel outside the urban centres was strictly controlled, the transport of foodstuffs was halted, and summary justice was introduced for those suspected of insurgent activity. Within ten months of the order, an estimated 400,000 civilians, representing almost one quarter of the entire population of Cuba, had been forcibly removed from the countryside and herded into the urban centres of the island.[17]

The adverse health effects of the reconcentration policy were to prove especially severe in the city of Havana (1899 population 235,981). Even in the absence of war, the sanitary conditions that prevailed in the city were notoriously bad.[18] Population reconcentration merely exacerbated the conditions. As the command centre and staging post for Spanish military operations in the island, Havana was already so overcrowded with Spanish soldiers and refugees that adequate shelter could not be found for the many thousands of *reconcentrados* newly arrived from the rural areas of Havana province. Sewerage systems, potable water and medical care were generally lacking, while, as the war progressed, food became increasingly scarce. By the summer of 1897, starvation, anaemia, intestinal and deficiency diseases were rife in the city. The health of the population continued to deteriorate throughout the remainder of the war, and only with the emergency relief that accompanied the US annexation of the island in 1899 did circumstances begin to improve.[19]

Graphic descriptions of the wartime conditions endured by the population of Havana are provided by medical officers of the US Marine Hospital Service (USMHS) who were stationed in the city at the time of the insurrection. Writing in October 1897, for example, USMHS Sanitary Inspector W. F. Brunner reported his observations on the accommodation provided for one group of *reconcentrados*:

An inspection of a pest hole, known as Los Fosos, was made by me on Thursday, October 14. This place has been set aside for the country people sent to Habana. Los Fosos consists of a large wooden building about 150 feet in length and 60 feet in width. . . . There were 500 people found in and around this building, and of that number over 200 were found lying on the floor sick and dying. I saw no child under 10 years of age who could be considered in good health. . . . The emaciation of their bodies was startling . . . the death rate is enormous.[20]

By the end of November 1897, no fewer than 1,190 of the 1,700 *reconcentrados* assigned to Los Fosos had died.[21] But the plight of the *reconcentrados* also spilled out onto the streets of Havana:

Just opposite to the office of the [US Marine Hospital] Service a wholesale grocery firm gives a pittance of rice to all who apply for it. . . . Hundreds of thin, emaciated people drag themselves there to partake of the bounty, and it is a gruesome sight to observe the condition, or rather lack of physical condition, of the crowd.[22]

In fact, by the autumn of 1897, starvation had assumed more general proportions in the city. With domestic food supplies all but exhausted, and the population increasingly dependent on foreign foodstuffs whose import duties were so high as to be 'prohibitive to the average customer', desperate citizens took to the disinterring of dead animals as a source of nutrition.[23] The hardships were exacerbated by the US naval blockade of Havana (22 April to 12 August 1898), and starvation continued into the post-war period; as late as December 1898, some four months after the cessation of hostilities, USMHS officials estimated the number who were still 'bordering on starvation' to be in excess of 3,000.[24]

Late nineteenth-century Havana was no stranger to the ravages of TB. In the five years, 1890–94, that preceded the outbreak of war, pulmonary and non-pulmonary TB accounted for a full 20 per cent of certified deaths in the city.[25] With the extreme deprivation, starvation and crowding that accompanied the onset of the war, however, TB assumed new, epidemic proportions (see Figure 4.2A).[26] Table 4.2 gives the total number of reported TB deaths for the war period, along with an estimate of the wartime increment in TB mortality; the equivalent information is also given for other infectious diseases and for deaths from all causes.

Although TB data are unavailable for the early months of the war, Figure 4.2 shows that the conflict was associated with a marked increase in TB mortality compared with all other years in the time series. From an average background level of some 100–120 deaths per month in the years that preceded the insurrection, mortality increased

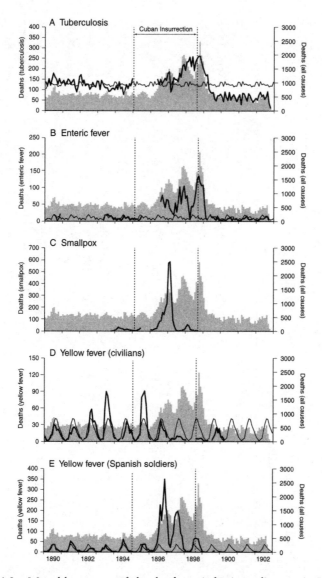

Figure 4.2 Monthly counts of deaths from infectious diseases in Havana, Cuba, 1890–1902. (A) TB. (B) Enteric fever. (C) Smallpox. (D) Yellow fever, civilians. (E) Yellow fever, Spanish soldiers. On each graph, disease-specific deaths (heavy line trace) are superimposed on the count of deaths from all causes (bar chart). For the three diseases endemic to Cuba (enteric fever, TB and yellow fever), the fine line trace plots the number of deaths as a seasonal average in the pre-war period (1890–94). The period of the Cuban Insurrection is indicated. Source of data: US Marine Hospital Service, *Public Health Reports*, Washington, DC: Government Printing Office.

Table 4.2 Periods of epidemic activity associated with sample infectious diseases in Havana, Cuba, 1895–98.

Cause of death	Deaths		Epidemic period[2]			Peak
	Recorded[1]	Estimated wartime excess[3]	Interval	Duration (months)		
Bacterial diseases						
TB	4,937[4]	1,500[4]	May 1896 – Mar. 1899	35		Sept. 1898
Enteric fever[5]	1,561	1,100	July 1896 – Feb. 1899	32		Sept. 1898
Viral diseases						
Smallpox	2,935	2,935[6]	Jan. 1896 – Jun. 1897	18		Feb. 1897
Yellow fever						
Soldiers	2,990	2,400	Apr. 1896 – Jan. 1898	22		Nov. 1896
			June 1898 – Dec. 1898	7		Aug. 1898
Civilians	596	–[7]	Apr. – Nov. 1895	8		Sept. 1895
			Nov. 1897 – May 1898	7		Feb. 1898
All causes	46,925	21,600	Feb. 1896 – May 1899	40		Oct. 1898

Notes: [1] War period, February 1895 – August 1898. [2] Defined as the phase of cause-specific mortality above the pre-war (1890–94) monthly average, and including the immediate post-war period. [3] Computed as recorded wartime mortality in excess of the pre-war average monthly mortality, 1890–94. [4] Estimates for the period May 1896 – August 1898. [5] Typhoid and paratyphoid fevers. [6] Estimate based on the non-endemic nature of smallpox in late-nineteenth-century Havana. [7] Recorded deaths fell below the pre-war expectation.

rapidly in the period that followed the reconcentration order of February 1896; by the end of 1897, TB deaths had reached almost 250 per month. The high mortality count continued throughout the remainder of the conflict, but was followed by a steep and sustained fall with the sanitary improvements that accompanied US occupation in 1899.[27] All told, Table 4.2 estimates the wartime increment in TB mortality at 1,500 deaths, equivalent to 7 per cent of the total mortality increment (21,600 deaths) associated with the war.

To place TB within a broader epidemiological perspective, figures 4.2B to 4.2E plot the monthly count of deaths from three further infectious diseases in wartime Havana. Table 4.2 gives an estimate of the war-related increment in mortality for each disease. In addition, the table gives the period(s) of the war for which each disease exhibited above-average (epidemic) levels of mortality, the duration of the epidemic period(s) and the month(s) of peak mortality.

While it is evident that the insurrection was associated with multiple epidemic events of unusual magnitude, Table 4.2 and Figure 4.2 identify important features relating to the differential effects of the insurrection on (a) levels of disease-specific mortality and (b) the timing of epidemic events.

Levels of disease-specific mortality. As judged by Table 4.2, the war had an unequal influence on levels of disease-specific mortality in the city. So, although TB ranks as the leading cause of death in Table 4.2, the estimated war-associated increment in TB mortality (1,500 deaths) lies well below the equivalent estimates for smallpox (2,935 deaths) and for yellow fever in Spanish soldiers (2,400 deaths). These findings remain substantially unaltered when corrected for missing data and suggest that, for the sample diseases included in the present study, high levels of susceptibility to viral agents (the smallpox and yellow fever viruses), rather than pre-existing or new infection with bacterial agents (including *Mycobacterium tuberculosis* and *Salmonella typhi*), represented the most important factor in the war-associated mortality increment of late nineteenth-century Havana.

Epidemic timings. Taken together, Figure 4.2 and Table 4.2 highlight a crucial epidemiological facet of the war–disease relationship: the tendency for different diseases, with different aetiologies, to assume prominence at different stages of a conflict. On the one hand, the two bacterial diseases (TB and enteric fever) developed to a peak in the latter stages of the war and reflected the gradual deterioration of socioeconomic and sanitary conditions as the hostilities progressed. On the other hand, the two viral diseases (smallpox and yellow fever), characterized by short incubation periods and lasting immunity in exposed but surviving individuals, spread rapidly with the population churning that accompanied the earlier phases of the hostilities; with many of those who were initially susceptible having already acquired the infection, there were insufficient susceptible people to support anything other than relatively minor outbreaks of the diseases in the later stages of the war.[28]

Although smallpox and yellow fever accounted for a relatively greater proportion of the wartime mortality increment in Havana, the significance of the substantial increment due to TB was not lost on contemporary commentators. In a brief, but candid, reflection on TB in late nineteenth-century Havana, the USMHS surgeon and chief quarantine officer of Cuba, H. R. Carter, could glimpse the epidemiological benefits that had accrued from the war. 'A great number must have died,' he observed, 'who would have otherwise lived a few years longer and would now be swelling our bills of mortality.' 'It was,' he concluded, 'a most cruel, but effectual method of lessening the presence of TB in the city.'[29]

World conflict and TB: the European theatre, 1914–18 and 1939–45

The social, physical and environmental conditions engendered by the First and Second World Wars were to have a severe, if geographically highly uneven, impact on TB activity in the European theatre of war.[30] Figures 4.3A and 4.3B show that the wars were associated with temporary interruptions – of a greater or lesser magnitude – to a long-term downward trend in underlying mortality. In Figures 4.3C and 4.3D, which examine the interruptions more closely (with the underlying trends removed) wartime mortality is manifested as major spikes of disease activity. Although the spikes are generally most pronounced for the belligerent states in a given war, it is also apparent that the epidemiological consequences of the conflicts spilled over to the non-belligerent states of Europe.

For each of the fifteen European countries included in Figure 4.3, Table 4.3 gives a percentage estimate of the increment/decrement in TB

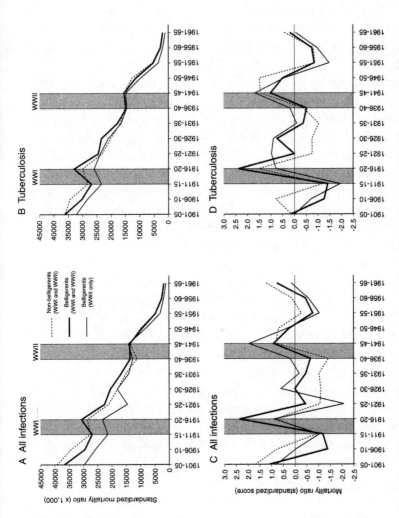

Figure 4.3 Mortality from infectious diseases in Europe, 1901–65. For sample European countries, grouped by belligerent status in the First and Second World Wars, the upper graphs plot the average standardized mortality ratio (SMR, formed to a factor of 1,000) by quinquennial period, while the lower graphs plot the detrended series of SMRs (expressed in standard Normal score form). (A) and (C), all infectious diseases. (B) and (D), TB (all forms). Countries are categorized by belligerent status in Table 4.3. Source of data: M. Alderson, (1981), *International Mortality Statistics*, New York: Macmillan.

mortality associated with each World War.[31] A relatively large and positive value indicates that the war period was associated with a proportionately large increment in TB mortality, while a relatively large and negative value indicates a proportionately large decrement. For reference, parallel estimates are also given for three non-European members of the Allied Forces (Australia, Canada and the USA).

While Table 4.3 underscores the epidemiological impact of the wars in many European states, geographical variations are evident and reflect the relative severity of the wartime conditions.[32] Among the belligerent states of the First World War, for example, the largest increments in TB mortality are recorded for the embattled states of Austria, Belgium and Italy; away from the scene of active hostilities, a more modest increment is recorded for England and Wales while, for Scotland, the long-term decline in TB mortality was largely unchecked by the war. Likewise, among the belligerents of the Second World War, stark increments in Italy and the occupied lands of northern Europe (Belgium, France and the Netherlands) contrast with mortality decrements in such countries as Bulgaria, Denmark and England and Wales. While the privations that contributed to these latter variations are outlined elsewhere,[33] three further features of Table 4.3 are also apparent. First, for many non-belligerent states, neutrality afforded little – if any – protection against the epidemiological consequences of war. In this context, the experiences of Denmark, Spain and the Netherlands in the First World War, and of Ireland in the Second, are especially noteworthy. Furthermore, although comparative data are limited, evidence for countries such as Belgium, Italy and the Netherlands suggests that the relative impact of war on TB activity was greater in the Second World War than in the First World War. Third, away from the European theatre, the wars had but little effect on TB mortality in the belligerent states of Australia, Canada and the USA.

Case study: England and Wales

While countries of continental Europe experienced the worst excesses of the war-related increases in TB mortality (see Table 4.3), the somewhat more modest – if still marked – experience of England and Wales is illustrated in Figure 4.4. The detrended series in Figure 4.4 yield a common signal. Regardless of gender or disease site, the First World War was accompanied by a steep rise in the mortality curve,

Table 4.3 Estimated impact of the First and Second World Wars on national-level records of TB mortality in sample European and non-European countries.

Country	Percentage impact of war on recorded levels of TB mortality[a]			
	World War I		World War II	
	Increment	Decrement	Increment	Decrement
EUROPEAN COUNTRIES				
Belligerents (WWI & WWII)				
Austria	9.3		No data	
Belgium	7.9		21.7	
Bulgaria	No data			−3.9
Czechoslovakia	No data		0.7	
France	No data		22.0	
Hungary	No data		4.0	
Italy	10.3			
UK				
England and Wales	2.3			−6.4
Scotland		−10.8		−0.4
Belligerents (WWII only)				
Denmark	5.3			−22.9
Finland[b]	No data		11.3	
Netherlands	26.4		47.4	
Non-belligerents (WWI & WWII)				
Eire	No data		16.9	
Spain	7.4		1.3	
Switzerland		−0.3		−6.1
NON-EUROPEAN COUNTRIES				
Belligerents (WWI & WWII)				
Australia		−8.0		−6.3
Canada		−6.5		−7.4
USA		−4.7		−7.5

Notes: [a] Formed as a percentage estimate of the increment/decrement in tuberculosis mortality associated with World War I and World War II. [b] Not classified as an independent state in World War I.

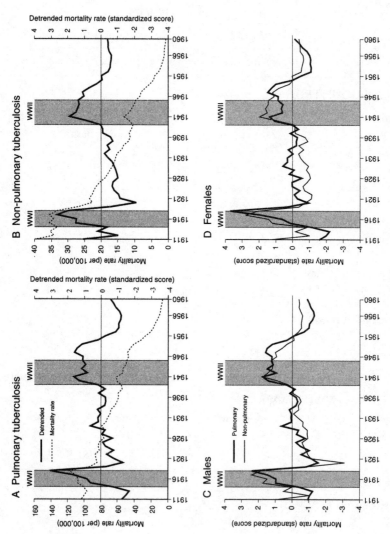

Figure 4.4 TB mortality in England and Wales, 1911–60. (A) Pulmonary TB. (B) Non-pulmonary TB. On both graphs, the broken line traces plot the TB mortality rate (per 100,000 population), while the heavy line traces plot the detrended mortality rate (expressed as a standard Normal score). The remaining graphs plot the detrended mortality rates for pulmonary and non-pulmonary TB for (C) males and (D) females. Source of data: Chief Medical Officer, *Annual Reports*, London: HMSO.

followed by an abrupt fall at the end of the hostilities. Minor interruptions to the relative epidemiological calm of the inter-war years were then replaced, from the onset of the Second World War, by a second, and more protracted, recrudescence in TB mortality; high mortality levels continued into the post-war period, only to begin a decline in the late 1940s. The complex of factors that could account for the sustained post-war effects of the Second World War relative to the First World War are uncertain but may relate, at least in part, to the adverse health consequences of the greater structural damage sustained in the second conflict.[34]

One prominent epidemiological feature of TB in the civil population of wartime Britain was the disproportionate increase in active disease among young adult women in the early years of the First World War. So, while the total number of TB-related deaths in England and Wales grew by about 7 per cent between 1914 and 1916, deaths among females aged 15–44 years grew by an average of 12.5 per cent, with the largest increases in those aged 15–19 years (22 per cent) and 20–24 years (14 per cent).[35] Spurred by speculation that the increases were attributable to working conditions associated with the wartime employment of females in munitions factories and other industries,[36] the results of a Medical Research Committee inquiry into the circumstances surrounding the mortality rise appeared in 1919 under the title *An Inquiry Into the Prevalence and Aetiology of TB Among Industrial Workers, with Special Reference to Female Munition Workers.*[37] While the report concluded that industrial employment had introduced a 'special factor' in the development of the disease,[38] a geographical examination of the data collated by the authors of the *Inquiry* reveals that the wartime rise in TB mortality among young adult females was characterized by a distinctive spatial pattern.

While Figures 4.5 and 4.6 confirm the general tendency for a wartime increase in proportionate mortality from pulmonary TB (formed as the ratio of deaths from pulmonary TB to deaths from all other causes), Figure 4.5 also reveals the marked geographical pattern to the increase.[39] In contrast to the boroughs of central and northern England, which are characterized by modest (0.10–0.19) or low (< 0.10) increments to a relatively high background level of proportionate mortality, the largest increments (> 0.20) are recorded in boroughs of southern England and Wales. So, with the notable exception of two northwestern towns (Warrington and Bootle), both adjacent to the

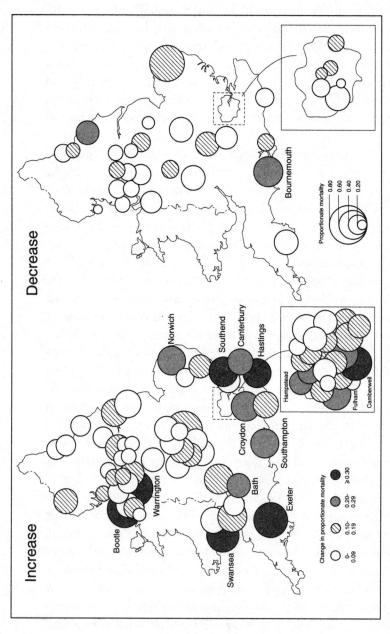

Figure 4.5 Changes in the proportion of deaths among adult females (aged 15–45 years) due to pulmonary TB in the county and metropolitan boroughs of England and Wales. Each borough is identified by a circle whose area is scaled to the proportionate mortality from pulmonary TB (i.e. deaths from pulmonary TB as a proportion of deaths from all other causes) in 1916. Boroughs are distinguished according to the change in proportionate mortality between the base year of 1913 and 1916. Source of data: Medical Research Committee, *An Inquiry Into the Prevalence and Aetiology of Tuberculosis Among Industrial Workers, with Special Reference to Female Munition Workers*, London: HMSO, 1919, Tables 18 and 19, pp. 39–42.

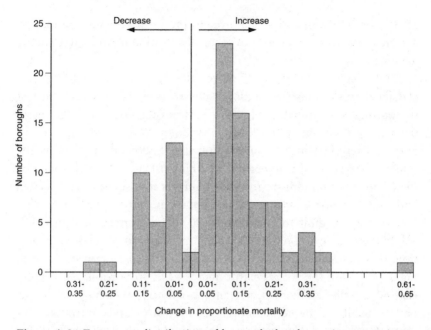

Figure 4.6 Frequency distribution of boroughs by change in proportionate mortality from pulmonary TB in adult females (aged 15–45 years) (county and metropolitan boroughs of England and Wales, 1913–16). Source of data: Medical Research Committee, *An Inquiry Into the Prevalence and Aetiology of Tuberculosis Among Industrial Workers, with Special Reference to Female Munition Workers*, London: HMSO, 1919, Tables 18 and 19, pp. 39–42.

port of Liverpool, the largest increments are identified in coastal/port towns, cities and proximal settlements of South Wales (Swansea) and southern (Bath, Exeter and Southampton) and southeastern (Brighton, Hastings, Canterbury and Southend) England. In addition, large increments are also identified in some boroughs of East Anglia (Norwich) and metropolitan London.

Although the authors of the *Inquiry* concluded that the wartime increase in TB mortality was linked to industrial employment, they emphasized that the association between the changes in proportionate mortality depicted in Figure 4.5 and the industrial status of the 106 boroughs was 'not very striking'.[40] The evidence presented in Table 4.4 concurs with their viewpoint. The table is based on the industrial/non-industrial categorization of boroughs adopted by the *Inquiry* and gives the average proportionate mortality for pulmonary TB in 1913 and

1916. For both categories of borough, the proportionate mortalities, and their associated increases over the observation period, are virtually identical.

While such a finding may reflect the need for a more detailed classification of industrial employment structure, we note that most of the boroughs identified in Figure 4.5 as having recorded large increments in proportionate mortality – including Bath, Brighton, Canterbury, Exeter, Hastings, Southampton and Southend, as well as the London boroughs of Camberwell and Hampstead – were classified by the *Inquiry* as non-industrial centres. Subject to instabilities associated with small disease counts in the less populous centres, therefore, other factors may account for the distinctive spatial pattern in Figure 4.5. While these factors could include such mechanisms as selective migration, it is noteworthy that the broad geographical pattern depicted in Figure 4.5, with the larger relative increases in proportionate mortality centred on the southern sector of the country, is analogous to the pattern exhibited by contemporary epidemics of other infectious diseases. Cerebrospinal meningitis, for example, spread widely with the southerly flux of both military and civil populations in the early part of the First World War;[41] further research is required to determine whether the same wartime population flux, centred on the settlements of southern England and Wales, contributed to the development of the TB pattern shown in Figure 4.5.

The enduring association of TB and war

Globally, no less than 350 wars, revolutions and *coups d'état* were staged in the half-century following the end of the Second World War.[42] Most of these clashes centred on developing countries; many were of limited extent and severity, and a bloodless few yielded little, or no, discernible effect on the health of the countries involved.[43] Many others, however, served to shatter local and national economies and infrastructures, leaving thousands or millions of dead, homeless or displaced people in their wake.[44] As far as the epidemiological evidence permits us to say, such conflicts, like their pre-1945 counterparts, were typically accompanied by a pronounced – sometimes dramatic and often protracted – increase in tubercular infection and disease. Five years into the 1965–75 Vietnam War, for example, estimates of the prevalence of active TB in some cohorts of the Vietnamese population reached as high as 20 per cent, with evidence of the circulation of multi-drug-resistant strains of *Mycobacterium tuberculosis* among both the civil population and US military returnees.[45] Subsequent wars with Cambodia and China, a US trade embargo and the rapid spread of the human immunodeficiency virus (HIV) merely served to compound the TB problem in late-twentieth-century Vietnam.[46] Likewise, the latter stages of long-running civil wars in the Lebanon and El Salvador were associated with marked increases in pulmonary TB while, among refugees, inflated levels of active disease have been reported in those fleeing conflicts in such places as Angola, Afghanistan, Bosnia-Herzegovina, Chechnya and Somalia.

In turn, the international flight of refugees, asylum seekers and other fugitives from modern conflicts has served to carry the TB problem beyond the borders of warring states, sometimes into territories where background levels of TB activity are relatively low.[48] Beginning with the Slovenian and Croatian wars of independence in the summer of 1991, for example, almost a decade of fighting in the former Yugoslavia has spawned the largest international movement of European refugees since the Second World War; in the years 1991–93, alone, an estimated 512,000 Bosnian and Croatian refugees entered the countries of Western Europe, with TB prominent among the anticipated health problems of these people.[49] TB screening by the recipient countries has underscored such health concerns, with exceptionally high levels of tubercular disease among Bosnian medical evacuees, assigned to the UK, serving to illustrate the problem.[50]

Although wars may promote the spread of all manner of infectious diseases, this chapter has attempted to highlight an important facet of the war–disease relationship: the tendency for different diseases to respond to the circumstances of a particular war in different ways. In the context of late-nineteenth-century Havana, for example, the gradual rise in mortality from bacterial diseases (enteric fever and TB) as the Cuban Insurrection unfolded contrasts with the rapid spread of viral diseases (smallpox and yellow fever) in the earlier stages of the war. While such differences in the timing of epidemic events associated with viruses and bacteria reflect fundamental differences in the epidemiological parameters of the disease agents involved, further research is required to establish the more general utility of a simple virus–bacterium model of epidemic timings in cities under the stress of war.

In an optimistic conclusion to his pathbreaking review of the spread of TB in Europe during the Second World War, Marc Daniels argued that the means for the elimination of TB were already in place. 'Given a long enough respite from mutual massacre,' Daniels commented, 'there is no reason why this disease . . . should not be almost eradicated before this century is out.'[51] Unfortunately, recent events have dashed such optimism and the epidemiological consequences of war, so far as TB is concerned, endure into a new century.

PART II

The 'New' Tuberculosis

5

The Present Global Burden
of Tuberculosis

Léopold Blanc and Mukund Uplekar

Nearly one third of the global population – that is, 2 billion people – are infected with tuberculosis and at risk of developing the disease. About 8 million people develop active TB every year, and 2 million die.[1] TB accounts for 2.5 per cent of the global burden of disease,[2] for 26 per cent of preventable deaths, and is the commonest cause of death in young women. Some 95 per cent of global TB cases and 98 per cent of deaths occur in the developing world, where 75 per cent of cases are in the economically most productive age group (15–54 years). There, on average, three to four months of work time are lost if an adult has TB. This results in the loss of 20–30 per cent of annual household income and an average of fifteen years' income if the patient dies.[3] In addition to the devastating economic cost, TB imposes indirect negative consequences. In India alone, for example, every year more than 300,000 children leave school because of their parents' TB, and more than 100,000 women are abandoned by their families because of their TB. TB impoverishes, and poverty attracts TB.[4]

Furthermore, co-infection with HIV significantly increases the risk of developing TB.[5] Countries with a high prevalence of HIV, particularly those in sub-Saharan Africa, have witnessed a profound increase in TB, with reported incidence rates increasing by two or three times in the 1990s.[6] Today, worldwide, 11 million people are co-infected with TB and HIV.[7] The TB/HIV co-epidemic is increasing and will continue to fuel the TB epidemic.

At the same time, drug resistance, which is caused by poorly managed TB treatment, is an increasing problem and many countries across the globe have seen a rise and spread of multi-drug-resistant (MDR-TB).[8] MDR-TB is much more difficult and much more expensive to manage than drug-sensitive TB.[9]

It was in the early 1990s that the world's attention was called to the growing TB problem, not only in developing countries but also in industrialized countries. In 1993 the World Health Organization (WHO) declared TB a global public health emergency and called for intensified support for TB control activities both by governments of the endemic countries and by the international community. In 1998 a meeting of experts identified as a priority for action the twenty-two countries that hosted 80 per cent of the total number of TB cases in the world. The Stop TB initiative was established in November 1998 and, since TB was recognized as one of the diseases of poverty which constitute a major impediment to the development of countries and their people, the WHO invited all agencies, groups and institutions to contribute to a new global movement.

This was well over a century after the TB germ was identified and over half a century after the introduction of effective drug treatment against it – a unique distinction of the TB epidemic.

Detecting and curing cases of TB is the most cost-effective way of arresting the spread of the disease. This is the aim of the directly observed therapy, short-course (DOTS) strategy, currently promoted by the WHO.[10] The extreme urgency of the need to tackle the global burden of TB cannot be overemphasized. There is hope nevertheless. Projections based on the epidemiology of the disease and the effectiveness of the DOTS strategy indicate that it is possible to reduce the number of new cases by half in fifteen years' time if the strategy is widely and efficiently applied.[11]

Assessing the global burden of TB

Making an accurate assessment of the TB burden poses problems. In many regions where the TB burden is high, disease surveillance is inadequate, while even in some developed nations notification and record keeping leave much to be desired. This explains the variation in the number of cases given in different sources. Case notification offers one way of assessing the TB burden, and it is the most commonly used one. In countries with effective TB programmes and optimal reporting systems, case notifications approximate the real number of TB cases. However, in countries with poor TB programmes and where access to health services is limited, detection and notification may be grossly inadequate.[12] During the 1990s, the introduction of the DOTS strategy, with its standard recording and reporting system for TB globally, has improved case notification, though reporting is still insufficient in many countries.

Of the 3.6 million cases of TB cases reported to the WHO in 1998, Southeast Asia and the Western Pacific regions accounted for almost 60 per cent of the global caseload, with India and China alone reporting more than 40 per cent of all notified cases. Although the Africa region contains only 10 per cent of the 5.9 billion global population, the region reported 18 per cent of total TB cases (Figure 5.1). Notably, the case notification rate for Africa (110 per 100,000 population) is greater than that for Southeast Asia (88 per 100,000 population) (Table 5.1).

But comparisons based on reported cases need to be interpreted with caution due to variations in reporting. In order to have a better assessment of the situation and a better picture of the worldwide distribution of cases, eighty-six TB experts and epidemiologists from forty countries and from the WHO published a consensus statement on the 'Global burden of tuberculosis'.[13] This gave systematic estimates of the incidence of TB (the yearly number of new cases), its prevalence (the total number of cases) and mortality by country, region and globally for 1997. The estimated global incidence of TB in that year was 7.96 million, of which 3.52 million (44 per cent) were cases of highly infectious pulmonary disease (sputum smear positive).[14]

Worldwide, only 45 per cent of the estimated total number of new cases and 40 per cent of the estimated total number of new smear-positive cases are reported.[15] There are wide regional variations in the proportion of cases that are notified. The European region, for instance, reports 80 per cent of the estimated cases there compared to the Eastern Mediterranean which reports only 38 per cent of estimated cases in the region.

From the data reported to the WHO, the global trend of new cases reported remained more or less stable at 60 per 100,000 population during the period 1980 to 1998.[16] Available data before 1980 are not comprehensive. In 1967, 1.16 million cases were reported from 145 countries, accounting for only 40 per cent of the world's population,

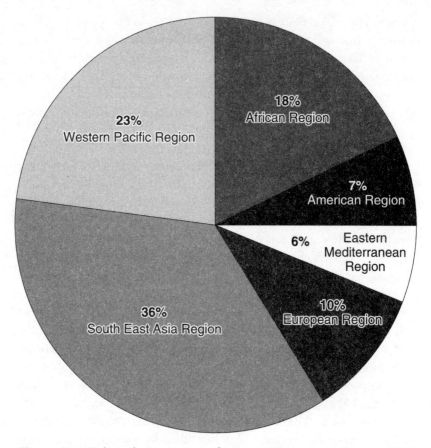

Figure 5.1 Tuberculosis case notification 1998, proportion by WHO regions. Source: World Health Organization.

while in 1998 the 189 countries that reported 3.6 million cases to the WHO represented 98 per cent of the global population.[17] According to crude estimates, in 1967 some 2.8 million cases should have been reported worldwide, a figure indicating that case notifications during the last three decades increased by almost 25 per cent.[18]

A more accurate analysis of trends is possible for selected countries within regions. While Western Europe showed a steady decline in case notifications of 4 per cent per year from 1980 to 1998, Eastern Europe observed a similar decline up to 1992 and then an unusual rise of 10 per cent a year (Figure 5.2). In fourteen African countries, case notifications were stable between 1980 and 1988. Thereafter, there has been a sharp increase at 10 per cent a year. The decline in eleven Latin

Table 5.1 The global burden of tuberculosis.

WHO region	No. of cases notified, 1998 (rate per 100,000 population)	No. of new cases estimated, 1997 (rate per 100,000 population)	% notification	Deaths estimated 1997 (rate per 100,000 population)	% of the population infected with *M. tuberculosis*
Africa	646,842 (110)	1,586,000 (259)	40	540,000 (88)	35
America	237,000 (30)	411,000 (52)	58	66,000 (8)	18
Eastern Mediterranean	235,042 (49)	615,000 (129)	38	141,000 (30)	29
Europe	351,521 (43)	440,000 (51)	80	64,000 (7)	15
South-east Asia	1,307,175 (88)	2,948,000 (202)	44	705,000 (48)	44
Western Pacific	839,019 (50)	1,962,000 (120)	43	355,000 (22)	36
World	3,617,045 (61)	7,962,000 (136)	45	1,871,000 (32)	32

Source: World Health Organization.

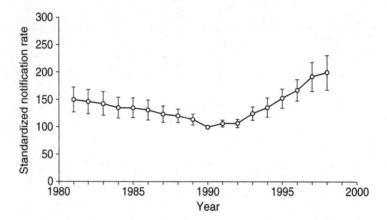

Figure 5.2 Trend in case notification in selected countries in Eastern Europe (Belarus, Estonia, Hungary, Kazakhstan, Kyrgyzstan, Latvia, Lithuania, Republic of Moldova, Romania, Russian Federation and Ukraine). To highlight trends in notifications within regions, the rates for all countries have been expressed to an arbitrary standard of 100 in 1990; error bars are 95% confidence limit on the standardized rates. Source: World Health Organization.

American countries has been steady at 2 per cent a year during the period 1980–98. In selected Asian countries, case notification rates increased by 1–2 per cent a year during the same period.[19] Overall, TB has apparently made a resurgence almost everywhere in the world.

The impact of HIV

The HIV pandemic has made a dramatic impact on TB in regions where TB and HIV infections are co-prevalent, for example, sub-Saharan Africa, some Southeast Asian countries – Thailand, Myanmar, Cambodia, China and Vietnam – and some states in India. In 1990, around 315,000 cases of TB worldwide were estimated to be attributable to HIV infection (Table 5.2).[20] In 1997, it was estimated that 640,000 cases would be attributable to HIV infection, double the number of 1990.[21] In developing countries in Africa, Latin America and Asia, where a large proportion of the population is already infected with TB bacilli, TB has emerged as the most common HIV-related disease. The proportion of patients developing TB during the course of

Table 5.2 Estimated TB incidents and HIV-attributable TB cases, 1990 and 1997.

Region	1990[e]			1997[f]		
	Total TB cases	Rate per 100,000 population	HIV-attributable TB cases	Total TB cases	Rate per 100,000 population	HIV-attribtable TB cases
Africa	992,000	191	194,000	1,586,000	259	515,000
America[a]	569,000	127	20,000	392,000	180	21,000
Eastern Mediterranean	641,000	165	9,000	615,000	129	16,000
Europe (Eastern)[b]	194,000	47	1,000	333,000	80	4,000
Southeast Asia	3,106,000	237	66,000	2,948,000	202	64,000
Western Pacific[c]	1,839,000	136	19,000	1,924,000	129	9,000
Industrialized countries[d]	196,000	23	6,000	166,000	18	10,000
Total	7,537,000	143	315,000	7,962,000	136	640,000

Notes:

[a] Includes all countries of the American Region of WHO, except USA and Cananda

[b] Eastern Europe and independent states of the former USSR

[c] Includes all countries in the Western Pacific Region of WHO except Japan, Australia and New Zealand

[d] Western Europe, USA, Canada, Japan, Australia and New Zealand

[e] From: Dolin PJ, Raviglione MR, Kochi, A: Global tuberculosis incidence and mortality during 1990–1995–2000, *Bulletin of the World Health Organization*, 1994; 72: 213–220

[f] From: Dye C., Scheele S., Dolin P., Pathania V., Raviglione M.: Global Burden of Tuberculosis, estimated incidence, prevalence and mortality by country, *Journal of the American Medical Association*, 1999; 282: 677–86

HIV infection was 20 per cent in Buenos Aires, in Mexico and in Haiti.[22] In many eastern and southern African countries (for example, Malawi, Uganda, Tanzania and Zambia), 30 to 60 per cent of new cases of TB are infected with HIV.[23] In Asia the proportion of TB cases infected with HIV has increased rapidly in some countries.[24] In 1994, Chiang Rai and Chiang Mai reported HIV sero-prevalence of 40 per cent among TB cases in Thailand.[25] In Phnom Penh (Cambodia) in 1994, no TB cases were reported to be infected with HIV, but in 1997 the proportion was 12 per cent and it rose subsequently to about 25 per cent.[26]

In 2000, the WHO estimated that globally about 36 million people were living with HIV infection, with Africa accounting for 60 per cent of the global total. In 1997, it was estimated that about 11 million persons worldwide were co-infected by HIV and TB.[27] The great majority of these persons live in sub-Saharan Africa (7.3 million) and Southeast Asia (2.4 million). The risk of progression to active TB among co-infected persons is 5 to 15 per cent per year, depending on the degree of immunocompromise, as compared to 10 per cent over the entire life for non-HIV-infected persons.[28]

The impact of HIV infection on the incidence of TB has not yet peaked. Figures from some sub-Saharan African countries, such as Malawi, Tanzania, Zambia and Zimbabwe, are frightening. In these countries notification rates for TB have increased two- to four-fold during the past decade (Figure 5.3) reflecting the spread of HIV infection. This rapid increase in the number of cases has posed a serious challenge to health systems and services in these countries.[29] The spread of the HIV epidemic in Asia is more recent. Northern Thailand is already showing alarming levels of HIV infection,[30] though since 1993, the prevalence has fallen in the country as a whole as a result of a vigorous health education campaign promoting the use of condoms.

Multi-drug-resistant TB

While the spread of HIV infection is increasing the number of TB cases, the spread of drug-resistant TB is worsening the TB situation by rendering cases unresponsive to the standard treatment, and some cases untreatable. A recent analysis of the treatment outcomes of patients treated with the standard WHO-recommended regimen in six countries reported that while the treatment success was 83 per cent for patients harbouring susceptible strains, it fell to 52 per cent for patients with MDR-TB.[31] The second-line drugs for treating MDR-TB cases are less potent, more toxic and enormously more expensive (up to 200 times more than the drugs usually used). The high price of second-line drugs is currently unaffordable by many developing countries.

To assess the magnitude of the problem of MDR-TB, the International Union against Tuberculosis and Lung Diseases (WHO and IUATLD) launched a Global Surveillance Project in 1994. As of 1999, the project had covered seventy-two geographical settings. Hot spots of drug-resistant TB have been identified in central and eastern Europe (Latvia, Estonia, some oblasts in the Russian Federation), Latin America (Argentina) and China (Henan). The second report of the project indicates that the occurrence of MDR-TB is high where the performance of the national programme to control TB is poor.[32] MDR-TB does not respect borders, and dissemination of the resistant strains is a reality in this era of frequent and fast travel. Although available information does not permit definitive conclusions, the current manageable pandemic of TB has the potential to become an unmanageable MDR-TB pandemic.

Several middle-income countries are particularly affected (Latvia, Estonia, the Russian Federation and Argentina), and in consequence urgent control measures are needed to address the problem of inadequate treatment of drug-susceptible patients.[33] Once these measures are successful, a specific management regimen for MDR-TB cases can be organized. An immediate response to MDR-TB without improving the treatment of drug-susceptible cases would result in the creation of more drug-resistant organisms and could make the containment of MDR-TB unattainable.

Developed and developing country perspectives

Most industrialized countries witnessed a profound decrease in the burden of TB over the twentieth century following improvements in social conditions, which accelerated significantly with the development of effective treatment regimens in the 1950s and 1960s. Several middle-income countries have been able to replicate these trends by introducing effective TB case management strategies on a wide scale, for example Algeria, Chile, Cuba, Jordan, the Republic of Korea and Sri Lanka.

However, most developing countries face a different situation. Rates of TB are static or rising, and drug resistance is increasing. Population growth, HIV, and stagnant or failing economies have contributed to this situation, which is exacerbated by failure to establish national TB control programmes delivering effective diagnostic and treatment services on a wide scale.

TB case notification declined steadily in the USA and Western Europe long before effective chemotherapy was introduced. Socio-economic improvement was certainly a major determinant in the decline, though the systematic removal of infectious cases from the community into sanatoria may also have played a role (see Chapter 1). Later, an effective use of chemotherapy accelerated the decline.[34] After thirty years of stable decline, however, in which TB case notification reached a level of fewer than 10 cases per 100,000 population, the rate increased steadily between 1985 and 1992 in the USA.[35] Among the factors that contributed to the reversal of the declining trend were increased poverty among the poor living in cities, and the impact of HIV. More important, laxity in the surveillance of cases reflected the inadequacy of the public health network to control the disease.

Countries in Western Europe, including Denmark, France, the Netherlands, Sweden and the UK, as well as other developed countries such as Australia and New Zealand, also reported a plateau or a rise in case notifications during the period 1988 to 1994.[36] (After 1995 the trend reversed in France, the Netherlands and Sweden among others.) The high proportion of these cases that were foreign-born (around 50 per cent in 1997 in most of this group of countries) underscores the importance of paying attention to the TB problem in their countries of origin (see Chapter 2).[37] This fact illustrates how much TB control is a global issue and cannot be limited to one or a group of countries.

Unlike other developed countries, notification rates in Japan are still high at 35 per 100,000 population, but they have declined steadily during the past twenty years.[38] Japan is a special case because it started to contain TB much later than European countries or the USA and has a large population of old people. As a consequence, there is a large pool of persons who were infected with M. tuberculosis at a time then TB was highly prevalent, and a proportion of these persons are developing their disease now.

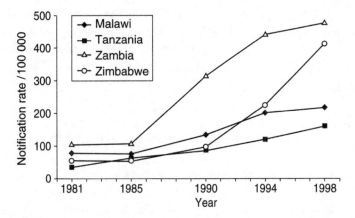

Figure 5.3   TB notification rates in four African countries with high rates
of HIV infection. Source: World Health Organization.

Following the Second World War, Eastern Europe showed a decline
in TB, but as a consequence of political and social instability and
economic crisis, health care infrastructures have collapsed in many
places. In many of these countries, TB started to rise again in the early
1990s at an average rate of 10 per cent a year. In the Russian
Federation, for example, notification rates more than doubled during
the period 1991–98.[39]

In developing countries, it is important to distinguish between
countries with a high prevalence of HIV infection and those with low
or very low HIV infection rates. After years of declining incidence of
TB[40] case notifications in some countries with high HIV infection rates
have doubled or quadrupled in less than a decade. Notification rates in
sub-Saharan Africa are very high, ranging from 41 cases per 100,000
population in Benin to more than 400 cases per 100,000 in Zimbabwe
and Namibia. Among forty-five countries of the African region, eighteen have a notification rate higher than 100 per 100,000 population.[41]
This burden affects not only the health services of these countries but
also their economies and development.

The second group of countries comprises developing economies in
Asia, the Americas, North Africa and the eastern Mediterranean
region. While the problem of TB persists in these countries, the HIV
epidemic is knocking at the doors of many of them. At the same time,
many countries are witnessing, as a part of wider structural adjustment programmes, a tightening of health budgets and turbulence

within ongoing programmes. Several countries in Asia have already introduced user fees for health care provision. Such measures fail to ensure guaranteed access for the poor to general health and TB services and could well prevent effective implementation of the DOTS strategy.

The economic and social impacts of TB

The major barriers to the successful application of the simple, safe and demonstrably effective tools available for TB control have been economic, social and behavioural. The relatively high costs of TB drugs, the social stigma of the disease, and the long duration of treatment needed are some of the important factors that have made the disease hard to tackle.

TB and poverty are closely linked. The probability of becoming infected with the disease and that of developing clinical disease are both associated with malnutrition, crowding and poor sanitation – factors associated with poverty. A vicious cycle is established. Poor people are malnourished and live in crowded, unhygienic conditions, where TB flourishes; the poor receive inadequate health care in which TB is not diagnosed rapidly; treatment, if received at all, is often inconsistent or partial. Resultant ill health and death worsen poverty.

TB and economic decline in a community seem to provide an example of reciprocal causation. The economic impact of TB results from the magnitude of the problem and the fact that it predominantly affects the economically active segment of the population – more than 75 per cent of cases occur among adults aged 15 to 54 years. TB accounts for about 20 per cent of deaths among this productive age group.[42] In Eastern Europe and the former Soviet Union, economic dislocation has contributed to an increase in TB. For example, the Russian Federation has reported a 69 per cent increase in annual new cases between 1991 and 1995. The Russian Federation now has the highest TB mortality rate in Europe.[43]

The costs to TB patients of having the disease can be crippling, especially for families. Not only do they lose income, they also often pay for treatment. In Uganda, for instance, the average income lost, based on a period of nine months without work, was US$161.[44] In Bangladesh, by the time patients presented for treatment at the public

TB clinic they had lost an average of fourteen months of work time and some had already spent US$130 for private sector treatment.

Part of the reason for the high direct treatment costs for patients and their families is delay in diagnosing the disease. Less than half of patients in poor countries are correctly diagnosed at the first source of help they approach; they are thus forced to 'shop around' for a diagnosis. For example, a study of adult TB patients in Thailand found that the delay between the onset of illness and diagnosis of TB was 61–76 days, even though one third of patients had sought care during that time at government hospitals.[45] Research in India showed that 20 per cent of rural patients and 40 per cent of urban patients had borrowed money to pay for expenses caused by TB.[46] In another study, these proportions were even higher: 67 per cent and 75 per cent respectively. The average amount borrowed was US$59, or 12 per cent of the annual household income. For the Indian economy as a whole, the costs of not controlling TB – loss of 50 million potentially healthy and productive years annually, loss of tax revenue, and loss of revenues diverted to public and private health expenditure on TB care – are enormous. These costs will rise if the problems of TB associated with HIV and multi-drug resistance grow unchecked.[47]

The non-monetary costs due to TB are also great. It is not only patients but also their families who have to bear these costs. Persistent social stigma remains an important problem. And often, as a result, women suffer more than men. A recent Indian study reported that 15 per cent of female TB patients were rejected by their families after they contracted the disease.[48] Married women with TB are more likely to experience divorce than other women and unmarried girls find it difficult to get married.[49] Social discrimination against both men and women is known to be associated with increased anxiety and depression, lower life satisfaction, higher unemployment and lower income. Children too suffer as a consequence of their mother's or father's illness. A study in Bangladesh found that a father's or a mother's death was associated with significant increases in child mortality. In India alone a parent's TB leads an estimated 300,000 children to drop out of schools, and a large proportion take up employment to contribute to the family income.[50] Social and emotional support does much to improve treatment adherence among patients. Without adherence to treatment, the likelihood of a cure is lower, relapse and death are more likely and disease transmission is enhanced.

The DOTS strategy: achievements and prospects

The package of services needed to control TB, based on diagnosis and treatment of infectious cases and incorporating the essential management tools, was developed by the International Union Against TB and Lung Disease in several developing countries in the 1980s, and packaged by the WHO as the 'DOTS strategy' and promoted as a global campaign in the early 1990s. It is based on five elements:

1. a political commitment to control tuberculosis
2. the diagnosis of cases based on sputum microscopy
3. standard treatment with short-course chemotherapy and directly observed treatment during at least the initial phase of treatment
4. regular drug supply to ensure uninterrupted treatment of patients
5. monitoring programme using a standard recording and reporting system that includes reports on treatment outcomes.

Many countries that have applied DOTS on a wide scale have witnessed remarkable results. Transmission has declined: Peru, for instance, has seen the fall in incidence double from 4 to 8 per cent per year over the last few years. Mortality has fallen: 30,000 deaths have been averted each year in districts implementing DOTS in China. Drug resistance has decreased: in New York in the 1990s the prevalence of drug resistance fell by 75 per cent following aggressive interventions to improve patient management as recommended in the DOTS strategy. With its potential for curing more than nine out of every ten cases of TB, it has been classified by the World Bank as one of the most cost-effective health intervention programmes.[51]

Despite widespread acceptance of the principles of DOTS, however, most developing countries have not been able to expand DOTS as rapidly as needed, and have failed to achieve the year 2000 global targets of detecting 70 per cent of infectious cases, and curing 85 per cent of those detected. The main constraints on rapid expansion were identified by an ad-hoc committee on the tuberculosis epidemic in London in 1998 as lack of political commitment, insufficient and ineffective use of financial resources, neglect of human resource development, poor health system organization and TB managerial capabil-

Table 5.3 Tuberculosis situation in the 22 worst-affected countries in the world, 1988.

Rank	Country	Population (million)	Estimated number of cases of TB (1997)			% New smear-positive cases with DOTS[a] 1998
			Total new cases	Incidence rate per 100,000 population	New smear-positive cases	
1	India	960	1,799,000	187	818,209	1.5[b]
2	China	1,244	1,402,000	113	636,066	30.1
3	Indonesia	204	583,000	285	265,522	12.2
4	Bangladesh	122	300,000	246	137,318	24.2
5	Pakistan	144	261,000	181	120,413	3.4
6	Nigeria	118	253,000	214	112,909	11.7
7	Philippines	71	222,000	310	100,609	10.2
8	South Africa	43	170,000	392	69,800	23.3
9	Ethiopia	60	156,000	260	67,295	28.0
10	Russian Federation	148	156,000	156	70,055	1.0
11	Vietnam	77	145,000	189	66,066	80.4
12	DR Congo	48	129,000	263	55,074	60.7
13	Brazil	163	122,000	75	55,160	4.0
14	Tanzania	32	97,000	308	40,915	58.0
15	Kenya	28	84,000	297	35,297	68.1
16	Thailand	59	84,000	142	37,378	21.3
17	Myanmar	47	80,000	171	36,426	27.7
18	Afghanistan	22	74,000	333	33,930	5.4
19	Uganda	21	66,000	320	27,316	66.7
20	Peru	24	65,000	265	29,442	94.1
21	Zimbabwe	2	63,000	538	24,531	59.1
22	Cambodia	11	57,000	539	25,890	53.6
	Total	3,658	6,368,000	174	2,865,621	19.7

[f] With DOTS: diagnosed and treated under the DOTS strategy. [f] Estimated 1999: 6.5%

Source: World Health Organization.

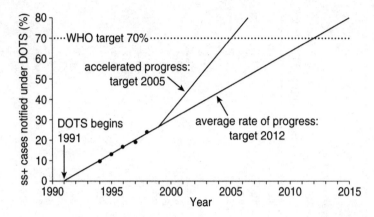

Figure 5.4 Current projected DOTS expansion rate compared with expansion needed to achieve the WHO's 2005 target. Source: World Health Organization.

ity, inadequate quality and regular supply of anti-tuberculosis drugs, and lack of information.[52]

Despite the dramatic increase in the number of countries adopting DOTS over the last decade from a handful in 1990 to 119 at present, including all 22 of the highest-burden countries,[53] only 21 per cent of people with infectious pulmonary TB had been treated in DOTS programmes by the end of 1998. With the current levels of efforts to control TB, it is expected that the global target for detecting and treating efficiently 70 per cent of cases worldwide will be reached only by 2012 (Figure 5.4). Accelerating DOTS expansion to achieve the same target by 2005 – an objective to which all countries committed themselves in March 2000 as part of the Amsterdam Declaration – will have a profound impact, saving 18 million lives by the year 2010 and preventing 48 million new cases by 2020 (Figure 5.5). This 'fast track' to DOTS will also mitigate the impact of HIV, reduce the prevalence of drug resistance, and avert the loss of 270 million working years over the next 20 years.

The window of opportunity for controlling TB – a window that widened remarkably with the discovery and development of effective drug regimens in the last forty years – is closing rapidly. The growing epidemic of HIV and the threat of drug resistance combine to form a major threat to any global containment of the disease. Yet treatment for TB is one of the relatively few cost-effective interventions currently

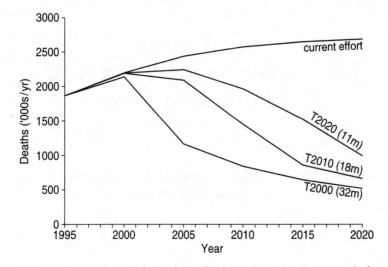

Figure 5.5   The projected number of tuberculosis deaths averted if WHO targets for case detection and cure are met in 2000, 2010 and 2020 compared with maintenance of current control efforts. Source: World Health Organization.

available for people with HIV in most developing countries, increasing both the quality and length of life. It is our view that all developing and developed countries must work in close collaboration to control TB. The DOTS strategy recommended by WHO should be expanded rapidly worldwide to contain the spread of the disease and to reverse the current trends in prevalence, and governments across the world, in collaboration with international, national and non-governmental organizations, need to increase human and financial resources to implement effective TB control. Without the urgent implementation of such measures, we risk the window of opportunity closing for a very long time.

6

Tuberculosis and HIV Infection in Sub-Saharan Africa

Anthony D. Harries, Nicola J. Hargreaves
and Alimuddin Zumla

The dual pandemics of tuberuclosis (TB) and human immunodeficiency virus (HIV) infection are destroying the quality of life and leading to the premature death of millions of people worldwide. Sub-Saharan Africa bears the brunt of these infections, which threaten to destroy the very fabric of its societies. This chapter focuses on the impact of HIV infection on the natural history, clinical features, treatment and control of TB in sub-Saharan Africa.

As the twentieth century drew to a close, the Joint United Nations Programme on HIV/AIDS (UNAIDS) estimated that 33.6 million men, women and children worldwide were living with HIV or AIDS (acquired immunodeficiency syndrome).[1] Given that AIDS was recognized as a disease syndrome only in 1982 and that the virus responsible for causing AIDS was identified only in 1983, the speed and extent by which HIV has spread globally is staggering. In the last twenty years an immense amount of knowledge has accumulated about HIV and AIDS. Two types of the virus have been identified: HIV-1 and HIV-2. HIV-2, largely confined to West Africa, is the less aggressive of the two viruses, and is associated with lower transmission rates, slower progression to AIDS and lower mortality.[2] Unfortunately, HIV-1 virus is by far the most widely distributed pathogen. Despite the accumulated knowledge of two decades, however, the world has been unable to contain the spread of this infection or the illness and death that result from suppression of the immune system. In 1999, 5.6 million people were newly infected with HIV and 2.6 million people died from AIDS.

Sub-Saharan Africa is the global epicentre of this pandemic, and

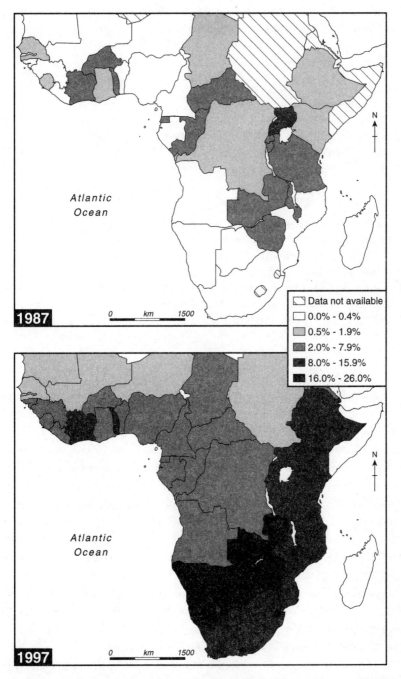

Figure 6.1 Percentage of people in Africa aged 15 to 49 infected with HIV or suffering from AIDS. Source: World Health Organization.

Table 6.1 Diagnosis and care for patients with HIV/AIDS: Best practices in industrialized countries.

Diagnosis of HIV

Informed consent sought for testing
Pre- and post-test counselling
HIV-ELISA screening test
Confirmatory tests (Western Blot/Polymerase chain reaction)
Base line CD4-T-lymphocyte count
Base line plasma HIV-Viral load estimation

Care of HIV patients

Care by a multidisciplinary team (e.g. specialist physicians, nurses, counsellors, pharmacists, palliative carers)
Combination anti-retroviral therapy
Chemoprophlaxis for opportunistic infection
Current best treatment for established opportunistic infection
Current best treatment for AIDS-related tumours
Excellent palliative care services

Source: Compiled by the authors.

continues to dwarf the rest of the world on the AIDS balance sheet. In 1999, 23.3 million Africans (close to 70 per cent of the global total of HIV-positive people) were estimated to be living with HIV or AIDS. Most of these people will be dead by the year 2010, more than doubling the current total of 13.7 million Africans already claimed by the epidemic and leaving behind shattered families and crippled prospects for development. Yet, despite these alarming figures, the HIV epidemic in sub-Saharan Africa shows no signs of coming under control. In countries in Southern Africa such as Botswana, Zimbabwe and Namibia, between 20 and 26 per cent of people aged between 15 and 49 are currently infected with HIV.

Enormous advances have been made in understanding the transmission of HIV, in improving the diagnosis of HIV and in managing and caring for HIV-related disease and AIDS (Table 6.1). In particular, the advent of combinations of effective drugs targeted against HIV (antiretroviral therapy) has been associated with a dramatic reduction in morbidity and mortality in patients with HIV-related disease and AIDS.[3] These advances have had their major impact in the rich countries of the Western world which can afford the very high costs of these drugs. Wards crowded with terminally ill patients or patients undergoing sophisticated treatment for advanced complications have emptied. What had been a terminal illness of one to two years' duration has been changed, with combination antiretroviral therapy, to a chronic illness like diabetes.

Antiretroviral therapy has had little or no impact throughout developing countries, where such therapy is unaffordable. Many African patients are diagnosed as having AIDS on clinical grounds, and blood testing to confirm HIV infection is not carried out. Denial and stigma are very widespread in southern Africa, and counselling services are few in number and variable in quality. These factors help to explain why nearly nine out of ten people with HIV infection in developing countries do not know their HIV status.[4] For the majority of Africans with HIV-related disease, there is no access to antiretroviral therapy, no routine use of preventive therapy against the infections that can occur when immunity is compromised (opportunistic infections), no facilities to diagnose some of the HIV-related conditions, particularly those that occur in the brain, and no specific drugs in the routine health service to treat common conditions such as fungal meningitis or HIV-related tumours such as Kaposi's sarcoma.

The spectrum of HIV-related disease in sub-Saharan Africa also differs greatly from that seen in industrialized countries, with TB, pneumonia, chronic diarrhoea and bloodstream infections being the commonest problems encountered.[5] Late-stage diseases that are commonly seen in industrialized countries are rare. Yet, even though TB, pneumonia and the other infections are potentially treatable, studies in Central and East Africa have shown considerable HIV-related adult mortality and substantial reductions in life expectancy in urban and rural settings. In rural Uganda, median survival from the time of diagnosis of HIV was four to five years and median survival after the onset of AIDS was nine months.[6] Life expectancy in the region has decreased from sixty-four to forty-seven years, and as more and more infected people become ill this trend will probably continue downwards.

The link between TB and HIV infection

HIV infection impairs the body's immunity to diseases such as TB. HIV infects cells which have specific markers on their surface such as CD4 antigens and receptors to which the virus can attach. These cells are principally a specific type of white blood cell (T-lymphocyte), which are the most important cells in the immune response against TB and some other infections. HIV infection causes a progressive decline in the number of T-lymphocytes, and those which survive do not perform their functions as well as they did before infection.

The impact of HIV on TB depends on the degree of overlap between the two infections. By mid-1994, 5.6 million people globally were thought to be dually infected with HIV and TB, 68 per cent of whom lived in sub-Saharan Africa.[7] In 1997, 10.7 million people were thought to be dually infected, with the proportion of those living in sub-Saharan Africa remaining unchanged at 68 per cent.[8]

One third of the world's population are infected with *M. tuberculosis*. Being infected usually means that a person carries TB bacteria inside the body, but the bacteria are in small numbers and are dormant. These dormant bacteria are kept under control by the body's defences, and the infected people are well. Under certain conditions, the bacteria start to multiply, become numerous enough to overcome the body's defences and cause disease. This process is called 'reactivation', and HIV is the most potent risk factor for it. The annual risk of developing TB worldwide is 5 to 10 per cent in adults co-infected with HIV and *M. tuberculosis*.[9] Conversely, at most 0.2 per cent of adults with *M. tuberculosis* infection alone develop TB each year. Reports from the USA and Europe suggest that HIV-infected persons may also be more susceptible to new TB infection, and once infected may rapidly develop TB disease.[10] US studies using techniques of molecular epidemiology have shown that in almost two thirds of HIV-infected persons TB is due to recent infection rather than reactivation of dormant infection.[11] Evidence is growing in sub-Saharan Africa that a significant number of both new cases of TB and recurrent cases result from recent TB infection.[12] Hot spots of TB transmission, fuelled by concurrent HIV infection, may occur in places where people are crowded together, such as prisons, refugee camps, boarding schools, bars and health care institutions.[13] In such situations, if there are long delays between the

Table 6.2   Annual tuberculosis notifications and case notification rates per 100,000: Malawi and Zambia 1983 to 1999.

Year	TB cases		TB cases/100,000	
	Malawi	Zambia	Malawi	Zambia
1983	4,707	6,948	70	113
1985	5,334	6,747	94	105
1987	7,581	11,525	95	171
1989	9,431	14,239	105	201
1991	14,322	23,373	147	316
1993	17,105	30,495	163	394
1995	19,155	35,958	180	445
1997	20,676	No data	188	No data
1999	24,396	No data	210	No data

Source: World Health Organization.

onset of symptoms and diagnosis or treatment the potential for the spread of TB is enormous.

In sub-Saharan Africa today, the first manifestation of disease in approximately one third of patients infected with HIV is TB, and for about one third of the HIV patients who have died, TB was the prime cause of death.[14] In many African countries, HIV infection among adult TB cases ranges from 20 to 70 per cent, and in some countries, including Burundi, Malawi, Uganda and Zambia, the rates are consistently above 50 per cent.[15] HIV infection is also associated with TB in children. In Zambia and Côte d'Ivoire, HIV infection in children with TB aged from one month to fourteen years is between 10 and 40 per cent.[16] In East and Central Africa, HIV-related TB is almost all due to infection with HIV-1, while in some West African countries HIV-related TB is due to HIV-1, HIV-2 or both.

Given the strong association between TB and HIV in Africa, it is no surprise that there has been an upsurge of TB in many countries in the region. The increase in the number of TB cases in the fifteen years to 1999 in two African countries with good notification systems is shown in Table 6.2. From a public health perspective, TB is the most important opportunistic infection observed amongst HIV-infected patients in Africa. Unlike most other opportunistic infections, TB can be highly infectious. There are therefore important reasons for controlling the disease: both to minimize morbidity and mortality in the individual patient and to reduce transmission of the infection in the community.

TB control in the face of HIV

In the last ten to fifteen years, TB case numbers have increased by 300 to 400 per cent in countries with a high prevalence of HIV infection.[17] This increase includes both an increase in the number of patients with smear-positive pulmonary TB and a disproportionate increase in the number of cases with smear-negative pulmonary TB and extra-pulmonary TB. (Smear-positive pulmonary TB patients are defined as those who cough up sufficient tubercle bacilli in their sputum to be seen under the microscope. Patients with smear-negative pulmonary TB have TB in their lungs, but do not cough up sufficient numbers of tubercle bacilli to be detectable by microscopy. Extra-pulmonary TB is TB outside the lungs in places such as the lymph glands.) In resource-poor regions of Africa, making a correct diagnosis of smear-negative pulmonary TB or extra-pulmonary TB can be difficult, and it is likely that a proportion of patients so diagnosed do not have TB but rather HIV-related disease. Nevertheless, all patients diagnosed and registered within the routine DOTS system are placed on TB treatment, and therefore consume resources.

Increased case numbers throw an immense burden on TB control efforts. First, there is a need for more staff, particularly TB programme officers to deal with the registration, recording and reporting of an increased number of cases and laboratory personnel to deal with an increased number of sputum specimens for smear microscopy. Second, there is a need for increased laboratory resources, drugs, sputum containers and stationery. Third, because many patients are hospital-ized for the initial phase of treatment (this often being the only way to ensure patients stick to their treatment), wards have become over-crowded rendering good nursing care impossible, and increasing the risk of hospital-acquired infection.

Moves are afoot in many TB programmes in Africa to decentralize treatment to peripheral health centres and the community.[18] This is a patient-friendly approach as hospital admissions tend to be costly both financially and socially to the patients and their families. However, the logistics of putting into effect observed drug administration, drug security (especially of rifampicin), supervision, monitoring and recording in the community are daunting, although not impossible. Any scheme of decentralization needs to be adapted to the local situation and carefully monitored in case there is loss of control. In Zululand, South Africa, TB treatment has been successfully decentralized to the community with responsibility for drug supervision being entrusted to non-health workers such as shopkeepers, teachers and work colleagues; reported results of treatment completion using this approach have been excellent.[19]

HIV infection increases the frequency of complications during anti-TB treatment. TB in HIV-positive patients responds as well to anti-TB treatment as in HIV-negative patients.[20] While they are on anti-TB treatment, however, HIV-positive TB patients often run a stormy course with other complications, for example fevers, chest infections and recurrent diarrhoea. The increased complications in HIV-positive TB patients are associated with increased prescriptions for antibiotics, antifungal agents, antidiarrhoeal agents and painkillers,[21] rendering the cost of care per patient more expensive than for HIV-negative TB patients.

Adverse reactions to anti-TB drugs are more frequent among HIV-positive patients, leading to interruptions of treatment and occasional fatalities. Of HIV-positive patients who are given 'standard treatment' (streptomycin, isoniazid and thiacetazone), adverse skin reactions may occur in 15 to 20 per cent; up to 5 per cent of these reactions may be severe with life-threatening peeling of the skin and ulceration of the mouth.[22] Adverse skin reactions appear to be even more common in HIV-positive children, in whom severe reactions are frequently associated with death.[23]

Thiacetazone, which was a useful and cheap anti-TB drug in the pre-HIV era, is the main cause of these adverse skin reactions, the frequency of which increase with more advanced degrees of immunosuppression. In many TB programmes in sub-Saharan Africa, the prevalence of HIV infection had led to the abandonment of thiacetazone in favour of other drugs such as ethambutol. This has led to an escalation of drug costs, and there are also concerns about the safety of ethambutol usage in children: visual impairment (an uncommon side effect) may not be mentioned by the child and may not be recognized by the health care worker.[24]

Unsurprisingly, HIV infection increases the mortality rate in TB patients.[25] In sub-Saharan Africa, approximately 30 per cent of HIV-positive smear-positive TB patients die within twelve months of starting treatment, and about 25 per cent of those who survive die during the next twelve months. The large numbers of HIV-positive, smear-positive TB patients and associated high death rates mean that treatment of TB in these countries is less cost-effective in terms of years of life saved than was previously calculated considering only HIV-negative patients.[26]

In the pre-HIV era, smear-negative pulmonary TB was a disease with a good treatment outcome. However, studies from Central Africa show that those HIV-positive patients with smear-negative TB who are more immunosuppressed than HIV-positive patients with smear-positive TB fare even worse than they do, with higher end-of-treatment and post-treatment mortality rates.[27] Yet these patients are often ignored by TB programmes, despite the fact that their numbers are high. In many countries, smear-negative TB cases are not routinely followed up, their treatment outcomes are not reported, and they are often given a cheaper treatment which does not contain rifampicin (a powerful anti-TB drug). The type of anti-TB treatment regimen may be important for survival: HIV-positive patients receiving rifampicin-containing regimens have a consistently lower mortality than patients treated with 'standard treatment'.[28] This improved survival may be due to the fact that rifampicin can treat many infections other than TB, and therefore may give added protection.

There has been little effort so far on the ground to combat the high mortality observed amongst HIV-positive TB patients in Africa. Despite the dramatic effectiveness of combination antiretroviral therapy, such therapy seems unlikely to become freely available for the vast majority of HIV-infected patients in sub-Saharan Africa because of the enormous expense, the complicated drug regimens and the difficulties of monitoring treatment. However, there are some alternative interventions which may be useful. A trial of the use of the antibiotic cotrimoxazole to prevent HIV-related complications in HIV-positive TB patients in Côte d'Ivoire showed a 46 per cent reduction in mortality and a 43 per cent reduction in hospitalization rates in patients treated.[29] This was probably because of a reduction in episodes of bloodstream infection and diarrhoeal disease. Some TB programmes in sub-Saharan Africa are now considering supplementary use of cotrimoxazole prevention as an intervention strategy in an attempt to reduce mortality.

There is also evidence that delay in the diagnosis and treatment of TB may compromise the chances of individual cure in HIV-positive patients. Untreated TB in HIV-infected persons may accelerate the decline in immune function and the progression to severe immunodeficiency.[30]

Another factor important in the survival equation is the capacity and quality of health care staff (TB officers, clinicians, nurses) available to care for patients. An added complication is that health care staff in many African countries are likely to experience the same HIV-seroprevalence rates as the general adult population,[31] which in some urban areas approaches 30 per cent or more. High absentee rates among health care staff due to illness or attending funerals, and high death rates due to AIDS threaten the capacity of many African countries to deliver good and effective health care. TB programmes are no exception to this serious threat,[32] and staff development needs to take these factors into account.

The aim of a DOTS TB programme is to identify and treat patients with TB, especially smear-positive infectious cases, thereby reducing the pool of TB patients and decreasing the risk of TB transmission in the community. In theory, in the absence of HIV infection, this strategy should result in declining numbers of TB cases. However, countries with a good DOTS TB control programme but a high HIV burden are seeing increasing TB case numbers.[33] Additional tactics may be needed if reductions in the incidence of TB are to happen.

What are these additional tactics? First, it is probably necessary not only to identify cases, but to find them as quickly as possible in order to interrupt transmission. The DOTS strategy emphasizes passive case finding, that is, waiting for patients to present themselves to the health services for investigation. In many African countries using passive case finding as the preferred method of identifying cases there may be long delays of up to six months between the onset of cough and diagnosis.[34] Universal active case finding is unrealistic, but targeting high-risk transmission environments such as prisons and households of diagnosed patients may be feasible and cost-effective. Second, it may be necessary to consider preventing the development of TB in HIV-positive persons. It now seems clear that isoniazid, one of the first-line essential anti-TB drugs, when given for six to twelve months to HIV-positive persons significantly reduces the risk of them developing TB.[35] However, translating these research findings into national policy and practice is not easy,[36] and no country in the region has yet adopted isoniazid preventive therapy as a strategy for TB control. Although it may be difficult to implement isoniazid preventive therapy as a country-wide control strategy, it could be used safely and selectively in certain situations such as in occupational health services for private businesses and factories, for personnel working in international agencies and missions, and amongst high-risk groups such as health care workers and prisoners.

The advent of HIV with large increases in the numbers of TB cases has threatened to overwhelm national TB control programmes in sub-Saharan Africa. Fortunately, in contrast to the situation in parts of the USA, HIV-related multi-drug-resistant TB has not yet emerged as a significant problem in Africa, for this would render TB once again an incurable disease.[37] Isoniazid preventive therapy may be useful in selected groups of people, and it may also be useful to prevent disease recurrence after an episode of TB has been successfully treated. At present, however, isonaizid preventive therapy is unlikely to have a major impact on TB control because of the difficulties of countrywide implementation. Novel TB vaccines to replace the BCG vaccine are being developed, but it will probably be at least another ten to fifteen years before any such vaccine finds its way into clinical use.

Thus, the current best way of trying to control TB in high-HIV-prevalent countries in sub-Saharan Africa is the WHO DOTS strategy. Countries need to be helped in implementing this strategy with particu-lar emphasis on quality microscopy-based diagnosis, health education, uninterrupted drug supplies and follow-up care. The DOTS strategy must also adapt to the challenges posed by the HIV epidemic if credibility is to be maintained, and research may be very useful in this setting.

Research should be relevant to the practical issues surrounding TB control. What are the important areas for this so-called operational research? Improving access to diagnosis and care requires social sci-ence, health systems and programmatic research. The difficult issue of how to best diagnose smear-negative pulmonary TB and extra-pulmonary TB must be addressed. Schemes to decentralize TB care to the community must be rigorously piloted and evaluated. Attempts must be made to reduce the high mortality during treatment, and this may involve the use of other drugs – in addition to the anti-TB treatment – which target HIV-related complications and the immune system. There has recently been international debate about bringing antiretroviral drugs, which specifically target HIV, into the public health sector in Africa. This is the intervention most likely to have a major effect in reducing complications and deaths from TB in HIV-positive individuals. However, it is also the intervention that is the most challenging because of the enormous costs and the difficulties of safely and securely providing such drugs in settings with weak health infrastructures. Ways to protect the health care workforce from TB and HIV, and ways to increase staff numbers in the health sector are other important areas upon which to focus.

TB programmes should collaborate more with AIDS control programmes, because it is now apparent that AIDS control is essential for TB control. Whilst an AIDS vaccine is unlikely to become available for another ten to fifteen years, much can be done to reduce the transmission of HIV by persuading young people to engage in safe sexual behaviour, by encouraging voluntary counselling and testing, and by removing the shame, silence and denial which characterize this infection in most countries in sub-Saharan Africa.[38] Countries that have aggressively tackled this problem, such as Uganda, have begun to see their efforts rewarded with a reduction in new HIV infections.[39]

Many countries in sub-Saharan Africa, in conjunction with the donor community, are embarking on reorganization of the structure of health service delivery. The aims of these reforms include a sector-wide approach to health and decentralization of power, services and financial control from ministry headquarters to individual districts. This includes a move to dismantle vertical programmes such as TB control and malaria control. These public health programmes currently have their own structures, with authority passing from central to regional to district level, and there is little, if any, cross-collaboration. Health sector reform emphasizes the need for programme integration and decision making at district level. Rapid implementation of health sector reform combined with an equally rapid dismantling of disease control programmes can be disastrous for specific disease control efforts. Zambia underwent health sector reform between 1995 and 1997, which resulted in the collapse of TB control, and an absence of anti-TB drugs at the district level.[40] It is important for control programme staff and health planners to work closely together in the reform process to ensure that regular drug supplies, supervision, monitoring, recording and reporting are maintained and continued in an uninterrupted fashion. Governments and the donor community also need to be persuaded and reminded that it is essential to invest in and support good TB control programmes, especially in the era of HIV infection.

7

The Recent Tuberculosis Epidemic in New York City: Warning from the De-developing World

Deborah Wallace and Rodrick Wallace

. . . [T]uberculosis might again become epidemic. It would only require some massive disruption of our social and economic systems, forcing human beings to live under crowded, unsanitary conditions. . . . [Historically] incidence and mortality from tuberuclosis increased markedly in those countries suffering the greatest dislocations in their economy and social structures. . . . Certain . . . areas . . . may become almost free of the disease, but the accumulation . . . of large numbers of susceptible persons may provide the basic requirements for future epidemics that, in turn, will restore tuberculosis as 'Captain of All the Men of Death'.[1]

The great mystery of the tuberculosis epidemic in New York City: 1975–92

We open with a mystery. For decades, TB had so declined in New York City by all measures that in 1968 the Mayor convened a task force to plan its elimination from the remaining small pockets.[2] In 1968, the city's governing and medical authorities envisioned a TB-free New York. Less than ten years later, in 1975–76, new case incidence rose two years in a row. In and of itself, this glitch would have been just a random fluctuation, but it was followed by an extremely rapid decline for two years (1977–78) and then a classic epidemic upward curve between 1979 and the present with an absolute peak of new cases and new case incidence in 1992.

The epidemic was completely unexpected even within the New York City Department of Health. In 1979 John Marr, Assistant Commissioner for infectious diseases, wrote:

> At present the highest case rate for TB is in the Lower East Side, followed by Central Harlem. The highest rate in the first instance is due to a mix of the Bowery population, the Chinese community (many of them recent immigrants) and the recent large influx of immigrants from Central and South America into large sections of the Lower East Side. Thus, in this instance, it appears that poor people gravitate towards the poorer sections of the city which are high-population-density areas, but the indigenous poverty of that area does not necessarily foster new indigenous cases of disease, that is, these people arrive already infected (as opposed to arriving as susceptibles). Similarly, in Central Harlem, the typical 'new case of TB' is an elderly black male who develops a reactivation of his primary infection which might have been five decades ago. Where that person lived 50 years ago was, in turn, the true source of his infection and not the community where he was living when he developed his reactive disease. And, he rarely infects his neighbors before discovery.[3]

Even after the incidence of TB rose throughout the 1980s and the epidemic could not be denied, no one dared address it openly: to keep the silence, Mayor David N. Dinkins forced Kevin Cahill, an expert on tropical diseases, off the Board of Health Commissioners when he determined that a health emergency should be declared in 1990. By 1990, the City Health Department had been aware of the epidemic for at least six years, possibly even a decade. Delaying public acknowledgment delayed demands for explanations of the roots of the epidemic and attention to those roots.

New York City is divided into thirty health districts. In 1978, the year in which new cases of TB and new case incidence were the lowest ever recorded in New York City, the two areas of heaviest concentrations of new cases were Central Harlem and the Lower East Side, both traditionally poor neighbourhoods of Manhattan. Other poor communities of colour also showed an elevated incidence of new cases. However, concentration of new cases and new case incidence was not extreme. In 1979, the top-ranking health district's incidence rose well above that of the others and signalled that the epidemic had begun. New case incidence had become unusually concentrated in large neighbourhoods of about 200,000 people. Unusual concentration of new cases implies that an epicentre has formed from which the disease will spread. As the epidemic unfolded, more health districts showed extreme concentrations of new case incidence, but the top-ranking district remained well above all others.[4]

During most of the epidemic, that top-ranking health district was Central Harlem, although the Lower East Side also served as a primary epicentre and, in one year, ranked first. Figure 7.1 shows the spread of high incidence and indicates two systems: Central Harlem dominating Upper Manhattan and the Bronx, and the Lower East Side dominating Lower Manhattan and Brooklyn. From Brooklyn and the Bronx, high incidence spread to Queens also. Thus, within New York City, TB re-emerged as an epidemic with the classical modes of spread: hierarchical and spatial diffusion.[5]

The establishment of a secondary epicentre from the primary Central Harlem epicentre across the Harlem River in the Bronx and one from the Lower East Side across the East River in Brooklyn illustrates hierarchical spread, namely the spread of high incidence to a popula-tion at a distance, a population with characteristics that ensure a high density of susceptible individuals. Contact between the primary epicen-tre and the potential secondary epicentre must be frequent and intense enough so that the potential secondary epicentre is seeded with enough new cases for its susceptibles to be exposed at a high enough rate to create a sustained contagious process. From all the epicentres, primary and secondary, the disease then spreads by simple spatial diffusion, the wine-stain-on-the-tablecloth effect.[6]

By 1990, as Figure 7.1 shows, all the Bronx health districts attained new case incidences above the 1978 citywide incidence and all but one of the health districts in Brooklyn also achieved that dubious distinc-tion. But the map is misleadingly optimistic. If one simply substracts the 1978 health district new case incidence from that of 1990, one sees that only one out of the thirty health districts escaped the epidemic and had an incidence in 1990 equal to or lower than that of 1978. This is an astounding fact: the disease penetrated all health districts but the very wealthiest. It bulldozed into middle-class neighbourhoods in Queens and Staten Island.

Figure 7.2 shows the time course of the epidemic from 1979 to 1990: the three-year running average number of new cases plotted against the middle of the three years. Thus the average annual number

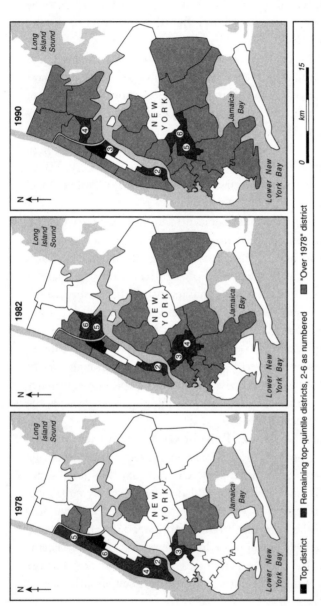

Figure 7.1 The geographic spread of high TB incidence across New York's four inner boroughs, 1978–90. The solid black health district is the top-ranked. The others in the top quintile (top fifth) are numbered according to rank for incidence. The stippled districts are those with incidence above the 1978 citywide average. In 1978, all districts but one in the top quintile were in Manhattan. Note the spread into the Bronx from the top-ranking district (Central Harlem) and to Brooklyn from the second-ranking district (the Lower East Side). From the secondary epicentres, high incidence spread through Brooklyn and the Bronx. The establishment of secondary epicentres in Brooklyn and the Bronx coincided with the change from slow to rapid increase in citywide numbers of cases. Source: D. Wallace and R. Wallace, *A Plague on Your Houses: How New York Was Burned Down and National Public Health Crumbled*, London and New York: Verso, 1999.

of new cases for years 1980, 1981 and 1982 is plotted against year 1981. This averaging smooths the little fluctuations and emphasizes the overall trend. The early years show a slow rise in the number of new cases. This period of slow rise is followed by a deflection point (1983) which begins a period of rapid rise. By mapping the new case incidences, we can identify the geographical changes which are reflected in the changes in the rate of rise of new cases. The early slow rise represents the early period of spatial diffusion from the two primary epicentres in Central Harlem and the Lower East Side before the establishment of any secondary epicentres. The deflection point marks the establishment of the secondary epicentres in the Bronx and Brooklyn. The period of rapid rise in new cases is that of spatial diffusion from both the primary and secondary epicentres.[7] The concentration of cases in a few neighbourhoods ensured rapid spread from those neighbourhoods and did not signify containment of the disease in those neighbourhoods.

In Central Harlem, the 1990 new case incidence (about 230 per 100,000 people) was essentially the same as that of South Africa. Another measure of concentration is the number of new cases per square mile. Central Harlem in 1978 had 43 new cases per square mile, and the Lower East Side 29. In 1990, they had 143 and 89 respectively. Indeed, all but one of the health districts in the top fifth for incidence had more than forty new cases per square mile in 1990, ensuring community transmission as well as household transmission.[8] Transmission in the community between households is necessary to sustain an epidemic. Density of cases determines the probability of exposure in the community. Density of susceptibles determines the probability that exposure leads to infection.

For obvious reasons, new TB cases among children under school age (under five years old) indicate household transmission. New cases in preschool children were strongly statistically associated with new cases in adults among African-Americans and Latinos during the epidemic. Transmission in African-American and Latino households can be inferred. By 1990, even white children under the age of five were showing elevated incidence of new cases, compared with earlier years. The epidemic had breached the colour barriers, and both community and household transmission occurred in white and integrated neighbourhoods.[9]

A research team from Montefiore Medical Center of Albert Einstein

School of Medicine described household transmission in the Bronx by analysing new cases among children under five.[10] By the use of the molecular biochemical markers for the particular strain of TB, this team showed that the adults in the household harboured the same strain as the child with active disease and that the child cases tended to arise in homes already harbouring one active adult case or more.

Thus, a high proportion of New York City health districts by 1990 had household and community conditions that supported infection transmission and progress to active disease. Different neighbourhoods, of course, showed differences in participation in the epidemic. Generally, health districts with 1978 incidence above the citywide 1978 incidence suffered from increases in incidence early in the epidemic and from greater acceleration in the rise in incidence than health districts with average or lower-than-average incidence in 1978. The time taken to reach the threshold case density for epidemic proliferation partly depended on the initial case density. We have identified approximately twenty-five new cases per square mile per year as the density required for an epicentre that sustains spatial contagion.[11] This was the case density achieved by the Bronx and Brooklyn health districts during the 1982–84 deflection point shown in Figure 7.2, when spatial diffusion commenced in Brooklyn and the Bronx. Thus, new case density per unit area of neighbourhood proved of vital importance in the progress of the epidemic, and reaching the epidemic threshold ensured rapid spread of the disease, just as the great disease mathematician Norman Bailey explained.[12]

Thresholds bring unexpected changes in rates and even in fundamental processes. That a disease increases at a given rate from year to year does not mean that it will continue this pattern in the future. Reaching an epidemic threshold may lead to accelerated increases and to leaps from one subpopulation to another. Nonlinear increase in new cases over time and hierarchical as well as spatial spread characterized the New York City TB epidemic and ensured that populations that had not experienced TB in decades became reacquainted with it.

The rise in new cases and new case incidence began slowing in 1991. By 1993, these two measures began to decline. Even now, the turn-around from increases in new cases to declines in new cases is not clearly explicable, although proponents of Directly Observed Therapy (DOT) wish to attribute the decline to the treatment. There is also the possibility that everyone in the path of the infection who was vulner-

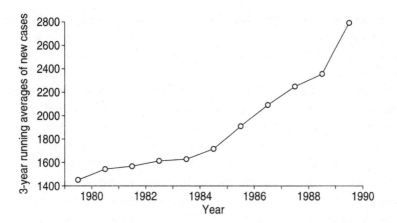

Figure 7.2 Each data point here shows the average of new TB cases for three years plotted against the middle year of the three. This method of plotting smooths the curve to reveal the overall trend. The year 1983 marks an inflection between slow and rapid annual rise in new cases, a characteristic of the S-shaped curve typical of an epidemic spread both hierarchically and spatially. The rapid rise occurred after the hierarchical establishment in 1982 of secondary epicentres in both Brooklyn and the Bronx from which cases spread spatially. Source: Wallace and Wallace, *A Plague on Your Houses.*

able had already come down with the disease, leaving too few susceptibles to sustain further epidemic rise.

Treatment with anti-TB drugs: a dubious control strategy

The 1968 Task Force recommended closing hospital beds reserved for TB patients and relying on the anti-TB drugs. Hospital beds were closed, but the resources for finding and following cases for drug treatment were barely adequate only for a very stable city. During the epidemic, these resources proved grossly inadequate.[13] Even so, large numbers of people were treated with anti-TB drugs: all reported cases and large numbers of their contacts. From 1978 through 1993, we estimate that about 50,000 people received anti-TB drug treatment, an estimate derived from the reported number of new cases and their treated contacts.

Of course, the number of people treated in each health district is proportionate to the number of cases and contacts. Thus, exposure to the highly toxic anti-TB drugs became a secondary health risk. In 1994, the Centers for Disease Control and Prevention reported on a series of cases of liver failure among the TB patients who had received treatment in New York City. From the number of liver failures reported for 1991–93 and the number of cases-and-contacts for that period, we can estimate the risk of liver failure. We can furthermore estimate the number of cases of liver failure during the epidemic – thirty-one to thirty-three, of which half were fatal. This number does not include cases of liver damage or of neurotoxicity or any other 'side effect' – only liver failure severe enough to merit application for a liver transplant. Risk of liver failures per 1,000 people treated far exceeded what the US Environmental Protection Agency terms an acceptable risk of serious disease from public exposure to useful chemicals. However, untreated TB poses a much larger risk of death.

The other outfall of massive treatment with inadequate resources to follow the patients was the generation of multi-drug resistance. Scandal arose from a highly publicized 1991 report that about two thirds of the cases in the shelters for homeless men had been treated before and had not completed the previous treatment.[14] Failure to complete treatment is, of course, the classic route to generating drug-resistant strains. As the epidemic proceeded, the TB Control Bureau found a larger and larger proportion of drug-resistant new cases. Indeed, a strain of MDR-TB (multi-drug-resistant TB) which arose in New York eventually made its way to places as far from its origin as Nevada, Colorado and Paris.[15]

The New York Academy of Medicine held a conference in 1992, 'Case Management and TB Control', which featured authorities in TB medicine who preached the gospel of DOT as the answer to the epidemic and to the generation of drug resistance. DOT is defined in different ways and has different standards, according to the administering organization, although most national health authorities accept the World Health Organization standards. Generally speaking, it refers to the observing by a health department employee of the patient's taking of the daily doses, observing in such a way as to guarantee that the pills were really ingested. The Health Department employee hunts down the patient and watches him/her take the required doses on the spot.

A well-funded programme of DOT was not initiated in New York until 1993, and did not begin working fully until 1994. Although most

TB medical specialists attribute the decline in new cases after 1993 to this programme, new cases began declining in 1993, before the programme was working in the field. The epidemic in fact began slowing in 1991. New TB cases may have begun declining in the same way that the number of new cases of chickenpox begins to decline after the epidemic crest because the number of uninfected susceptibles drops below the density threshold required for epidemic proliferation. As Figure 7.1 shows, the disease swept through the city and became incident in most health districts at levels above the 1978 citywide incidence. Saturation could not be far behind.

Even if the DOT programme did defeat the epidemic, the failure to institute such a programme in a timely way, as soon as the new case incidence began rising obviously in the 1979–82 period, means that many more people were infected and/or diseased and required treatment than would have been necessary had the Health Department fulfilled its responsibilities competently. Thus, unnecessarily large numbers of people had to take the toxic anti-TB drugs and risk liver damage and even liver failure and death. Unnecessarily large numbers of people had to risk the generation of resistant infection, even within the DOT programme, since several control programmes have reported that even patients who had never been treated with anti-TB drugs before occasionally incur drug resistance.[16] The research team reporting from San Francisco noted that HIV infection and other infections that hinder absorption of the drugs in the digestive tract are associated with drug resistance arising even during DOT.

When the decline in new cases became an annual feature in the TB Control Bureau's annual report, the authorities proclaimed that the city had 'turned the tide' and attributed this new order to the measures put in place in 1993–94: DOT, expanded searches for contacts of new cases, and hospital detention of those who do not take their drugs.[17] The present plan for TB control is increased screening of immigrants for latent infection, as well as for active cases, immigrants accounting for a disproportionate number of new cases in the post-epidemic period.

Even in the context of DOT, however, sole reliance on anti-TB drugs to control TB at the population level, rather than to cure individuals, increases the probability of generating multiple drug resistance. The TB bacillus has been with humans for tens of thousands of years, maybe even before *Homo sapiens* existed. Its tokens appear in ancient mummies from widely separated civilizations – from the Middle East to Central Asia to the Andes. It must, therefore, have the capability of rapid evolution to survive in changing conditions. Antibiotics are merely another environmental challenge to this evolution machine. Even though DOT minimizes the chance of MDR-TB arising, it does not render the probability zero. Therefore, the large numbers of people treated will eventually accumulate and raise to certainty the generation of MDR-TB even in the DOT context. Understanding the roots of the recent epidemic is absolutely vital to the task of designing a responsible primary prevention programme that minimizes the number of active cases that have to be treated with the toxic, evolution-stimulating antibiotics.

Even if treatment programmes could prevent new cases, which they cannot, proclaiming the New TB Order ignores the recent history of the epidemic. Here in the largest city, the financial and cultural capital of the wealthiest nation on earth, a disease characteristically tied to conditions of poverty and social disorder terrified the populace for over a decade. People of nearly every ethnicity, class, age and educational attainment eventually became ill from it. Only the wealthiest, most economically diverse neighbourhoods escaped this epidemic. Literally tens of thousands of people had the active disease between the beginning of the epidemic and its end (between 1975 and 1993). Unless we understand how and why the epidemic began and why the authorities ignored it for years, we cannot conclude that we have 'turned the tide'.

Unravelling the mystery of TB in New York: the roots of the epidemic

According to Guy P. Youmans, the great TB physiologist and epidemiologist, a resurgence of the disease in an industrialized society requires a massive upheaval, essentially a social, economic and political process of de-development.[18] In seeking the roots of the lengthy New York epidemic, we must look for an event or condition that brought disruption, forced migration, mixing of populations and severe material deprivation (like that experienced during war or natural disaster) to city neighbourhoods. Although the Health Commissioners who served during most years of the outbreak, under Mayor Koch, noted that infection with the AIDS virus (HIV) predisposed toward easy infection with TB and immediate progression to active disease, the TB epidemic cannot be attributed solely to the spread of HIV infection. In 1975/76, when the first signs of loss of control over the disease showed up as consecutive increases in annual incidence, HIV infection was concentrated in the middle-class, largely white homosexual community and had not widely penetrated the African-American and Latino communities. Additionally, children under five years of age without paediatric HIV/AIDS and elderly Asian women were clearly part of the TB epidemic. Finally, the conditions of social and economic marginalization that foster the spread of HIV infection also foster the spread of TB. Even if the TB epidemic could be attributed to the spread of the AIDS virus (and it cannot), this attribution does not absolve the public health authorities from addressing the forces driving both epidemics. Eventually, the two epidemics became entwined, but only after they had both gathered steam and spread widely in the poor neighbourhoods.[19]

TB has historically depended on overcrowding for household transmission. In their study of cases in the Bronx among children under age five, the research team from Montefiore Medical Center found that those children almost without exception resided in dwellings with two or more persons per room, much more crowded than the US Census Bureau's definition of extreme housing overcrowding (1.51 persons per room or more).[20] If housing overcrowding was a factor in the epidemic, it must have shown drastic changes between 1975 and 1990. Indeed, it did. As housing overcrowding declined between 1975 and 1978, new cases declined; as housing overcrowding increased between 1978 and 1990, new cases increased. In fact, by 1990, the number of extremely overcrowded housing units was about double that of 1970, before the epidemic.[21] New TB cases declined and increased as the proportion of extremely overcrowded housing declined and increased, not as HIV seroprevalence increased.

In a sense, attributing the epidemic to changes in patterns of housing overcrowding begs the question as much as attributing it to the spread of the AIDS virus. Both TB new case incidence and the prevalence of extreme housing overcrowding had been declining in New York City for decades. Why was the healthful trend reversed? Figure 7.3 shows the geography of extreme housing overcrowding prevalence in New York in 1970, 1980 and 1990. Some immense event shifted population massively between 1970 and 1980 and then resulted in large numbers

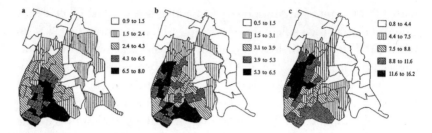

Figure 7.3 Proportion of extremely overcrowded housing units by health area of the Bronx in 1970, 1980, and 1990. Figure 3a: 1970; 3b: 1980; 3c: 1990. Note the changes between 1970 and 1980: the geographic shift from the south-central to the western edge of heavy overcrowding and the general decline in proportion of overcrowded units. In 1990, however, the top-ranking health area for overcrowding had twice the percentage of over-crowded units as in 1970, and the area of worst overcrowding was the western edge. Clearly massive shifts in population had occurred between the censuses. Source: Wallace and Wallace, *A Plague on Your Houses*.

of housing units changing from being non-crowded to extremely over-crowded by 1990. This figure shows that something akin to a war or a natural disaster did occur, affecting hundreds of thousands of people.

To illustrate further that something immense occurred between 1970 and 1980, we offer the following two facts. First, the health areas (groups of 1970 census tracts with roughly 20,000 people and similar socioeconomic characteristics) of the traditional ghettoes lost 33 to 84 per cent of their populations. These people moved to adjacent areas, a vast internal migration. Second, 1.3 million white people left New York City.[22] Between the internal migration of poor people and emigration of middle-class white people, almost 2 million people moved in about five years, a massive population instability.

The internal migrations resulted from sudden, rapid destruction of housing units, primarily in poor communities of colour (African-American, Latin American and Chinatown). Approximately 600,000 people were uprooted directly by the housing destruction, and the loss is estimated at 150,000–200,000 units.[23] The neighbourhoods most heavily affected were the South Bronx, Harlem and the Lower East Side in Manhattan, the poverty belt of Brooklyn (Fort Greene, Williamsburg, Bedford-Stuyvesant, Bushwick, Brownsville, East New York), and Jamaica and the Rockaway Peninsula in Queens. These neighbourhoods had existed stably for many decades. Much of the housing had been built during the early twentieth century and main-tained in use continuously and in a chronically overcrowded condition. The sudden loss of housing units simultaneously in all these neighbour-hoods indicates a new citywide public policy, not isolated events.

During the 1970s, two intertwined epidemics destroyed the housing: fires and landlord abandonment. Fires behaved like a parasitic disease on the housing stock and, as a population, could be described with the mathematics of disease epidemics.[24] Landlord abandonment also behaved like a contagious parasite on the housing stock.[25] One plague (abandonment) followed the other (fire) in a given neighbourhood. Figure 7.4 shows the index of fire damage, a combination of the number and size of fires, and new TB cases, plotted against year. Clearly, the latter followed the former. Since TB is associated with extreme housing overcrowding and the number of housing units is a prime determinant of extreme housing overcrowding for a given popu-lation, this figure is easily understood. We have here a synergism of plagues: fire and TB.

Landlords during this time of spreading high fire incidence and large damage per fire would watch the approach of the fire front to their property. They would often withdraw maintenance from the buildings as the fire front neared because of the futility of investing in an at-risk property. After collection of rent became difficult because the tenants found the building in decay, the landlord would stop paying the taxes and the building superintendent's salary. Essentially, the landlord walked away from the building in the path of the fire front.

The contagious nature of building fires and landlord abandonment in US cities is counterintuitive and difficult to understand. The dynam-ics of the epidemic in the relatively small Brooklyn neighbourhood of Bushwick, population about 130,000, illustrates contagion. At the height of Bushwick's local epidemic, about one hundred fires occurred in that little neighbourhood in a single month, when 80 per cent of the fires were occurring in clusters of five or more on a single block.[26] This extreme clustering in time and space, like the clusters of chickenpox cases during an epidemic, was responsible for the massive, concentrated housing destruction, and indeed community destruction. Contrary to assertions by public officials, even at the height of the Bushwick fire epidemic, less than half the fires were even suspicious, much less proven arson.[27] The epidemic cannot be blamed on arson. A large proportion of a neighbourhood would be destroyed in a short time (six months to

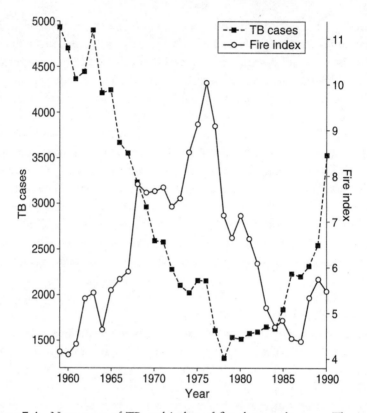

Figure 7.4 New cases of TB and index of fire damage by year. The index of fire damage melds the number of fires and the number of alarm assignments needed to control them, an indicator of fire size. The pause in decline of new TB cases during 1975–76 coincides with the peak in fire damage index. The TB epidemic, however, followed the fire epidemic, partly because of lags in effects and partly because the housing crisis was delayed by the mass emigration from the city between 1974 and 1978. Source: Wallace and Wallace, *A Plague on Your Houses.*

two years) because of the clustering and the geographical spread of clustering as a fire front.

In the late 1960s, the contagious nature of building fires in New York City (and other large American cities) was known, even to the operations researchers of the New York City–Rand Institute, a quasi-governmental organization created by Mayor Lindsay's administration in the late 1960s and given unprecedented extra-governmental authority over Fire Department policy. The fire service unions, under intense membership pressure because of the growing workload, had forced the

opening of about sixteen fire companies in the ghettoes during
1968–69, companies that stabilized the number and size of fires, the
way a good immune system keeps an infection controlled. Reports by
such line officers as Division Chief Kirby of the Bronx showed that the
Fire Department was informed internally of the contagion and geographical spread of high fire incidence.[28]

The NYC–Rand Institute, by 1969, was working closely with Daniel
Patrick Moynihan, the urban policy adviser to President Nixon. Moynihan received fire alarm data from NYC–Rand and an extremely
misleading interpretation of these data.[29] He used both the data and
the interpretation in his infamous January 1970 'Benign Neglect' memo
to Nixon to brand poor black neighbourhoods as pathological and
criminal:

> You are familiar with the problem of crime. Let me draw your
> attention to another phenomenon, exactly parallel and originating in
> exactly the same circumstances: Fire. Unless I mistake the trends, we
> are heading for a genuinely serious fire problem in American cities.
> In New York, for example, between 1956 and 1969, the over-all fire-
> alarm rate more than tripled from 69,000 alarms to 240,000. These
> alarms are concentrated in slum neighborhoods, primarily black. In
> 1968, one slum area had an alarm rate per square mile 13 times that
> of the city as a whole. In another, the number of alarms has, on an
> average, increased 44 percent per year for seven years.
>
> Many of these fires are the result of population density. But a
> great many are more or less deliberately set. (Thus, on Monday,
> welfare protectors set two fires in the New York State Capitol.) Fires
> are in fact a 'leading indicator' of social pathology for a neighbor-
> hood. They come first. Crime, and the rest, follows. The psychiatric
> interpretation of fire-setting is complex, but it relates to the types of
> personalities which slums produce. (A point of possible interest: Fires
> in black slums peak in July and August. The urban riots of
> 1964–1968 could be thought of as epidemic conditions of an
> endemic situation.)

At this time, a similar policy was gaining popularity among New York
City's ruling oligarchy (known as 'Permanent Government'): whose
principal strategy was Planned Shrinkage. This policy also branded
poor communities of colour as bad beyond salvation: 'uncivil'.[30]
Planned Shrinkage means withdrawing essential services from 'sick and
dying' neighborhoods. Thus, both Benign Neglect and Planned Shrinkage supported the withdrawal specifically of fire control services from

the ghettoes. Under the guise of increasing fire service efficiency, the NYC–Rand Institute was assigned the task of creating mathematical models that would designate fire companies to be closed. *Mirabile dictu*, almost all the designated companies that were closed between 1972 and 1975 were in ghettoes and many were the same ones opened in 1968–69 under labour arbitration, the ones that had stabilized the fire damage. Taking the fire companies away from the ghettoes is the opposite of John Snow taking the handle off the Broad Street pump during the London cholera epidemic. It is the fire equivalent of making people drink the cholera-tainted water from the Broad Street pump. It was an act of war on domestic populations viewed as internal colonies.

About 10 per cent of all the fire companies in New York City were removed, largely from poor neighbourhoods of colour. The triggering of the 1972–78 fire epidemic coincided in time with the removal of fire control resources from the ghettoes. The geography of housing destruction also coincides geographically with the removed companies and with companies made grossly overworked by the removals. So it would appear at first glance that the strategy of targeting these neighbourhoods for destruction did work. However, contagious phenomena have a way of spreading to non-targeted populations.

When fire companies in a neighbourhood are out working for extended times (two hours), the dispatchers temporarily relocate companies from other neighbourhoods to cover for the busy ones. By this mechanism of temporary relocation, the company closings changed the fire service from essentially many independent neighbourhood fire departments into one big, overstretched network. Each large fire strained the whole system. Thus, non-target neighbourhoods suffered a degraded fire service and were drawn into the fire epidemic.[31] Even middle-class neighbourhoods lost some housing units to fire during the epidemic. The decline in the condition of middle-class neighbourhoods and of the city in general motivated the white middle-class emigration.

Similarly, contagious diseases like TB and AIDS did not remain within the targeted populations but spilled over into middle-class and even upper-class neighbourhoods. Figure 7.1 shows the spread of TB from the epicentres across the city. Other diseases and contagious behaviours such as substance abuse and violence spread in similar fashion, and for similar reasons: the destruction of the physical and social community and the loss of social capital, social structure and political power.

Unexpected consequences

The spread of TB did not respect the city limits. All the counties of the New York City metropolitan regions (24 counties, including the five boroughs) were drawn into the TB epidemic. The daily commuting pattern is an index of contact between counties and between the city and its suburban counties, and the county-level poverty rate is an indicator of local TB vulnerability. When we combined the commuting pattern and county-level poverty rate into a composite index, we could predict TB incidence across the counties of the metro region (Figure 7.5) with very high accuracy.[32] Figure 7.5 also shows that as the new case incidence of the inner boroughs rose between 1985–88 and 1989–92, the entire line rose as a single system, including the farthest counties. Thus, the TB incidence of even the wealthiest, most distant county in the metro region, Hunterdon County in New Jersey, was determined by the TB incidence of Manhattan, the Bronx and Brooklyn.

It is a simple arithmetical operation to calculate the number of TB cases that arose between 1985 and 1992 in the suburban counties as a result of the New York City epidemic. Since as the incidence rose in Manhattan, the Bronx and Brooklyn the whole system of counties' incidences also rose *en bloc*, the difference in the number of cases in the suburban counties between 1985 (778 new cases) and 1992 (1,244 new cases) may be largely attributed to the epidemic in the city: 466 excess new cases.

TB was not the only condition showing metro regional diffusion. The incidences of AIDS, violent crime and low-weight births also showed this 'regionalization'. TB and these other public health and public order conditions are markers for contagious urban decay.[33] In seeking to segregate and disempower poor black communities, the policies of Benign Neglect and Planned Shrinkage spread the previously contained and soluble problems of the ghettoes over the whole metro region.

We examined violent crime and AIDS cases on a national level as we did metro regional TB, AIDS, violent crime and low-weight births. Instead of commuting as an index of connectedness between the major metro regions, the migration within and between the metro regions of the twenty-five largest cities was used. Instead of the poverty rate, we

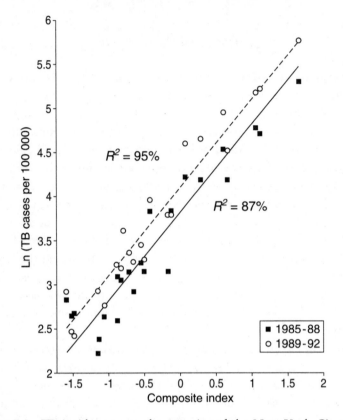

Figure 7.5   TB incidence over the counties of the New York City metro region. This graph plots the logarithm of county TB incidence for two periods 1985–88 and 1989–92 against a composite index which includes the county vulnerability to TB (its 1989 poverty rate) and its socioeconomic embeddedness in the metro region indicated by its commuting pattern. Note how the line rose as a unit as the new case incidence in the top-ranking counties rose (Manhattan, the Bronx, and Brooklyn). Source: Wallace and Wallace, *A Plague on Your Houses.*

found that the violent crime rate indicated the metro regional vulnerability to AIDS. According to this analysis, the numbers of AIDS cases in the major metro regions of the USA depended on their connectedness with New York City and San Francisco and on their local violent crime rate. We found that violent crime also diffused along the network of metro regions and depended on the migration pattern within and between the metro regions.[34]

Locally we found that one serious violent crime (homicide) is closely associated with the unemployment rate.[35] Therefore we took a look at AIDS and the factor possibly underlying the violent crime wave, namely changes in manufacturing employment between 1972 and 1987. This later analysis proved as powerful as the first one, yielding associations just as strong.[36] The log of the AIDS cases in the metro regions was highly associated with the logs of probability of contact with New York (based on migration pattern), number of violent crimes in 1991, and the ratio of manufacturing jobs in 1987 to those in 1972.

Although we did not examine TB on a national level as we did AIDS and violent crime, new cases of TB arise in similar circumstances of marginalization as new HIV infections. It is reasonable to hypothesize that TB infection also diffused along the national network of major metro regions, depending on similar vulnerabilities to provide high densities of susceptibles.

The future of TB in New York

No major improvement in living conditions in poor New York communities of colour has occurred since the end of the fire epidemic of the 1970s, although the economic boom of the 1990s has eased unemployment rates. Despite the basic lack of improvement, the incidences of TB, AIDS, violent crime and infant mortality declined greatly even in the epicentres, beginning around 1993. Although the municipal administration takes credit for these declines, the likely cause is the social reknitting of communities after the end of rapid housing destruction and forced migration.

Because middle- and upper-class neighbourhoods were dragged into the TB epidemic, the Health Department finally applied for funding from the federal government to pour resources into case finding, screening, DOTS, and contact finding and treatment. However, medical treatment can remove only the cases and contacts that can be found, and not the latent infections or the well-hidden cases and contacts. We have calculated that the rate of disease reactivation and the time between reactivation and treatment are the most important driving forces in determining whether TB increases or decreases in incidence over time.[37] Also of vital importance is the density of susceptible individuals in a community. The treatment of active cases and of named contacts may reduce incidence, but cannot drive the disease steadily downward over the long term in the context of deteriorating physical and socioeconomic conditions.

Population ecologists who study endangered species have analysed the role of rare catastrophes in driving local populations to extinction.[38] TB is the negative of an endangered species. Because of latent infections and the sensitivity of these infections to both physiological and emotional stress (continued encasement of the infection depends on the immune system which, in turn, is sensitive to stresses), TB blooms in the aftermath of catastrophe. The intensity and extent of that blooming depend on the initial conditions on which the catastrophe is imposed: the prevalence of latent infections, the areal density of latent infections, and the density of susceptible individuals.[39] Healthy, happy people fight off infection consequent on exposure and, if faced with a heavy infecting exposure, quickly render the infection latent and avoid active disease until stressed.

Under normal conditions, TB has a particular threshold of active case incidence and areal density necessary to support the contagious processes of an epidemic (the increase over time in new case production). This threshold depends partly on the density of susceptibles.[40] If the population is healthy, there will be few susceptibles, mainly the very old. Exposure will only rarely lead to infection and infection to active disease. So the threshold of active case incidence and density for entering an epidemic will be high. However, background conditions that stress the population lead to high densities of susceptibles both directly from the stresses and indirectly from the risk behaviours that are adopted to cope with the stresses (such as substance abuse and violence). So an active TB case will lead to many new infections and active cases under stressful conditions.

The context of the population stress may be debated but our work on AIDS and the incidence of violent crime within the network of major metro regions implicates both the loss of manufacturing jobs and the instability of social and political structures consequent on rapid mass migration at local, regional and interregional levels. The waves of multi-rooted catastrophes (factory closures, the redirection of federal funding – the so-called Southern strategy, national adoption of Rand Corporation and other mathematical models to destroy poor neighbourhoods, and diversion of resources to the military adventures first of the Southeast Asian war and then of the Cold War intensification/ New World Order) left large proportions of the nation, particularly the areas of great loss and great gains in population, economically precarious and socially individualized, without normal social networks or normal densities of linked social networks. There is no buffer to further catastrophes and, indeed, events that in the past would have been mere blips are now likely to assume the stature of catastrophes. The proportion of the populace that is susceptible to TB infection and to coming down with active disease is probably much larger than during the 1960s when New York City dreamed of leading the nation to TB elimination.

The breadth of this susceptibility has generated great fear of exposure, fear that is reflected in the calls for massive resources to reduce TB incidence in developing countries.[41] These calls arise not merely from the fact that TB incidence has grown in those countries to the point that travellers from those countries to the USA pose a threat of exposure to Americans. During the great immigration of 1880–1930, large numbers of TB infections also arrived in the USA, but the improvements in living and working conditions due to the Great Reform produced a healthy, happy, hopeful and involved population. TB mortality and incidence during the great immigration continued to decline nationally, even in New York, a major receiver of immigrants.[42] Hence, it seems clear to us that reliance on investment in TB treatment on a massive scale without any pretence at primary prevention – removing the fundamental causes – allows neocolonialism in developing countries and both civil and international local wars to continue without attention to these underlying catastrophes. This massive secondary prevention is seen as a way to retain de-development in the USA without causing the kind of outcry that arose among the middle and upper classes during the epidemic of the 1980s to early 1990s.

When pesticides are used as the primary means of preventing insect damage to agricultural crops, the target pests often evolve resistance to the chemicals. The chemicals kill off the susceptible individuals and leave the few resistant ones who then can reproduce without competition from the large population of pesticide-susceptible conspecifics. Under the pressure of pesticide use, the great preponderance of the pest population becomes resistant. Similarly, bacteria that are treated with antibiotics become resistant to the drugs. This is especially true for rapidly mutating species such as the TB bacillus. Use of chemical means of secondary prevention in place of primary prevention is begging for evolution of resistant forms. The general problem of antibiotic resistance has loomed so large that antibiotic-resistant forms of *Streptococcus pneumoniae* have become notifiable diseases in the USA, that is, diseases requiring frequent, reliable and regular reporting to the Centers for Disease Control and Prevention. Although vancomycin-resistant forms of enterococci have not yet become notifiable, by 1998 about 22 per cent of all enterococci sampled from patients in hospitals were resistant, up from only 0.3–0.4 per cent in 1989, a nearly hundredfold increase.[43]

Thus, we find that the production of MDR-TB consequent even to directly observed therapy bodes evil. Long-term reliance on anti-TB drugs will produce MDR-TB even under the best directly observed therapy programme. In addition to the general problem of antibiotic resistance, another contributing factor in this is individual differences in ability to absorb these drugs. Indeed, the populations treated most frequently are also those most likely to have gastrointestinal abnormalities: HIV-positive people, alcoholics, drug users and residents of overcrowded housing – the ulcer bacterium *Helicobacter pylori* is found most frequently in residents of overcrowded housing.[44] MDR-TB will become a massively emergent disease in the USA under the circumstances of repeated catastrophe, lowered threshold for what is a catastrophe, and grossly increased density of susceptibles which lowers the threshold for the density of diseased, infectious individuals required to trigger a contagious epidemic.[45] To minimize production of MDR-TB, public health authorities must minimize the number of people treated by applying primary prevention measures such as reducing housing overcrowding, assuring food security and proper nutrition, and enforcing anti-sweatshop laws.

De-development in the USA is not merely losses of manufacturing capacity and manufacturing employment. It is a severe distortion of social, political and economic relationships at all levels of organization and scales of population and geography. Because of the place of several US cities in the hierarchy of international cities, US de-development is a known international AIDS spreader.[46] We predict that US de-development will similarly contribute to the international spread of MDR-TB, as the USA becomes known in the twenty-first century as the 'Sick Man of the Americas', in much the way as the declining Ottoman Empire was called the 'Sick Man of Europe' at the beginning of the twentieth century.

8

Private Wealth and Public Squalor: The Resurgence of Tuberculosis in London

Alistair Story and Ken Citron

The global resurgence of tuberculosis is now apparent in the UK. London, once a world centre for the proliferation, export and dissemination of TB, has again become a significant producer in its own right. Since 1997, there have been more new cases in London annually than in New York (see Figure 8.1). More than 50 people in the city develop TB every week, and approximately one in twenty of those will die of the disease.[1] Notifications have increased dramatically over the last decade, and in some boroughs rates of the disease have risen threefold.[2] London is home to 40 per cent of all cases in England and Wales and 50 per cent of all drug-resistant cases.

The determinants of TB in the UK today are multifactorial: increasing wealth inequality and social deprivation, homelessness, co-infection with the HIV virus, migration, the neglect and consequent failure of public prevention and control services have together provided a fertile environment for our most ancient and devastating airborne adversary. This chapter will examine these determinants and describe the changing social epidemiology of TB in London at the start of the twenty-first century.

Historical background

At the beginning of the twentieth century, TB claimed more than 20,000 lives annually in the UK. With the exception of the two world wars, rates of disease continued to decline rapidly, mainly as a result of

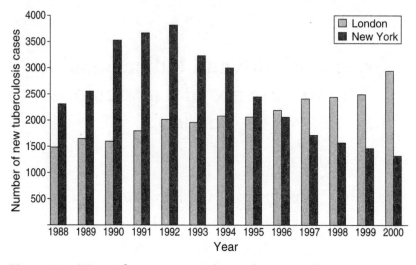

Figure 8.1   TB notifications in London and New York, 1987 to 2000.
Various sources including Public Health Laboratory Service, London.

improved nutrition and better standards of housing and health care,
before levelling off in the late 1980s. The use of antibiotics heralded the
advent of effective drug treatment, and the pioneering work of the
Medical Research Council's Tuberculosis Unit in South India soon
afterwards showed that patients could be effectively treated and cured
in their homes. The UK's TB sanatoria were closed, with an estimated
annual saving of £30 million,[3] and patients were managed predominantly by hospital doctors on an outpatient basis. But as the rate of
disease declined so did the expertise in its management. Patient numbers
dwindled to levels that could not justify sustaining specialist services,
and TB management was incorporated into general respiratory clinics
in most centres, or scattered throughout hospital outpatient services.

   The widely held belief that TB had been conquered in the UK
fostered a climate of complacency and a lack of vigilance that enabled
insidious, yet fundamental epidemiological changes to occur without
response. Its declining prevalence masked a significant concentration of
disease in specific groups, particularly in London. This delayed
response to the changing epidemiology of TB has resulted in current
services often failing to reach the worst affected. Rates of disease are
now highest in people who are marginalized and those who experience
serious difficulties accessing mainstream health care – new and recent

entrants to the UK, homeless persons, alcoholics and the mentally ill. To conceptualize the current TB situation in London around specific high-risk groups is, however, potentially misleading and discriminatory. Whilst undoubtedly certain social and cultural groups are now disproportionately affected, placing emphasis on this fact does little more than reinforce negative stereotypes and draws attention away from the bigger public health issues.[4] TB develops as behavioural, biological and environmental risk factors – influenced by powerful social forces including poverty, wealth inequalities, lack of rights and racism – interact to exacerbate one another and increase vulnerability.[5] Thus unless UK health policy makers and planners can embrace the full spectrum of determinants driving the epidemic there is little chance of achieving an appreciable impact on the rates of disease.

Widening wealth disparities

Disparities in wealth have become extreme within the capital: the city contains most of the UK's richest people and many of its poorest. Fourteen of the country's 20 most deprived wards are in London, more of its households receive some type of benefit than in any other area in the UK, and nearly 40 per cent of women in manual work earn less than £200 a week.[6] Moreover, the polarization of wealth continues and the gap between the relative health in the richest and poorest areas of London is increasing: current health inequalities between social classes are the greatest ever recorded in British history.[7]

Numerous studies have highlighted poverty as a major reason for increasing TB in the UK.[8] National data show that there has been an increase in the notification rate of TB since 1988 in the poorest 30 per cent of the population of England and Wales but no increase in the remainder.[9] In London, TB is particularly prevalent in the poorest, most ethnically diverse communities.[10]

One of the major reasons for the increase in wealth disparity has been the reduction in public housing investment over the last twenty years, and the concomitant increase in support for private homeowners and the private rented sector. The social housing sector shrank from some 6.4 million dwellings (31 per cent of all UK housing stock) in March 1979 to 4.3 million (21 per cent of stock) by the end of 1997.[11] Two thirds of the most deprived housing estates in the UK are now in

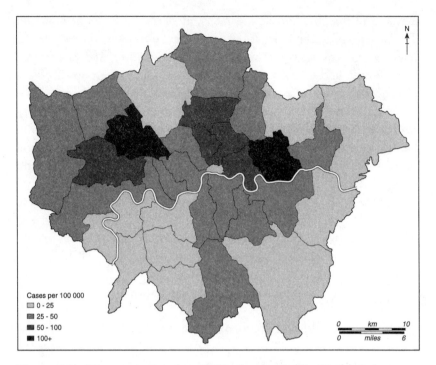

Figure 8.2 TB rates in London, 2000. Source: Public Health Laboratory Service, London.

London, with 20 per cent of homes considered unfit for habitation in some boroughs.[12] The link between poor-quality housing and health is long established. Respiratory problems have been related to damp housing conditions, and TB specifically is strongly associated with overcrowding, particularly in women.[13] Between 1984 and 1997, levels of overcrowding in London rose by more than 40 per cent.[14] The current acute shortage of affordable accommodation in the capital primarily impacts upon the poor who have quite literally been priced out of the housing market, pressured into overcrowded, temporary and substandard accommodation or rendered homeless.

The role of immigration

Immigration is often cited as a reason for the return of TB in London and undoubtedly plays a part. However, to focus specifically on

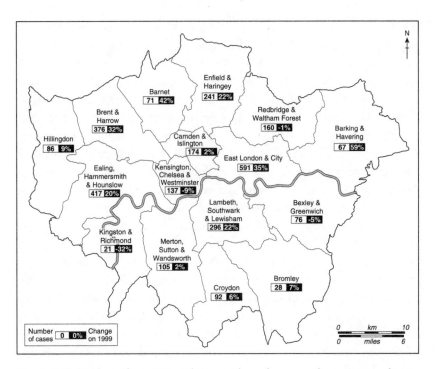

Figure 8.3 Tuberculosis in London; number of cases and percentage change by area, 2000. Source: Public Health Laboratory Service, London.

immigration diverts attention from two key issues. The first is that movement between London and areas where TB remains endemic is two-way: the current volume and reach of travel are unprecedented, and increasing numbers of people are spending extended periods in endemic areas exposing themselves to an appreciable risk of TB infection.[15] Second, the capital's environment is now conducive both to the development of disease from latent infection and to the acquisition of new disease following exposure to infectious Londoners, making a clear distinction between TB as an imported or an acquired phenomenon increasingly problematic. A study among the Asian community in east London, for example, found that almost half of TB cases had been infected by contacts in the UK, compared to only one in three who had been infected abroad.[16] This state of affairs makes paradoxical the current regulations governing the requirement for immigrants to undergo TB screening on entering the UK. Currently, anyone planning to live in the UK for more than six months who arrives from an area where TB is common, defined as more than 40 cases per 100,000 population, should be screened by chest X-ray at the port of entry.[17] Although arguably worthwhile, this seems ironic when many will end up living in areas of London where rates of disease are twice that considered common by port health authorities. Given the relative risks, should we also be screening people on their way out of London? Pointing the finger at immigrant communities to explain the resurgence of TB in London does little more than fuel xenophobic political thinking against persons already segregated from society, confined to menial jobs or unemployment and relegated to the worst housing in the least desirable areas of the capital.[18]

Chronic insecurity, war, environmental disaster, famine and widespread violation of human rights caused massive displacements of people in the latter quarter of the twentieth century.[19] The London boroughs are currently supporting over 50,000 destitute asylum seekers, and another 9,000 asylum seekers have been provided with temporary accommodation.[20] (There are, however, no routine UK data sources at local level that give even the most basic information such as numbers of refugees within a given area.)[21] They are among the most vulnerable and excluded people in UK society experiencing high levels of material and social deprivation. Given the massive global resurgence of TB in most resource-poor countries, people in search of asylum are now arriving from areas where the disease is epidemic and access to health services is extremely limited or virtually non-existent.[22] To compound this problem, refugee communities continue to receive poor health care and suffer poor mental and physical health after arriving in the UK. There is some evidence to suggest that the health status of new entrants may become worse in the two to three years after entry to the UK.[23]

Actively screening populations for TB is only practical and cost-effective if rates of disease are high and the number of cases detected justifies the effort and intrusion. The process itself can be stigmatizing and stressful, particularly if the rationale for screening is not well explained and understood. The existing port-of-entry screening system in the UK for people arriving from endemic areas into London reaches only a small percentage of those who fit the criteria and was recently described as both incomplete and random.[24] To screen only new entrants when a significant number of cases occur in established UK communities is also discriminatory.[25] More effective and comprehensive approaches to reaching infected migrants in London are required.

An obvious solution would be to include TB screening for new arrivals when they register with a general practitioner, and in some areas of the capital pilot schemes have demonstrated this to be effective at detecting cases early.[26] However, there are difficulties with this approach. Refugees and asylum seekers arriving in London have serious problems getting registered with a general practitioner (GP) despite their entitlement to the full range of National Health Service treatment free of charge.[27] Registration is also only temporary for many, includes no basic new patient health check and is often not local to their place of residence. Significant barriers to GP registration and consequent access to health services exist for a variety of reasons. Many GPs have little experience or confidence in dealing with the wide-ranging social, psychological and physical needs of refugee communities, and some are unaware of refugees' entitlement to free health care.[28] Reluctance to admit refugees and asylum seekers onto patient lists is also motivated by GPs' perception that cultural and language barriers will result in lengthy and time-consuming consultations.[29] Refugees and asylum seekers themselves are commonly unaware of their rights to free health care, have no practical knowledge of how the system works and feel culturally isolated from mainstream health services.

The consequences of ineffective TB screening services and poor access to health care for new arrivals to London are delayed seeking of medical help after the onset of disease, increased TB transmission, more serious morbidity and poor uptake of preventative initiatives including BCG vaccination and prophylactic treatment. Refugee health is afforded a low priority on the UK health agenda, and access to care is unlikely to improve significantly without institutional reform and investment in appropriate services. Health initiatives targeted at new arrivals at risk of disease must offer reassurance that TB screening is not a manifestation of a xenophobic bureaucracy but a means of protecting the immigrant, their family and community.[30] Additionally, negative public perceptions of new arrivals, fuelled by recent media reports of bogus asylum claimants, must be countered to present a more realistic and balanced image of valuable people who are resourceful and capable survivors.[31] The government's 1998 white paper on immigration and asylum makes no reference to tackling current health inequalities experienced by asylum claimants, who can wait years for approval or rejection of their application.[32] It proposed a system to disperse refugees throughout the country and afford them no access to cash-based benefits. This increased isolation and poverty will lead to worsening health and even less access to what community-based support and specialist health services have developed in areas that have traditionally housed asylum seekers.[33]

Another social group commonly arriving in London from areas where TB remains endemic have no right to free health care, welfare support or employment. They are termed illegal immigrants. Their number is hard to quantify, but a recent United Nations report cited human smuggling as the fastest-growing criminal business in the world. The exploitative treatment of the victims of trafficking often amounts to new forms of slavery.[34] Many arrive destitute and at the mercy of organized gangs of racketeers who supply workers for the burgeoning UK low- or no-pay job sector. Over half of the prostitutes working in central London are said to be illegal immigrants.[35] In terms of TB prevention and control, people with no legal right to remain present a significant challenge. Most live in constant fear of detection and are extremely reluctant to engage in any contact with state authorities – including health workers. They are at risk of latent disease due to their birth origin and also at risk of progression of the disease and primary infection due to their social environment and often poor mental and physical health. TB services in London do see a significant number of patients who have no right to remain in the UK, but there is no information on how many similar people the TB services are unable to reach. The UK demand for extremely low-paid workers seems set to continue to rise, and this, coupled with the huge numbers of people desperate to migrate in search of a better life, will mean the issue is unlikely to go away despite stricter border controls and harsher treatment and penalties.

It is up to TB service providers to ensure that services are accessible to those most at risk. Health workers are in no way obliged to inform on patients' immigration status and must respect confidentiality. If TB services are perceived as organizations in league with the authorities, people on the margins of society will continue to arrive at hospital emergency departments with advanced and infectious TB. There are no simple solutions to this dilemma and there is a distinct lack of published work and debate on the subject. The Blair administration continues to flounder with such issues for fear of appearing soft on illegal immigration. The incorporation of the Human Rights Act 1998 into UK law, although a significant step in the UK's democratic development, did not enshrine health – or access to health care – as a basic and enforceable human right.[36] Without humane legislation to protect the rights of illegal immigrants to seek medical attention without fear of persecution, incarceration or deportation, it will be very difficult for TB services to begin to establish trust and initiate effective outreach activities with the communities worst affected.

The impact of homelessness

The UK has one of the highest levels of homelessness in Europe.[37] The sight of people – often young people – sheltering under cardboard and plastic ramshackle structures, sleeping in shop doorways, lying comatose on pavements and crouched begging in public places has become commonplace in the capital, and indeed most major UK cities, over the past two decades. London has the highest concentration of homeless households in England, though the actual numbers are unknown.[38]

Homelessness is becoming increasingly prevalent among younger people and people from minority ethnic groups, including refugees and asylum seekers of whom the majority are young males. In 1997, members of minority ethnic groups were over 3 times as likely to be amongst the statutory homeless than white people.[39] Minority ethnic groups are also overrepresented among the single, or hidden homeless, particularly in inner London.[40]

A recent survey showed that 25 per cent of people sleeping rough are aged between 18 and 25.[41] In part this is because of social changes over the past twenty years that have seriously disadvantaged many young people in the UK.[42] Factors include high unemployment, fundamental changes in the labour market with loss of job security, and the withdrawal of social security benefits to persons under eighteen. In addition, the traditional support mechanisms of family and community have been severely disrupted with more young people leaving home to escape physical and emotional conflict and abuse: 86 per cent of young homeless people had been forced to leave home. In 1999 the homeless charity Crisis reported that 40 per cent of young homeless people had been in local authority care at some point in their lives; one third of those sleeping rough had mental health problems, and half abused alcohol.[43] Three in four of those sleeping rough have done so for at least two years. The life expectancy of someone who sleeps rough in London is 42 years compared with the UK average of 74 for men and 79 for women.[44]

But people who are genuinely roofless and sleeping rough on the streets comprise only a small fraction of the total numbers of people who are actually homeless. Estimating the actual number of homeless persons in London is extremely difficult due to the limited amount of data collected, the varying definitions employed and the complexities of attempting to count the hidden homeless. These are a highly mobile population of people sleeping rough, living in squats, hostel accommodation and temporary shelters or on the floors and sofas of friends and relatives.[45] There is no universally accepted definition of homelessness because any definitions currently in existence are, to some extent, based on ideological views about the conditions in which people should be expected to be responsible for their own lives.[46] Government statistics are based on the 1977 legal definition of homelessness that gives local authorities responsibility to house those homeless people deemed to be in priority need – usually families with children and others considered to be especially vulnerable. Official homeless statistics consequently exclude most single homeless people. For the purposes of examining the relationship between homelessness and TB we need a broad definition that incorporates all those persons whose housing circumstances could predispose them to a significantly greater risk of disease.

Tackling TB among homeless people poses particular difficulties. Like other UK socially excluded groups, homeless people not only experience more health problems than the general population but also have greater difficulties accessing health services.[47] A 1995 survey revealed that only one quarter of GPs would fully register a homeless person seeking treatment.[48] The following year, a study by Shelter found that 37 per cent of homeless people were not registered with GPs.[49] Prejudice, stereotyping and bureaucracy are formidable barriers between the homeless and health care. TB services in London located in tertiary referral hospitals must seem very distant and remote when viewed from a 'sickbed' on the street.

Many homeless people have profound and multiple problems. In an environment where high levels of stress, drug and alcohol abuse, violence, insecurity and poor mental and physical health are the norm, TB can often seem a low priority. Homeless people suffering from TB who manage to access medical care are likely to present with more advanced and often more infectious disease resulting in higher rates of transmission. It is also well documented that significant numbers of homeless people who are diagnosed as having TB fail to complete treatment.[50] Directly observed therapy (DOT) is recommended for all patients in the UK who are likely to experience difficulty in taking prescribed TB drugs. Despite the complexities of supporting homeless persons through TB treatment, studies in London have demonstrated that it is possible to provide an effective service. With highly skilled outreach workers, incentives and a well-coordinated interdisciplinary approach, 80 per cent can attain cure.[51]

Whilst TB is curable, the treatment is not only long (at least six months), but also complex. Some drugs must be taken with food, some on an empty stomach and all cause side effects that range from mild to life-threatening. Taking TB treatment intermittently, however, or in insufficient doses, can rapidly result in the emergence of drug resistance, whereby the most usual, or first-line drugs become useless. Once sensitivity to the most effective first-line drugs, particularly rifampicin and isoniazid is lost, treatment options are limited, the prognosis is poor and side effects are considerably worse, medication must be taken daily for two years or more and costs, when compared to standard six-month therapy, are much higher. Unlike what happened in New York, rates of multi-drug-resistant TB in London remain comparably low at less than 2 per cent but the threat is growing.

Further evidence of an advancing epidemic of TB now affecting socially excluded people living in London is drawn from recent research using DNA fingerprinting to study transmission; this study found that homeless people were often involved in unrecognized outbreaks of TB.[52] The study findings suggest that uncontrolled and previously undetected transmission both within the homeless population and between the homeless and the larger London community is now taking place. Studies of transmission among the urban homeless in London and elsewhere show that the majority of cases are due to recent infection,[53] highlighting the importance of early diagnosis and effective treatment. Overcrowded and poorly ventilated hostels are an important focus for TB transmission. Thus the current efforts to remove rough sleepers from the street into hostels could increase the transmission of TB unless effective screening and preventative measures are enforced. Moreover, removal of rough sleepers from public view should not be allowed to conceal the fact that there is an increasing population of vulnerable single people, among whom TB develops often near the end of a long history of self-abuse, neglect and poor health.

The impact of HIV infection

Around one third of the 30,000 people in the UK who are infected with HIV live in London. HIV-related mortality has become the largest single cause of death among young men living in inner London and the third-biggest cause in young women.[54] HIV infection was a major factor in the epidemic of TB in New York, but its contribution to the current London epidemic remains unclear. Previous studies in the UK have shown little evidence of a major overlap between HIV infection and TB.[55] However, there is evidence both of significant undernotification and of considerable local variation in rates of co-infection likely to be missed by national surveys and diverse local testing procedures.[56] By 1998 at least 3 per cent of TB cases in the UK were estimated to be HIV-infected.[57] Approaches to the care and clinical management of AIDS-related TB in London vary greatly between different centres. In some areas, effective programmes for voluntary HIV testing and counselling appear to identify most people at risk of co-infection prior to them developing TB, whereas in others the uptake of testing and counselling services is poor and the sero-status of TB patients is known in only a small fraction of cases. This has restricted the use of prophylactic treatment to reduce the risk of HIV-infected individuals developing TB and made it difficult to assess the true impact of HIV on rates of TB in the capital. In most cities in the USA, the overlap between HIV infection and TB has been evident and the approach adopted has been to offer all patients presenting with TB an HIV test.

Shared care between specialist services remains the exception rather than the rule in London with a majority of co-infected patients not accessing TB nursing services. This is, in part, due to a shortage of specialist nurses, as compared with HIV/AIDS services, and is another example of how underinvestment has compromised the ability of TB services to adapt to the changing needs of those affected. There is considerable common ground for shared learning between TB services and HIV/AIDS services. Both deal with diseases that are heavily stigmatized in the UK, necessitating a strong information and advocacy role for health and allied professionals. Both services are attempting to engage and meet the needs of people who are often socially marginalized. Both require a broad and inclusive community base to their activities, involving a wide variety of allied agencies in delivering coherent and integrated care to persons with diverse and complex needs. Additionally, both services aim to support patients through long and often complicated programmes of drug therapy with significant associated risks of side effects and poor adherence.

Whilst there are many commonalities, TB services and HIV/AIDS services have had different perspectives. The emphasis with TB has been on a medical approach centred around case detection, appropriate treatment and cure whereas, in the absence of an effective cure, HIV/ AIDS services have commonly adopted a more holistic approach with an emphasis on primary prevention, care and support. The advent of more effective antiretroviral therapies has brought these perspectives closer, with the ability to tolerate and adhere to a complex drug regimen now being the most important factor determining the prognosis in HIV infection. Developing collaborative links and shared care between TB services and HIV/AIDS services in London should be seen as a priority and might also present opportunities to temper the biomedical emphasis on disease still dominant in London's TB service model.

Rethinking tuberculosis control in London

As an infectious disease, TB raises many ethical issues in balancing the rights and responsibilities of the individual against the need to protect the society in which they live. There are two diametrically opposed positions on the appropriate public health response to this disease.[58] Sections 37 and 38 of the UK Public Health Act, which relate to the detention of patients with notifiable diseases such as TB 'who pose a serious risk of infection to others', are seldom enforced and are considered controversial. In New York, however, legislation was amended in 1993 to enable the city's commissioner for health to detain persons 'who cannot be relied upon to participate in and/or to complete an appropriate prescribed course of medication for TB' irrespective of whether or not they are an infection risk to other persons. Incarceration of 'potentially' non-compliant patients has been cited as a factor that contributed to the reduction in TB seen in New York, where over 3 per cent of patients with TB received regulatory orders between 1993 and 1995.[59] However, without prior investment in efforts to engage and support those most vulnerable to TB there is little or no justification for a more coercive approach culminating in loss of civil liberty.[60] To date, that investment has been lacking in the UK.

Efforts are now under way to examine critically London's current TB services and to improve quality and standards.[61] The available data necessary to steer the process of reforming London TB services are not substantial, but there is considerable consensus on where services are lacking and what is required, and a significant body of experience from other cities exists. What happened during the 1990s in New York clearly demonstrates that it is possible to turn the tide against TB. New York has spent in excess of $1 billion, implemented arguably draconian reforms to public health legislation, and put TB back on the front pages of newspapers and the lips of politicians, and in the minds of its people.[62] These measures have reversed and contained the epidemic but are probably still beyond the material and political means of most countries, including the UK. In London, the policy debate is now poised at a crossroads. What is increasingly clear is that, to be effective, a TB programme must reach beyond the clinic and actively engage those worst affected in the community. Equally, it must combat the stigma and prejudices that enable the world's richest countries to tolerate preventable deaths among their poor. TB is a barometer of social justice and equity, the solution to which cannot be found in medicine alone.[63] Those contributing to current efforts to develop TB services in London and the UK should recognize the inherent flaw in reform dominated by biomedical thinking that tends to focus on the disease and not the person. This narrow focus has resulted in a failure to recognize the importance of social, economic and environmental factors that perpetuate the cycle of infection among the poor and socially disenfranchised.

Social science research on TB in countries where it is endemic indicates that policies and programmes that take *control* as their primary focus may fail to meet the health needs of patients and their communities.[64] We should be conscious of how language affects attitudes among health and allied professionals, laypersons and sufferers and ensure that control is not achieved at the expense of care, and that treatment supervision is not imposed in place of support. TB service delivery in London is focused within referral hospitals. There is an increasing body of evidence from community-based care initiatives that decentralizing TB control measures beyond health facilities can, by harnessing the contribution of the community, improve access and outcomes to treatment.[65] The medical treatment of TB in vulnerable communities can be successfully accomplished concurrently with patient-focused care that seeks to address the broader contextual issues of disease such as housing, mental illness and substance abuse.[66]

London has a great deal to learn and perhaps a limited time to do so. The number of persons failing to complete treatment is unknown as no routine data is collected on outcomes.[67] There is no comprehensive strategy to deal with TB, and current services are under-resourced, poorly coordinated and highly fragmented, being delivered from nearly fifty hospitals in the capital.[68]

It remains unclear how policy initiatives can be implemented in London given the current organizational complexity and fragmentation, and the absence of any clear commitment to inject additional resources.[69] Prior to the creation of a single NHS Executive for London in January 1999 and more recently the London Health Commission, launched by the newly created Greater London Authority (GLA), there was no specific London-wide health planning capacity or framework for linking public health policy across the whole city. This severely compromised efforts to take a strategic view of London's public health and, from a structural perspective, resulted in TB services functioning largely in isolation from one another, adopting no consistent set of standards or operational criteria. The formation of a London-wide NHS executive and the GLA's independent London Health Commission afford a real opportunity to bring together disparate public health services and to develop a coordinated and strategic response to the current TB epidemic.

The effectiveness of TB service delivery in London is hampered by a lack of operational research resulting both in poor recognition of the limitations of the TB service and in limited evidence to promote policy and planning initiatives. There is a particular need to explore locally those factors that promote access and adherence to treatment and to tailor the service to the specific needs of those worst affected.

Within national government, the Department for International Development (DFID) has demonstrated a major commitment to supporting TB control internationally and a clear recognition of the severity and implication of the current global pandemic. Through

DFID, the UK government is directly funding the World Health Organization's TB control efforts. Given its encouraging international stance, it is paradoxical that the UK government has yet to demonstrate a similar level of commitment to combating TB in London.

9

The Social Impact of Multi-drug-resistant Tuberculosis: Haiti and Peru

Paul Farmer and David Walton

Introduction: emerging resistance to antituberculous drugs

Resistance to antituberculous agents was described shortly after the 1944 introduction of streptomycin.[1] As new drugs were developed, so too did resistance to them: cases of highly drug-resistant disease were described in the 1960s.[2] But multi-drug-resistant tuberculosis (MDR-TB) is of more recent vintage, since by convention the term is used to mean disease caused by strains of *Mycobacterium tuberculosis* resistant to at least isoniazid and rifampicin, the two most powerful agents, and usually the basis of first-line chemotherapies for TB. The first cases of MDR TB were described in the early 1970s, shortly after the 1966 introduction of rifampicin,[3] but cases were rare and epidemic transmission was not documented until much later. MDR-TB came to more widespread attention in the 1980s, when a number of epidemics were registered in North America and Europe. Outbreaks became increasingly common in the latter part of the decade and in the United States especially, were often associated with HIV. Many were nosocomial, centred on hospitals, with prisons and homeless shelters also serving as the settings for institutional outbreaks, most of which were associated with loss of life.[4]

In the subsequent decade, these scattered outbreaks were eclipsed by evidence of a much more widespread problem. MDR-TB epidemics were documented mostly in North America and Europe because it was there that laboratory capacity was robust. Beginning in 1994, however, the World Health Organization (WHO) and the International Union

Against Tuberculosis and Lung Disease (IUATLD) inaugurated a multi-site survey of resistance to first-line antituberculous agents. Their first report, issued in 1997, revealed that resistance to first-line drugs was found in every country studied.[5] The more one looked, the more one found. In 1999, Harvard Medical School's Program in Infectious Disease and Social Change began combing the medical literature, and found reports of drug-resistant TB in over 100 countries.[6] The second report of the WHO–IUATLD survey was issued in the spring of 2000 and revealed MDR-TB cases in those settings in which it had not previously been a problem.[7] MDR-TB has arisen as a significant global health problem in the space of a single generation.

The development and spread of MDR-TB has outpaced our ability to respond. In most MDR-TB 'hot spots', case finding and effective therapy are non-existent. What is to be done about MDR-TB in resource-poor settings? This question has provoked a good deal of controversy. The backdrop for the debate is one of scarcity of effective TB treatment. It is of note that the majority of those who die of TB die not of drug-resistant disease, but of lack of access to any effective antituberculous therapy. By one estimate, less than half of all cases even come to medical attention,[8] even though the diagnosis and treatment of most cases of smear-positive pulmonary TB is straight-forward, inexpensive and highly effective. For this reason, since the early 1990s those charged with defining policy for international TB control have championed DOTS – directly observed therapy, short-course – as the cornerstone of TB control.[9] Partly in response to the therapeutic chaos that reigned in several countries where there is a high prevalence of TB, leaders in international TB control began to push DOTS as the sole strategy worthy of support by national TB control programmes and their funders. That the World Bank classed DOTS as one of the world's most 'cost-effective' public health interventions was significant, because the Bank has emerged as the world's leading funder of TB control in resource-poor countries.[10] By the late 1990s, DOTS uptake could be described as 'rapid' by the WHO, even though at the century's close only a minority of the world's TB sufferers had access to DOTS-based therapy.[11]

The advent of MDR-TB led to bitter debate, since patients with MDR-TB are by definition resistant to the drugs used in the DOTS strategy. When advocates argued for effective therapy for MDR-TB, many TB control experts responded negatively. They argued that because we have failed to diagnose and treat drug-susceptible disease, we cannot hope to treat MDR-TB in poor countries.[12] Others went so far as to claim that short-course chemotherapy (SCC) – based on isoniazid and rifampicin – will cure patients with MDR-TB.

To clinicians, the idea that therapies based on isoniazid and rifampicin could cure patients resistant to precisely these two drugs seemed far-fetched, at best. But the logic underpinning such claims was other than clinical. Universal DOTS was a managerial and public health strategy that attempted to preserve scant funds by using the least expensive drugs and bypassing use of laboratory data in resource-poor settings. That SCC is an ineffective therapy for MDR-TB has recently been acknowledged by the WHO. A six-country study of the use of SCC among patients with MDR-TB showed that it failed in most patients.[13] Cure rates varied from between 11 to 60 per cent, depending on the quality of the national TB control programme. The highest rates of cure were in Hong Kong and Peru, which have excellent TB programmes; the lowest rates were in Russia. But the real rates of cure can be far lower. The Centres for Disease Control and Prevention, working in Russia's Ivanovo Oblast, cured only 5 per cent of primary MDR-TB cases (that is, cases infected from the start with a drug-resistant strain of *M. tuberculosis*) with SCC, even though their regimen included a fifth agent, streptomycin.[14] This seems closer to the expected figure when one learns, as we have, that many patients who are smear-negative after treatment – and thus declared 'cured' by DOTS criteria – are in fact only transiently suppressed. They may remain culture-positive throughout therapy, becoming smear-positive after SCC is stopped. Some of the Peruviuan 'cures' reported in the Six-Country Study were in fact referred to us after they relapsed. In the course of DOTS therapy, many had recruited additional resistance. We have termed this the 'amplifier effect of short-course chemotherapy'.[15] Whether acknowledged or not, the driving force behind the pressure for a single treatment strategy that did not rely on laboratory and radiographic data was its low cost.

In summary, globally, the proportion of prevalent TB cases that are due to MDR strains of *M. tuberculosis* ranges from extremely small to a substantial minority. But the majority of these patients will fail SCC, and as their number grows we will need new strategies that can cure them in resource-poor settings. To fail to do so carries a substantial social and economic impact.

MDR-TB in Haiti and Peru

In order to appreciate fully the social impact of MDR-TB is it necessary to look at the ways in which the disease is experienced. As our own experience in Haiti and Peru shows, the costs of failing to treat MDR-TB are in some ways far greater than is appreciated, just as the cost of responding effectively is lower than may be believed.

The Joseph Family, Haiti

The Josephs might be termed a typical lower-middle-class Haitian family, if not for MDR-TB. They live in a small house in Carrefour Feuilles, a poor neighbourhood in the sprawling city of Port-au-Prince. Mme Joseph is a street vendor; her husband is an irregularly employed construction worker. Although by the standards of the West, they live in poverty, theirs was a household in which it might be expected that all eight children would attend school; one or two of them might even find jobs.

One of their most talented children is Jean, in 1997 a 21-year-old student. The way Jean recalls it, his family's problems began when he started to cough. At first he sought to treat his persistent hack with herbal teas. But when his cough worsened, he began to think he might have something other than an ordinary cold. In the second month of his illness, with new back pain and a fever, Jean took himself to a TB hospital in Port-au-Prince. 'It's not that I thought I had TB,' he recalled recently. 'Not at all. It's rather that I knew they could take a chest X-ray.' But Jean did indeed have TB, and he was started that day on a four-drug regimen that included not only rifampicin and isoniazad but also streptomycin, a drug that is injected intramuscularly. 'I took all my medications,' he recalled, 'but I kept coughing.'

Towards the end of the year, Jean's fears were heightened by an episode of haemoptysis. Coughing up bright red blood terrified the young man, as it did his entire family. 'I knew I was getting worse, so I went to a pulmonologist.' The specialist referred Jean to the national TB sanatorium in January 1998. There Jean was found to be floridly smear-positive – he had evidence of heavy infection on routine study of his sputum – and was admitted for further therapy.

Jean was an in-patient for almost three months, during which he received directly observed therapy with the same drugs he had taken previously. He remained smear-positive throughout his time at the sanatorium. 'I was discouraged, I wanted to stop [taking the medications]. I was sure these medicines wouldn't do anything for me, since I had taken them for over a year and been smear-positive the whole time. I stopped taking them and went to an herbalist (doktè fey) for a few weeks.' At the herbalist's, Jean was treated with various concoctions containing the bark and leaves of trees held, it was said 'to cure TB and other lung disease'. But his symptoms persisted, and when he again began to cough up blood, he returned to the sanatorium. Again he was prescribed the same first-line drugs. During that time, he recalls, he was placed in an open ward with other patients, many of them, he knew, with drug-resistant disease. 'None of them were getting better. They started talking about other medicines that were better, but they said that the government either didn't have the medicines or wasn't going to distribute them.'

The names of these better drugs are kanamycin, cycloserine, ethionamide and levofloxacin. They are more expensive, more toxic and less effective than are rifampicin and isoniazid. There is little reason, then, to take them – unless you have the misfortune to have MDR-TB. In that case, such 'second-line' drugs often hold the only real hope of cure. Once Jean's parents had the names of the drugs, and a prescription from one of the pulmonologists, they started selling off assets – furniture, livestock, a parcel of land – in order to buy the medications. 'I started taking [second-line] medicines inside the sanatorium, and I was soon [smear-]negative. In July, I went home. But after five months of treatment, my parents couldn't buy any more medicines, and so I had to stop. I became positive again.'

Jean soon had fevers every night and drenching sweats. He coughed incessantly, and lived in fear of haemoptysis (he had learned during his sanatorium stay that this symptom could prove rapidly fatal). But the situation was to become even worse. 'Even though I had stopped coughing blood, my sister Maryse began coughing in about October, and then she started coughing up blood.' One after another, the Joseph children became ill: after Maryse, the oldest, came Myrlene, who had for years suffered with sickle cell anaemia. Then Kenol, the youngest, and, finally, Shella started coughing.

The Joseph family found itself in the middle of an international controversy: what was to be done for patients with MDR-TB who happen to have the misfortune to live in 'resource-poor countries'? The argument from the international public health community was clear. DOTS, based on first-line drugs, should be the sole TB treatment strategy in the Western hemisphere's poorest countries. Furthermore, this line of thinking went, patients with MDR-TB had acquired their disease through 'non-compliance' or 'poor national TB program (NTP) performance'.[16] But neither of these aetiologic hypotheses was correct: the Joseph family had not been 'non-compliant', nor had the Haitian NTP treated them contrary to international guidelines. In fact, the siblings had been infected with an MDR strain of M. tuberculosis. The SCC treatment could not cure them, but it could complicate their condition significantly.

One by one the Joseph siblings began treatment with first-line drugs. None of them improved. 'I felt terrible,' Jean recalled. 'I was getting sicker, but I mostly felt guilty. I just knew they had drug-resistant TB, and that's why they weren't getting better. I knew it was my fault.'

Because the Joseph children did not get better on first-line drugs, the nurse who was administering their streptomycin injections referred them back to the non-governmental organization that had originally diagnosed Jean with TB. 'She knew we were failing therapy,' recalled Jean, 'and she knew it was MDR-TB. But she said the government could not buy the drugs for patients with MDR-TB, it could only buy first-line drugs. So she referred us to [the non-governmental organization].' There, Jean was asked to submit a sputum sample for culture and drug susceptibility testing. 'I never got the results. I kept going back every couple of weeks, and they kept telling me to come back again in a couple of weeks.'

Jean worsened. Recurrent haemoptysis and coughing kept him sleepless and on edge. He woke before dawn on those mornings he'd been lucky enough to sleep. He became wasted, gaunt. His sisters knew that Jean was deeply depressed. 'He blamed himself for making us all sick,' said Myrlene. 'We tried to reason with him, but he didn't listen. He still blames himself.'

But Jean didn't give up. 'I had heard that there was one place in the country where we could be treated, and couldn't believe it. It seemed even more strange that it would be out in the middle of nowhere when the big hospitals in Port-au-Prince didn't have the medicines for anyone but people who could pay for them. So I came to see for myself.'

In October 1999, Jean left for central Haiti in a crowded truck –

what the Haitians call 'public transport'. He was coughing and short of breath, drawing the attention of the people among whom he was sandwiched. Once at the clinic, he spoke to none of us involved in treating MDR-TB: 'I just spent the morning looking around.' He liked what he saw, evidently, because in November all the Joseph siblings came to the Clinique Bon Sauveur and, following the requisite laboratory work, began therapy for MDR-TB. All became smear-negative within two months, and remain so after completing therapy.

Blanca, Andrés, and the Familia Tebeceana, Peru

Subtle as her initial symptoms may have been, Blanca Pérez had little doubt what was coming when, in July 1995, she began having fever, chills and a productive cough. Blanca and her husband Andrés, both then twenty-two years old, were living in her mother's house with Blanca's six siblings, two of whom were being treated for active TB. But they alone were not the reason that the Pérez family had been labelled a *familia tebeceana* – a TB family. Blanca was in fact the fifth in her family to be diagnosed with the disease – from which two of her nine siblings had already died.

It all started in 1987, when Blanca's older sister Sonya tested positive. Sonya received numerous treatments, all unsuccessful despite what she described as 'religious' compliance. Because TB treatment in Peru is supervised, there is a high likelihood that Sonya had primary drug resistance: that is, she had been infected with a drug-resistant strain from the start, which is why her treatments failed. In any case, she remained smear-positive for years, living in a small house in the hills of Carabayllo with her mother, nine siblings, and a changing cast of partners and children.

It was only a matter of time before others in the household began to cough. Pablo, the family's only son, was diagnosed with TB in 1990. Pablo was a teenager at the time, but was already the main breadwinner in the family. He worked as a street vendor, which entailed a pre-dawn ride to Lima's central market to collect old limes from the trash, then return to sell them in the Carabayllo market. The trip in a crowded bus took almost two hours each way. Responsible for feeding his siblings, Pablo often missed his medications on days when he was unable to leave work. For years, he was in and out of treatment and was considered a classic 'problem patient' by the health centre. As more and more of his lungs were destroyed, Pablo became increasingly short of breath. Eventually, he was unable to work. In late November 1994, Pablo was referred, following his repeated requests, to a pulmonologist. Although he eventually did see a specialist, and was diagnosed presumptively with MDR-TB, Pablo was never able to follow the pulmonologist's advice. He died the following day, still receiving first-line antituberculous drugs.

In 1991, Sonya's husband Raúl was diagnosed with TB. Sonya continued to have positive smears throughout her directly observed therapy, but it was not until 1993 that she was recognized to have MDR-TB; Raúl's resistance was not confirmed until mid-1996. Sonya and Raúl made heroic efforts to buy second-line drugs, but they could do so only intermittently, since their work as street vendors could barely feed them and their daughter. Both remained smear-positive for years, and Sonya was terrified by life-threatening episodes of haemoptysis.

Luisa, another older sister, was also diagnosed with TB in 1991. She followed the same pattern of unsuccessful treatment and retreatment as her siblings. After she saw Pablo die, Luisa gave up hope, and refused any further treatment. She often said to Sonya, 'Why do you go through all that to get those pills, when you know we're both going to die just like Pablo?' Luisa died one year after Pablo, in November 1995.

Rosa was diagnosed with TB in the first months of 1995. While receiving her anti-tuberculous treatment, she became pregnant but miscarried. Since completing her treatment, Rosa has been symptom-free. Blanca's mother was also treated for TB, and her symptoms have also disappeared.

For all of these reasons, then, Blanca suspected she, too, was ill with TB when she began coughing in July 1995. Initially, however, she sought neither diagnosis or treatment. But one morning in August, about a month after her symptoms began, Blanca had an episode of massive haemoptysis. Blanca's sisters, by this time experts, rushed her to the local health post, where her sputum was found to be abundantly positive for the tubercle bacillus. In spite of her known MDR-TB contacts, Blanca began receiving the *esquema único*, the standard six-month treatment regimen sanctioned by the Peruvian national TB programme.

In patients with fully drug-susceptible TB directly-observed therapy with these four drugs leads to rapid response; patients usually feel better within a couple of weeks. Most are usually smear-negative – and thus non-infectious – within the first month of treatment. By mid-September, a full month into treatment, Blanca's symptoms had failed to improve. Her chest X-ray looked worse, and her sputum smear remained positive. In fact, during every month of treatment, Blanca had a repeat smear; every month, it was positive.

During this entire period, the local health workers who gave Blanca her daily medications were concerned that she might be resistant to these drugs. They knew about her family history: it was they, in fact, who coined the term *familia tebeceana* to describe the Pérez and other families laid waste by TB. Fearing MDR-TB, the health workers collected a sputum specimen from Blanca in November and sent it for culture and susceptibility testing.

In early January 1996, Blanca's drug sensitivity results finally revealed that her TB strain was, like that of her sister, resistant to isoniazid and rifampicin, the two most powerful antituberculous drugs. Despite these laboratory results, and to the dismay of the health workers who visited her each day, Blanca was told by the health authorities that she must complete the *esquema único*, even though it consisted, at that point, of precisely the two drugs to which she had confirmed resistance. Discouraged, indeed frightened, Blanca did as she was told. Her symptoms worsened.

In late January, after completing the daily six-month regimen, Blanca's sputum continued to show abundant tubercle bacilli. She was wracked by fevers and coughing, and had experienced life-threatening haemoptysis; she now weighed less than 80 pounds. In keeping with the rules of Peru's national TCP, Blanca was evaluated by a programme pulmonologist, who placed her on an 'alternative' three-drug regimen approved by the national programme. In addition, this physician prescribed Blanca two third-line drugs, ciprofloxacin and ethionamide, explaining that if she could obtain these drugs, her treatment would be even stronger. Blanca recognized the names of these drugs, as they had been prescribed to Sonya and Raúl, too. Since these drugs were not part of the standard programme's regimen, Blanca knew that she would have to buy them herself. But the $200 a month that would be necessary to buy the drugs was well in excess of her entire family's monthly income.

The extended family pulled together enough resources to purchase one week's worth of the drugs for Blanca. This only made her feel worse, she recalled, since she could see that it was not possible for her family to sustain the economic burden and survive. Blanca announced that she would find another way of getting the drugs. Desperate for effective treatment, and thinking of her small children, Blanca changed her name and moved to another catchment area in order to be accepted by another health centre. Under an alias, she began a standard retreatment regimen in February 1996 – despite the laboratory documentation that she was resistant to the most powerful of the drugs she was receiving. Her symptoms improved, but she remained smear-positive throughout this second treatment as well. After completing this regimen, Blanca's symptoms returned, then worsened. Without further treatment options, she spent the next two months bedridden, losing weight, and coughing blood – the classic picture of galloping consumption.

Just when things seemed as if they could not get worse, Blanca's husband fell ill. Andrés worked as a street vendor, selling books, but he had also taken on all the cooking and housekeeping as well. So the increased fatigue and muscle pain he felt were initially attributed to overwork. In August 1996, though, he began coughing, and soon he too was diagnosed with TB. Given his multiple MDR-TB contacts, Andrés was reluctant to begin standard therapy with the drugs to which his wife, sisters-in-law and brother-in-law were resistant. But he, too, was pulled into the official regimen; he, too, remained smear-positive for most of his treatment.

In October, Blanca's nineteen-year-old sister Ana was diagnosed with TB. She was in the first trimester of her first pregnancy. She was the sixth Pérez child to fall ill with TB.

The Pérez family did receive some good news, though: in October, Blanca, along with Sonya and Raúl, began receiving a treatment regimen with drugs to which their strain of TB had demonstrated susceptibility. These drugs were being provided, along with nutritional support and daily community health worker visits, by Socios En Salud, a community-based organization. On 18 November, Blanca's sputum test was negative for the first time since she had been diagnosed with TB. Raúl and Sonya were also soon smear-negative.

By the end of 1996, Andrés and his family were sure that he, too, had MDR-TB, and he was angry that he was being forced to complete the standard regimen. The advent of therapy for MDR-TB had engendered a certain amount of tension in the local 'TB community', since many of the patients who had failed the official regimen understood, as did some of their providers, that they might have 'knocked off' other potentially effective drugs in the process: Sonya, for example, had become resistant to five drugs, although she had initially been resistant only to two; the same was true of Blanca. Still other patients had died while waiting, as one patient put it, 'to be liberated from *esquema único*'. The drugs made her nauseous. 'Why should I take drugs that make me sick if they're ineffective?' she asked.

Laboratory studies done by Socios En Salud revealed that Andrés did, in fact, have resistant disease. In January 1997, a few days shy of completing *esquema único*, Andrés refused to take his medications. He was forced to sign a statement acknowledging that he was 'abandoning treatment'. For this reason alone, Andrés will never figure in national data as a case of primary MDR-TB. Instead, he will be mislabelled, as were all the Pérez family, as having acquired MDR-TB though erratic compliance. They were 'problem patients'.

DNA fingerprinting of Andrés' infecting strain shows, of course, that he is sick with the same strain that almost killed his wife. He too is now improving on appropriate therapy, which he began in late January 1997.

The global burden of drug-resistant TB

Estimating the global impact of MDR-TB is difficult for several reasons. First, we have no reliable method of measuring the burden of disease. The few assessments we have are quite discrepant.[17] Although some underline the relative insignificance of MDR-TB, data from global surveys suggest that already-identified hot spots of MDR-TB transmission will account for hundreds of thousands of new infections in the short term – and millions of new infections if patients with active pulmonary MDR-TB are offered no effective therapy.

Second, the analytic challenge extends beyond resistance to isoniazid and rifampicin: the argument that other forms of drug-resistant TB can be cured by SCC is also problematic, since any resistance to first-line drugs confers a comparative disadvantage when empiric SCC is used.[18] Third, projecting the cost of laboratory expenses and, especially, drugs is difficult: rapidly changing drug prices characterize the second-line drug market, even though almost all of these drugs are no longer under patent and therefore subject to monopoly pricing.

These difficulties, when linked to various ideological positions, have led to TB costings that are stranger than fiction. For example, the popular press has noted that MDR-TB treatment 'costs about $250,000 per patient'.[19] In fact, the cost has not been documented. An expert in the management of the disease once remarked that costs can 'run as high as $250,000 per patient', a statement that was transformed into a treatment cost per MDR-TB patient and compared to the low cost of SCC, which itself is wildly disparate from place to place. To give an idea of the dimensions of the variations in costs, we can compare some of the routinely heard figures. First, our own experience has shown that second-line drug prices can drop rapidly in response to advocacy and to changes in perceived demand.[20] In Peru, where we have treated MDR-TB since 1996, we saw drug prices drop from as high as $10,000 per MDR-TB patient to as little as $600 per patient in the space of less than three years. As for the low cost of DOTS, although the WHO claims that a full course of first-line drugs can cost as little as $13 in China, it costs more than $20,000 to treat a single case of pan-susceptible TB (that is, TB that is susceptible to all antituberculous agents) in New York City.[21] Thus context is everything, and confident claims about how much it costs to treat MDR-TB – or even pan-susceptible TB – must be viewed with a great deal of scepticism, as should claims about cost-efficiency or the lack thereof.

The debate might have remained academic were it not for the resurgence of TB in Russia and other parts the former Soviet Union. In the wake of significant social and economic changes, this is a region in which TB incidence has risen sharply. Although the epidemic may have begun in the penitentiary system, it has spread rapidly to the civilian population. TB prevalence in the former Soviet Union trebled in the 1990s, but the rub is this: many, and in some cases *most*, patients are ill with strains resistant to at least one first-line drug. Throughout Russia, the use of universal SCC has led to low cure rates, an outcome attributed to many factors but one due, in large part, to the fact that MDR-TB cannot be cured with SCC. The ensuing debate about the effectiveness of SCC has hobbled effective responses to the world's first significant outbreak of drug-resistant TB.[22]

The cost of inaction

The cost to families of doing nothing – or, more commonly, of doing something ineffective or noxious, such as repeated courses of SCC – is evident from the case studies presented above. It is clear that a single smear-positive family member can rapidly transform a cramped dwelling into a setting of daily bombardment with viable MDR bacilli. Universal infection can be fairly confidently predicted in such households.[23]

The costs, to care providers, of inaction are poorly understood. In settings throughout the world, we have met physicians and nurses who are highly uncomfortable – at times, distraught – about the lowering of standards of care on the grounds of 'cost-effectiveness'. Giving SCC to new cases when they are close contacts of patients with known MDR-TB is viewed as dimly in Haiti or Peru as it is in Russia. The administration of SCC or 'isoniazid for life' to patients with documented MDR-TB is regarded by many as a violation of the social contract between patient and healer.[24] When the world's leading authority on MDR-TB argued that patients with MDR-TB 'are in so many ways our own children', he was referring to the fact that patients acquire resistance to antituberculous drugs during the course of poorly supervised or incorrect therapy – or that they are infected after contact with someone who has been inappropriately treated.[25] In the eyes of many within and outside the medical profession, patients with MDR-TB have moral claims on all of those charged with treating the sick.

These patients also have claims on those charged with protecting public health. Failure to treat patients with infectious MDR-TB means the ongoing spread of drug-resistant strains. In relation to this phenomenon, a number of ideological positions have been taken: allegedly scarce resources and vested interests have led, once again, to highly confident claims regarding the spread of drug-resistant organisms. Scant evidence of 'variable fitness' or 'decreased infectiousness' has already engendered projections in which MDR-TB epidemics 'burn themselves out'. Such exercises would be merely wishful thinking if they did not lead to complacency and ill-conceived policies.

Discrepant claims regarding the transmissibility and treatment of MDR-TB erode faith in TB control and public health in general. In setting after setting, patients with MDR-TB are denied access to effective therapy on the grounds that such treatment is neither 'cost-effective' nor 'sustainable'. Alas, the epidemic itself is sustainable as long as different standards of care are applied on the basis of the ability – of the affected – to pay for effective therapy.

If SCC is ineffective and second-line drugs are difficult to procure and use, what should be done to respond to MDR-TB? Certainly, prevention is critical. We know that MDR-TB acquired through poor TB programme performance can be prevented by effective treatment of pan-susceptible TB with DOTS. New vaccines and new drugs are also needed, as are effective infection control practices. But in settings in which MDR-TB is already present, we must expand the DOTS strategy to include effective management of patients already sick with drug-resistant TB. Elsewhere, we have presented DOTS-Plus as a DOTS-based strategy that relies on drug susceptibility testing and second-line drugs in order to bring patients with MDR-TB to cure.[26] The history of the idea is recent: the term was coined in April 1998 to describe the successful grafting of such projects on to a robust DOTS programme in Peru. Since that time, the demand for DOTS-Plus projects has grown rapidly, in large part because there are several hot spots of MDR-TB in precisely those settings in which effective therapy is scarce.[27] The WHO and affiliates have led the call for pilot projects that can meet both demand and also stringent criteria regarding the use of second-line drugs.

Key sites for DOTS-Plus expansion include Peru, where such programmes are now being scaled up to a national level; Tomsk Oblast in western Siberia, where both prison-based and civilian projects were inaugurated in 2000; and Bangladesh and South Africa, where standardized MDR-TB regimens are proving more effective than inaction in regimens based on SCC.[28]

Future expansion of DOTS-Plus is critical if we acknowledge the suffering of those already sick with MDR-TB. The incidence of global hot spots must also be the map of our engagement with a novel threat to public health. As the global era leads to an increasing awareness of the suffering of others, it has not led to a more just partition of the fruits of science and technology. If we are to prevent the ongoing spread of MDR-TB, *global health equity* must become a central component of wise policy in the coming years. Anything less than this promises to lead to poor outcomes for the poor and better outcomes for the non-poor. This has been the rule for the past several decades, and the health inequalities documented at the outset of the antibiotic era have become further entrenched with time. The emergence of drug-resistant microbes will always be favoured by the imprudent use of antibiotics. But their impact on the health of people living in poverty will be further accentuated by any policy that fails to insist on equity as the central concern of modern TB control.

10

The House of the Dead Revisited: Prisons, Tuberculosis and Public Health in the Former Soviet Bloc

Vivien Stern

> [The] ... unregulated, frequently packed, assemblage of unwashed, verminous, often starving and diseased prisoners in ill-ventilated and badly sewered rooms was a spontaneous breeding-ground of typhus.[1]

Prisons have long been associated with epidemics. Perceived as reservoirs of disease, they have often been deemed to concentrate infection and to threaten those outside. As early as 1666 an English Act commented that judge and jurypersons often caught diseases from prisoners.[2] In towns where the courts held sittings, the public became alarmed at the danger they were exposed to from having a prison in their midst.[3] In 1750 an outbreak of gaol fever led to the deaths of some of the Old Bailey judges and provoked discussion of alterations to Newgate prison to make it less prone to spread disease.[4] The Health of Prisoners Act of 1774 laid down requirements for prisons to be cleaned, ventilated and provided with sickrooms, a bath and a surgeon,[5] but the accounts published in 1777 by prison reformer John Howard of his visits to many British and European prisons showed that little improvement had been made. He recorded in great detail the squalor and disease that he found.[6] A visit to a prison gave his clothes such a disgusting smell that he could not travel by coach with other people but had to travel on his own on horseback. He also had to disinfect his notebook in front of a fire before he could use it. On the basis of what he saw, he argued in his writings the case for prison reform. One of the reasons why prisons should be improved was, he said, ethical. Prisons needed to be improved because the suffering that current conditions imposed on prisoners was unacceptable within a Christian framework. But there was another argument too, an argument about public health. Society had an interest in improving prisons because bad prison conditions led to disease, and disease spread from the prisons to the citizens living in the towns and villages surrounding the prison.[7] Eventually John Howard died from his dedication to penal reform. On a visit to the Ukraine he contracted typhus after visiting a sick prisoner, and died in 1790.[8]

Howard's arguments are still relevant today: the ethical and human rights questions about keeping people in inhumane prison conditions are regularly raised, and prisons still constitute a risk to public health. In most countries in the world those in prison come from the poorest sections of the population.[9] These are people who have already had little access to good health care and who are then often crammed into a disease-producing environment. Moreover, the prison healthcare service is usually inferior to that available in the community, and is sometimes only on offer to those prisoners who can pay. In some countries it is non-existent.

For these reasons epidemics and communicable diseases are concentrated and amplified in prison. A study carried out in Puerto Rico in 1999, for example, showed that 94 per cent of the prisoners were infected with hepatitis C.[10] In the prison system of the state of São Paulo in Brazil, over 14 per cent of the prisoners in 1995 were HIV-positive.[11] It is not surprising therefore that in the mid-1990s, after half a decade of disruption and impoverishment, a tuberculosis epidemic struck the prisons of Russia and other former Soviet bloc countries.

TB in Russia's prisons is not new. In his classic work *The House of the Dead*, Dostoevsky described everyday life in a Tsarist prison. The prison hospital had its TB patients and every year a certain number of prisoners met a sad end, dying of consumption with their legs still swathed in chains till the moment of their death. Writing about the Russian Federation in *The Global Impact of Drug-resistant Tuberculosis*, Paul Farmer, Mercedes Becerra and Jim Yong Kim of the Harvard Medical School point out that Tsarist Russia had an enormous TB problem but no coherent state public health policy. TB mortality rates prior to the First World War reached 400 per 100,000. Whilst 1.7 million Russian soldiers were killed in the First World War, during the same period some 2 million civilians died from TB.[12]

Whilst the upheavals that followed the war and the revolutions led to increased risks of TB, part of the embryonic Soviet state's drive to centralize and control was the establishment of a nationwide network of anti-TB institutions. Even in the prison camps of Stalin's gulag, where many millions met their deaths, TB care was organized. Following the Second World War, resources continued to be devoted to TB control. There were more dispensaries and sanatoria, BCG vaccinations and mass screening programmes. By the 1970s, instances of TB were rare. By 1989, just at the end of the Soviet era, the TB rate was 44.7 per 100,000.[13]

All that has now changed. The 1998 rates indicated by the World Health Organization (WHO) are 82.4 per 100,000 for the Russian Federation, 126.4 for Kazakhstan, 96.4 for Georgia, 122.9 for Kyrgystan, 81.3 for Latvia, 114 for Romania and 89.1 for Turkmenistan.[14]

The causes of the new epidemic are well documented. One major cause was the sudden drop into poverty of millions of people and a consequent reduction in their living standards. As the World Bank points out in its study of world poverty, the former Soviet countries maintained a moderate standard of living for most of their citizens. Employment was readily available; children were educated, and very few people went without basic foodstuffs. The loss of that standard of living was very sudden.

In addition to poverty the end of Soviet Communism brought massive social disruption. In the dismantling of the planned economy and the transition to a market economy millions of people lost their jobs. Many in the state sector were kept employed but not paid their salaries for months on end. In Georgia, Armenia and Tajikistan, armed conflicts and civil wars added to the upheaval.

The effects were not just economic either. Workplaces had earlier provided welfare and health services for employees, and had also exercised some degree of control. In the health field, for example, the workplace enabled mass screening to be done. It provided sanatoria, and enabled workers to keep their jobs even if they had to stay for several months in a sanatorium.[15] The new market-oriented enterprises provided none of this. Thus whilst rates of infection were increasing because of social problems, the efficiency of the TB control system was simultaneously reducing rapidly.

Once state budgets for health services were reduced and ideas of 'value for money' were introduced into the public sector, it became clear how far the Soviet TB control system had been a model from an earlier age. Peter Davies, Director of the Tuberculosis Research Unit at the University of Liverpool, writing on the history of TB treatment, notes the way that treatment changed when drug therapy was introduced:

> By the end of the 1950s the introduction of drug therapy for tuberculosis was considerably reducing the need for sanatoria beds in most developed countries. It was also realised that drug treatment, which could be given at home, might be able to eliminate the need for hospitalisation for all but the sickest tuberculosis patients.[16]

These changes had largely passed the Soviet Union by. The Soviet TB infrastructure was based on individualized treatment, isolation, a stay in a sanatorium, diagnosis by X-rays, and sometimes surgery. In Tomsk, for instance, an administrative region of Siberia with a population of 1 million, there were in 1996 seven TB institutions with over 1,000 beds and 1,000 staff, and a specialized TB hospital. The clinical staff followed methods of TB control that included 'multiple BCG vaccinations, flurographic surveillance, prolonged stay in hospital and a range of unusual treatments'.[17] Furthermore, medical personnel in Russia and Central Asia had an interest in keeping the system that way since their jobs were dependent on the existence of TB beds and the carrying out of operations. A move to the DOTS system recommended by the WHO – with a nurse giving out medication in a clinic or another setting – was very unsettling to them.[18] It threatened not only their jobs but also their professionalism: they had believed in what they were doing, and with some justification. Before the economic collapse they had indeed been successful in achieving high cure rates.[19]

Imprisonment in the former Soviet bloc

Once TB rates began rising again in the former Soviet bloc, it was predictable that the prisons would become the site of an epidemic. Prison conditions deteriorated in parallel with conditions in outside society, and prison populations were drawn largely from amongst the poor and the rootless. But to understand fully the epidemic it is necessary to put the prison situation in context.

The history of imprisonment in the Russian Empire and later in the

Soviet Union is one of banishment and hard labour. The novels of Dostoevsky and Tolstoy give a picture of the prisons of Tsarist Russia, of journeys into exile and treatment in faraway prison camps. In Soviet society the Tsarist system continued and was even developed and refined. A crime was seen as a political act and criminals were enemies of the state.[20] Prisoners were not citizens; indeed once they were committed to the gulag they lost their citizenship and joined a different world, a world run by the Ministry of the Interior, the MVD.

A prisoner in the Soviet Union progressed through two main stages: the pre-trial prison and then the camp. The pre-trial prison held suspects for periods of up to several years pending their trials. Most pre-trial prisons were built to hold several thousand prisoners, who lived in large dormitory-like cells holding any number from perhaps twenty to over a hundred. Once the trial was over and the prisoner was convicted, the long journey began to the final destination, which might be thousands of miles from his or her place of origin, often to the far north, or to Siberia or to Karaganda in what is now Kazakhstan. The prisons where these exiles ended up were not prisons in the Western sense but labour camps, sometimes huge factories or mines, with barracks attached where the prisoners lived. The slave labour meant that certain large projects, such as the building of strategically important canals, could be carried out even though no free citizen would voluntarily participate in them due to the harshness of the conditions.[21]

With the end of Communism a process of change in the systems of criminal justice began in the countries of Eastern Europe and Central Asia, to bring them into line with international human rights standards. But at the same time as reforms of the legal and prison systems were instituted, the prisons came under new pressures. Economic crisis and the collapse of the old structures had their effects not just on the health and welfare systems but also on the criminal justice system. First, widespread and sudden poverty led to an increase in crime.[22] Second, economic insecurity led to a fear of crime and a public demand for greater protection. So, the number of arrests rose, tripling between 1988 and 1995. Most of those arrested ended up in the pre-trial prisons, many of them for the most trivial of offences. (In an interview in 1998 the Vice-Minister of Justice, Yuri Ivanovitch Kalinin, described two prisoners he met in the pre-trial prison in Chelyabinsk, one being held because he was accused of stealing two bottles of vodka and a box of chocolates, the other for fighting with a school friend.) These social upheavals put enormous pressure on a prison system in the throes of fundamental change.

The first pressure was the sheer number of prisoners. In the late 1980s during the period of glasnost and perestroika the prison population had fallen, but as the economic crisis developed, the number of prisoners increased causing extreme overcrowding, particularly in the pre-trial prisons. By the year 2000, the Russian Federation had the second highest imprisonment rate in the world – 678 per 100,000.[23] Other former Soviet countries also had some of the highest rates in the world.[24] (The United States had the highest with a rate of 682 per 100,000 population. The comparable median rate for southern European countries was 70; that in England and Wales was 125.)[25]

So in spite of substantial reforms in the treatment of prisoners and their entitlements, prisoners still suffered appalling conditions because of the high imprisonment rate and consequent massive overcrowding. In the dormitories of the pre-trial prisons the prisoners slept in shifts because of the shortage of space to lie down. In 1999, Kresty prison in St Petersburg, built to hold 3,000, was holding 10,000 people. Prisoners not only slept in shifts on three-tiered bunks but they also slept in the daytime on the floor under the lowest bunks, with barely an inch between their face and the bunk above.[26] In 1994 the head of the prison service reported to the Russian parliament that overcrowding was so intense in some pre-trial prisons that prisoners had died of suffocation. In April 2000 Radio Free Europe reported that

> The average inmate in Russia's jails has a living space smaller than the size of a coffin – about 60 square centimeters. Prisoners take turns lying or sitting on bunks. . . . In St Petersburg's Kresty jail last year, 56 inmates died of asphyxiation in packed, stuffy cells.[27]

The problems of overcrowding were compounded by the difficult economic position of the prison administration, which changed considerably after the end of Communism. During the Soviet era the Ministry of the Interior, which was in charge of the labour camps, was very powerful economically. Work was the basis of the system, but the labour of the prisoners did not just provide income for the state. The prisons were also dependent on that income. Whilst the salaries of the prison employees were paid by the state, other costs, such as food, heating and medicines, had to be met from the profits of the industrial enterprises run by the camps.

With the advent of the market economy the prison industrial enterprises lost their customers. The state was no longer contracting with the prisons to build roads or railways. Nor was there a market for the vast range of goods – including tractors, aeroplane seats, engine parts, office furniture, household goods, shoes – produced by the Ministry of the Interior in its prisons. The routine in Soviet labour camps was for prisoners to line up and march off in the morning, go to an adjoining factory area and work till evening. Now the factories were idle. The break-up of the Soviet Union has brought an added problem. The high level of specialization in the Soviet gulag manufacturing arm meant that parts of the same machine were made in labour camps that were now in different independent countries. Of the parts of a tractor for instance, the wheels might have been made in Ukraine, the tyres in what is now Russia, the body in Kazakhstan and the engine in Armenia. Huge wheel or engine factories therefore now lay idle. So there was no work for the prisoners and no money for prison running costs. In addition, the money available to the prisons from the state was greatly reduced. The staff were sometimes not paid for months on end. Buildings crumbled. Food quality was reduced.

Then, in the mid-1990s, information began to emerge about dangerous levels of TB infection. The International Committee of the Red Cross, which visits prisoners in countries involved in war or internal conflict, revealed high levels of TB among prisoners in Azerbaijan. In 1995, therefore, the International Committee of the Red Cross started a TB treatment programme in the central prison hospital in Baku. Also in 1995 the medical director of a special prison camp in Marinsk, Siberia, for prisoners ill with TB asked Médecins Sans Frontières (MSF) for help. The following year Hans Kluge from MSF started a DOTS programme in the prison.[28] In July 1997 a mission from the international non-governmental organization, Penal Reform International, and the Royal Netherlands TB Association visited the prisons in Pawlodar, Kazakhstan, at the invitation of the authorities there who were concerned about the high level of TB amongst prisoners. The two organizations subsequently set up a combined TB treatment and prison reform programme in Pawlodar.[29]

In 27 October 1998, at a Moscow press conference organized by three non-governmental organizations active in the medical field, it was announced that almost 100,000 prisoners, one in ten of the Russian prison population, suffered from active TB and that an estimated

20,000 had multi-drug-resistant TB. Echoing the arguments of John Howard two centuries earlier, Tine Demeulenare of MSF told journalists, 'The TB epidemic in Russian prisons is not just a far-away humanitarian disaster. It is a threat to us all since the infection does not stop at fences and borders.'[30]

The role of prisons in the epidemic

Commentators regard the prison system as a key element in the epidemic, a bridge and a reservoir. Generally TB is reported to be 100 times more common in prison than in civilian populations.[31] The WHO reports a Brazilian study of 1992–93 giving a rate of 5,714 per 100,000 for the prison population and a rate of 55.9 in the civilian population. A similar study in Rwanda in 1996–8 gives a figure for prisons of 5,142 and for civilians of 79.3.[32] These high figures reflect a combination of factors. First, many people come to prison already infected. Second, the infection is readily transmitted in prison. The Harvard Medical School/Open Society Institute Global Report notes that 'it is clear that many detainees become infected during pre-trial detention'.[33] The WHO lists a number of factors that contribute to the spread of TB in prisons: late case detection, lack of isolation, inadequate treatment of those who are infectious, high turnover of prisoners, overcrowding and poor ventilation. The low nutritional value of prison food also acts to weaken the prisoner and makes him or her more prone to disease. The physical and psychological stress of imprisonment also makes a contribution.

According to official reports, in Russia 'the number of incidences of TB among prisoners has doubled over the past five years and the mortality rate has quadrupled (it is 40 times higher than the national average mortality rate)'. In May 2000 there were 90,786 infected prisoners and the figure was predicted to rise.[34] In 1999 one third of all Russian TB cases were estimated to be in prisons.[35] In Russia there are separate prisons for convicted prisoners suffering from TB. In May 2000 these 'TB colonies', as they are called, held 43,118 people and were significantly overcrowded. The rest of the infected prisoners are held in the pre-trial prisons and in ordinary labour camps. Moreover, according to the Public Health Research Institute, the penal system in Russia had at its disposal only 15 per cent of the medical equipment and facilities necessary to cope with the epidemic. In 1999, for example, only 20–30 per cent of the requested budget was made available for drugs.

In Georgia in 1997–98 there were an estimated 7,437 smear-positive prisoners, comprising 26 per cent of all estimated TB cases in the country.[36] In Azerbaijan the prisons are estimated to hold 4,600 cases of TB per 100,000 of the prisoner population, a rate which is 47 per cent higher than the national average. TB is thought to be responsible for up to 80 per cent of deaths in Azeri prisons.[37] In 1997 it was estimated that over 20 per cent of Kazakh prisoners were suffering from some form of TB.[38] Between January and August 1998, 962 of the 1,290 deaths there were TB-related.[39] In the first eight months of 1997, 90 per cent of all deaths in Mongolian prisons were from TB.[40] It is not only prisoners who suffer. Prison staff are also very vulnerable. In 1997, 428 staff in Russian prisons were diagnosed with active TB.[41]

Much of the publicity since 1998 has been concentrated on the spread in Russian prisons of MDR-TB. This form of TB occurs in two ways. The infected person has either taken enough antibiotics to strengthen the infection but not enough to eliminate it or has become infected with a form that is already resistant. Whilst TB generally can normally be dealt with by an inexpensive course of treatment, the drugs needed to deal with the MDR TB variety are much more expensive, costing between $4,000 and $10,000 per patient. The danger this form of the illness poses to Russians not in prison and to the world more generally has been a source of much comment. In a typical piece, in March 2000 the *Boston Globe*, under the headline 'TB, Rampant in Russian Prisons, imperils Country at Large – Resistant Strain Stirs Fears Illness will Jump Borders', stated that, 'From behind the crumbling yellow-brick walls of the Holding-Cell No.1 prison complex [in Moscow], a deadly epidemic is slowly being loosed upon an unsuspecting world.'[42]

Estimates differ on the actual level of MDR-TB amongst Russian prisoners. The medical charity Merlin suggests the rate is 40 per cent.[43] The Harvard Medical School/Open Society Institute Global Report suggests 'at least 20%'.[44] The Institute of Tropical Medicine in Antwerp reports laboratory findings from the projects in Baku and Marinsk of rates of 24.6 per cent MDR TB amongst newly enrolled cases and 92.1 per cent amongst non-responding cases.[45] In other states the figures are also high. In Georgia a figure of 13 per cent is quoted by the WHO. For Azerbaijan the figure is 23 per cent.[46]

The arrival of MDR TB was predictable to those with experience of TB epidemics amongst poor populations and people in institutions. The Soviet Union was not an underdeveloped country and drugs were available. But the supply was intermittent and complicated by the realities of prison life where everything was traded, where families visited and would bring some tablets with them, or where prisoners might pass their medicines on to family members outside. Laboratory facilities were not available to test for resistance. Infected people were often not isolated.

A further complicating factor has arisen with the spread of HIV infection in the prisons of the region. The connections between HIV infection and TB have been well documented. The annual risk of developing active TB for those infected with the tubercle bacillus is increased 40 times for those who are HIV-positive.[47] According to UNAIDS the fastest growing rate of HIV infection is to be found in the former Soviet Union countries. In Russia at the end of March 1999 there were 12,332 reported cases of infection. By January 2000 the figure had grown to 26,414 and by the beginning of August 2000 it was 52,427 – the number had more than quadrupled in less than a year and a half.[48] Just as in the general population, HIV infection rates inside Russian prisons are increasing rapidly. In fact it is estimated that in prisons HIV infection is 75 times more common than in the community at large.[49] Official figures showed 3,500 HIV-positive prisoners in Russia at the end of May 2000, compared to 2,661 a year previously.[50] Whereas Médecins Sans Frontières reports that there were 7,541 people who were HIV-positive or living with AIDS in the prisons of the Russian Federation on 1 August 2000.

Responses to the epidemic

In the five years since the TB epidemic became big news, much has been done in some countries to take the steps needed to deal with it. At first, however, the system in a number of countries struggled to come to terms with it. Early initiatives such as the intervention in Pawlodar and the project in Mariinsk were the result of middle-ranking officials taking risks and going outside their own hierarchy to ask overseas agencies for help.[51] The International Committee of the Red Cross project in Baku, for example, encountered many difficulties in its early stages as the Azeri authorities tried to come to terms with the implications of outside intervention,[52] and in Ukraine on the other hand the penitentiary adminstration was very slow to respond to the epidemic. In Latvia, however, where the numbers were small, a concerted effort and help from an outside donor ensured that treatment was in place. The number of infections began falling in 2000.

In Russia in 1998, in a move to break with many decades of history, the management of the penitentiary system was transferred from the jurisdiction of the Ministry of Interior to the Ministry of Justice. Afterwards the administration became more open about the TB situation, the gap between needs and available resources, and the dangers the epidemic posed to those in outside society. In autumn 2000 the WHO issued a new manual, *Tuberculosis Control in Prisons*, which set out how to deal with TB in prisons where there was a high incidence and scarce resources. On the wider penal reform front, the Russian Parliament approved an amnesty in May 2000, which made up to 90,000 prisoners eligible for early release.[53] The administration hoped to reduce the prison population to 300,000.[54] The author visited the TB wards in Mattroskaya Tischina prison in Moscow in May 2000. The staff reported on a much-improved situation with a reduction in the number of prisoners held there from 6,000 to 4,000, a drop they attributed largely to the speeding up of the trials in the Moscow area. The medical staff also reported that they were now able to test patients for resistance before commencing a course of treatment. Other countries in the region had also reduced their prisoner numbers.

The future

Maybe the corner was turned by the end of 2000. But the price has been high, both in numbers of deaths and in human suffering. Unless the spread of HIV can be slowed and the project to treat prisoners with MDR-TB expanded the prospects are bleak for many prisoners in the region.

The epidemic raises several issues about the relationship between prisons and public health, about social policy and about justice and human rights. One issue is the conflict inevitably generated between the imperatives of a criminal justice system and the imperatives of public health. This conflict can be seen in many aspects of prison life. One example very relevant to the TB epidemic is the question of shutters, or *jalousies* as they are called in Russian. By law, all pre-trial prisons throughout the former Soviet Union have heavy metal shutters on the outside of the already-small cell windows. The shutters are there because it is a prosecution requirement that prisoners should have no contact with others involved in the same case in order to prevent collusion. The shutters prevent prisoners shouting to each other. The shutters also prevent access to light and fresh air. When combined with overcrowding this leads to an almost total lack of ventilation and results in very poor air quality. Yet in spite of the TB epidemic these shutters remain. The prosecutors are more powerful than the doctors. Preventing collusion is more important than preventing a deadly infection.

Measures to manage the prisoners also take precedence over health requirements. If there are security problems and some prisoners have to be transferred out to other prisons where there is no treatment, will the doctors be able to ensure that prisoners in the middle of a course of treatment will not be transferred? The answer is that probably the doctor will not be consulted. What is the right decision to be made when the prison sentence is shorter than the course of treatment? To withhold treatment is harsh. To commence treatment when there is no guarantee that it can be continued on the outside is to risk creating drug resistance. To continue to hold prisoners for treatment reasons once their sentence has been served is a human rights abuse.

Serious questions of equity and human rights emerge. If there are not enough antibiotics for everyone, how will allocation be determined? Will the doctor decide on medical criteria or will the prison management decide? Will the medicines go to the most powerful prisoners, because they threaten violence unless they get them? Or will they go to the informers, as a reward from the authorities for information provided? Or will corruption be the decider? Prisons with their secrecy are prime sites for corruption. If prison medical staff are poorly paid or not paid at all for long periods, and if some prisoners can organize violence against those who cross them, then there is potential for selling drugs. The prisoners who have money or power will get the treatment.

Another issue of great importance is the structural question about the organization of prison health services and the relationship between the prison and the outside world. The prison health service is not part of the national health service in many countries, including all the countries of the former Soviet Union. In the Soviet era, prisoners were subject to a different law, and received their medical services from the Ministry of the Interior. Even now there is still separate documentation for civilian TB cases and what are called 'others'. 'Others' refers to prisoners, refugees, homeless people. The prison administrations have their own medical directorates, career structures, budgets, rules and requirements. Yet, there is considerable traffic between the prison and the community. Prisoners have visits from their families. Prisoners will leave prison at the end of their sentences (300,000 prisoners leave prison every year in Russia) and go to another area, perhaps halfway through their treatment, perhaps with a note for their local dispensary giving the details of their treatment, perhaps not.

Then there are social policy and human rights questions about the use of imprisonment. It is well known that TB is a disease of 'poverty, malnutrition and overcrowding'. Commentators argue that changing these social conditions is an essential part of TB control. And indeed reforming those factors in prisons in the former Soviet Union is essential. Otherwise, new cases will be created as fast as the old cases are treated. Prison reform should be an essential part of any TB control programme. In the Pawlodar project in Kazakhstan it was a prerequisite of the involvement of both Penal Reform International and the Royal Netherlands TB Association that TB treatment and a prison reform project should go hand in hand, and halfway through the three-year programme a major international conference on alternatives to prison was organized to highlight the need to reduce the prison population and the ways it could be done.[55] At the end of 2000 Kazakhstan was pressing ahead with the development of alternatives to imprisonment and with prison reform. To improve conditions for those prisoners who cannot be dealt with in other ways some prisons have started to grow food and market prisoner-made products, using the proceeds to refurbish the prison. In Azerbaijan the law requiring pre-trial prison cells to have shuttered windows has been repealed.[56]

It is clear that the TB epidemic will not be contained unless action is taken on a broad front. Organizations will have to work together. Criminal justice and health policy will have to be brought together and the old rigidities will have to go. But there are wider lessons. The TB epidemic highlights the human rights dilemmas posed everywhere by imprisonment. Article 6 of the International Covenant on Civil and Political Rights states: 'Every human being has the inherent right to life. This right shall be protected by law. No-one shall be arbitrarily deprived of it.' Governments have a duty to protect from harm and disease those whose liberty they have taken away. Sentencing a prisoner to spend a prolonged time in an environment where he or she is up to 40 times more likely to contract a lethal disease clearly contravenes this principle. A custodial sentence may be tantamount to an extrajudicial sentence of death. The situation in the former Soviet Union is extreme, but not that extreme. Public health advocates need to question the mass use of incarceration everywhere. In the United States for instance, where the use of imprisonment is now higher than it is in Russia, resources are available to prevent the sort of epidemic that will strike poor countries. But mass incarceration can lead to other ills, family breakdown, violence and mental ill health.

The TB epidemic in the prisons of Eastern Europe and Central Asia reinforces many of the points made by John Howard in 1777 and by prison reformers subsequently. Prison reformers argue for prisoners to be treated as citizens, for prisons to be closely connected to the community, and for imprisonment to be used as a last resort. These are ethical arguments. But as John Howard noted more than 200 years ago, they are also good public health arguments.

PART III

Advocacy and Action

11

Rethinking the Social Context of Illness: Interdisciplinary Approaches to Tuberculosis Control

Christian Lienhardt, Jessica Ogden and Oumou Sow

Over the past thirty years, many articles about TB control have emphasized the importance of poverty and social justice in the fight against the disease[1] and some local efforts at control have attempted in various ways to take these factors into account in their design and implementation.[2] Surprisingly, however, the same factors were not taken into adequate consideration when an international strategy for TB control was first developed at international level in the mid-1990s. In this chapter we argue that in order to control this disease, it is imperative that the strengths of all of the public health disciplines are brought into practice. We show that the social sciences, which have in the past been marginalized within public health, have important contributions to make to this effort. A framework for integrating a social science approach into operational research on TB control is offered, which can support current efforts internationally to make TB control a global reality.

Those working in the classical public health disciplines of medicine and epidemiology have established the foundations for diagnosis and treatment of TB, and the conventional TB control model encompasses many aspects of medical science, such as microbiology, pharmacology, immunology and genetics. These foundations are essential for efficient TB control programme operations. Microbiology and genetics have contributed to the understanding of the bacteria and the development of appropriate drugs; immunology and molecular biology address the issue of the response to infection, and research is presently being conducted actively on the search for new vaccines against TB; epidemiology helps to understand both the transmission of TB in populations and the factors influencing transmission. While these disciplines address issues of the microbe in relation to an individual or a population, social science looks at the dynamic relationship between the disease, the individual and society. The aims of social science approaches to understanding TB are not to measure the effect of disease on individual bodies, but to understand how the person and the disease interact within the context of everyday life.[3] By taking into consideration the social dimensions of disease and well-being, an interdisciplinary approach considers the individual as part of a community and addresses questions that are fundamental to control, such as access to health care, recourse to treatment, delivery of care, and completion of treatment. Much more than the approach of any other discipline in medical research, the contribution of social sciences is directly oriented towards the concept of operational research because it can answer the 'why' questions that often arise when programmes are established (Why don't patients come to us for treatment? Why do they only come when it's too late to help them? Why don't patients complete their therapy?) and the 'how' questions that arise when programmers and policy makers realize the need to change the way they deliver services (How can we make our programme more accessible and acceptable to patients? How can we better meet the health needs of the community?).

The international strategy for TB control developed by the World Health Organization (WHO) in the early 1990s relied on classical public health paradigms: a broad 'political commitment' by governments to its acceptance as national policy, and a focus on the treatment of individual patients without consideration of their social environment or the economic and political context in which they live.[4] After a brief overview of TB control objectives, we discuss this strategy and outline what we perceive to be its primary weaknesses. We also outline some ways in which these weaknesses may be overcome, for instance by paying closer attention to the varied, multiple and sometimes conflicting needs of individual patients, the communities in which they live, and the health service structures that are charged with their care. It is our assertion that, in the twenty-first century, it is time to move towards a concept of control that views the sick individual as a *participant* and his/her well-being as an *objective*.

Conventional TB control

The aim of TB control is to break the cycle of transmission, either by interrupting human transmission of infection or by protecting individuals against infection/disease. There are various levels of intervention along the line of the natural history of TB, where different methods can be used.[5] However, as most transmission occurs from those with infectious pulmonary TB, the specific objective of TB control is to detect and cure these cases as early as possible so as to cut the chain of transmission.[6] Most TB control programmes in developing countries use 'passive' case-finding (relying on suspect TB cases to present spontaneously to health services) rather than 'active' case-finding (where people with symptoms of TB, such as cough and fever, are sought in the population and brought in for diagnosis). It is generally accepted within TB control that the former is more cost-effective.[7] In all cases, however, the key element is to establish contact with the TB case who must be diagnosed and fully treated. Access to health care is thus the cornerstone of TB control programmes, which must ensure that patients developing the signs and symptoms of TB are able to seek help for their condition, that proper diagnosis is made, and that drugs are effectively provided to patients during the full course of treatment.

Problems of access to care are illustrated by the delay often observed between the onset of symptoms and diagnosis. This delay is a problem both because of the prolonged suffering it causes the patient, and because of the increased possibility for the illness to be further spread in that person's household and community. Extensive research has taken place in recent years to measure delay in diagnosis and treatment of TB and to try to identify factors contributing to this delay. Delays in diagnosis have been reported both in developed and in developing countries and vary considerably in duration, from an average 6.2 weeks in Australia to 12 weeks in Botswana and 16 weeks in Ghana.[8] Factors that have been reported as influencing delay include the individual's perception of the disease, severity of the disease, differential access to health services, age, gender, social deprivation, economic burden, and the attitude and expertise of health personnel.[9] In the USA, social deprivation was shown to reduce access to healthcare services, thus increasing TB morbidity and mortality. In several countries in Africa, a striking difference in health-seeking behaviour patterns was observed between urban and rural areas. This can be explained by a poorer access to health care in rural areas, lack of training of village health workers, lack of supervision of health staff at the peripheral level, and differences in education levels between rural and urban areas. In Zambia, the economic burden on patients resulting from lost income, transport and food expenditures was an important contributing factor to delayed diagnosis and, hence, continued spread of the disease within the community. Few studies, however, have measured the impact of specific social factors on the delay to treatment, and attention to the patient's perspective has mainly come so far from anthropological case studies.[10]

Another key aspect of control is to ensure that patients take the full course of treatment, in order to achieve clinical cure and reduce the development of drug resistance. Much research has been conducted over the last forty years to improve TB treatment by shortening its duration, so as to favour proper and complete drug intake. Numerous regimens have been tested, leading to the recommendation of using highly effective short-course treatment regimens of six to eight months' duration. Although this sounds like – and is – a long time to be ingesting tablets, previous regimens, with less powerful drugs, lasted for eighteen months or more. Efforts to improve the range of drugs at the disposal of doctors in treating TB, to shorten the duration of medication and reduce the drugs' side-effects go hand in hand with efforts to make services more accessible and acceptable to patients.

Thus patient adherence to treatment is an important area of overlap between the social and biomedical sciences. In an influential article about adherence to TB therapies, Esther Sumartojo, a behavioural psychologist, points out that adherence issues are not only multifaceted and complex, but range from characteristics of the individual patients to qualities of the social and economic environment.[11] This resonates with Paul Farmer's insistence that 'in most settings where TB is prevalent, the degree to which patients are able to comply is significantly limited by forces quite beyond their control'.[12] For Farmer, compliance is a problematic concept, not only because it implies docility and subservience of patients relative to providers, but also, and even more insidiously, because it assumes that all patients are equally able to comply – or to refuse to comply – with anti-TB therapies. The profound effects of poverty and/or economic inequity, racism, gender inequalities, drug use, homelessness, overt political violence, civil disturbance and war are all key factors in the inability of patients to obtain, maintain and complete therapy. These forces, Farmer argues, are everywhere more important in shaping 'patient compliance' than are illness beliefs or the patient–provider relationship. In relation to multi-drug resistant (MDR) TB, for example, it is these social-structural factors that will influence whether or not appropriate drugs are available and properly prescribed as well as the presence and accessibility of adequate care facilities.

Issues of access and adherence raise our awareness of the relationship between TB treatment and social vulnerability. If social-structural factors are largely to 'blame' for treatment failures in TB, as Farmer suggests, which of this myriad of factors are most important, for whom, and who is willing and able to do something about them? Clearly not all people with TB will face problems of access and adherence. Some will be more vulnerable to slipping through the net, or to falling out of care once they have been put on to treatment, than others. Indeed, despite the dramatic overall drop in TB notifications in New York City in the early 1990s, 'tide pools' of infections remained in 'some of the poorest sections of the boroughs of Brooklyn and the Bronx'.[13] Furthermore, evidence from Delhi indicates that those 'most able to comply', even among the economically marginalized (the 'poor'), will be those who are well supported by their families and communities. Conversely, those 'least able to comply' will include those who are economically and socially marginalized: those who lack both the support of their families and the support of the wider community or polity.[14] This finding is echoed in a number of qualitative studies, conducted around the world, showing that household and family support are positively associated with anti-TB treatment completion: patients who receive the support and care of their families are significantly more likely to adhere to therapy and achieve cure.[15] Thus the social context of illness is important, not only to help us understand its spread, but also to give us important insights into its management. Yet, TB control programmes are slow to take up this challenge, as the next section will show.

The international strategy

In the early 1990s, a model for global TB control was developed by the International Union Against Tuberculosis and Lung Disease (IUATLD) and the WHO, with the objective of reducing mortality, morbidity and transmission of TB worldwide. This model was based on research conducted by the IUATLD in several countries in Africa.[16] The objective of this model is to cut the chain of transmission by treating infectious TB cases as early as possible so as to render them non-infectious. Prior to this work, there were concerns in the international community about the introduction of effective short-course treatment regimens in developing countries. This was largely because of fears that the lack of strong healthcare structures in many of these countries would make it difficult to monitor drug taking and, therefore, might lead to the emergence of drug resistance, particularly to one of the drugs in the regimen, rifampicin.[17] For this reason, the model developed on the basis of the IUATLD experience included the recommendation to ensure direct observation of treatment intake (directly observed therapy, or DOT) by a trained healthcare worker, at least during the first two months of intensive phase treatment.

In 1994, the WHO defined specific targets for TB control (to cure 85 per cent of newly detected infectious TB cases and detect 70 per cent of existing infectious cases) and introduced the DOTS strategy as the main tool to reach these targets.[18] DOTS was set up as a comprehensive strategy, with the following five features: (1) a strong government commitment towards TB control; (2) case detection through passive case-finding using sputum smear microscopy; (3) treatment using standard short-course chemotherapy regimens containing rifampicin, administered under direct observation for at least the first two months of treatment (DOT); (4) a secure and regular supply of essential anti-TB drugs; and (5) a monitoring, recording and reporting system for programme supervision and evaluation. This strategy has been launched widely and marketed as the best tool currently available in the fight against TB. Early reports showed that, in 1995, 23 per cent of the world population had access to DOTS; the proportion reached 56 per cent by 1998.[19] Based on a mathematical model, the potential effect of DOTS on TB in developing countries was reported to be 'even greater than the results achieved in industrialised countries when drugs became available in the 1940s'.

DOTS does not, however, offer guidelines on its implementation. The diversity of patients' attitudes towards the disease and the extreme variability of access to care in the world are two of the many factors of social context that will profoundly affect the ability of governments to implement the policy effectively. In addition, the DOTS strategy has been marketed widely without strong evidence of the efficacy of DOT in improving patient adherence to treatment and cure, as compared to alternative methods.[20] Three randomized control trials of directly observed *versus* self-supervision of treatment have been reported so far – in South Africa, Thailand and Pakistan – and they show conflicting results.[21] The South African trial showed no difference between self-supervision of treatment (collection of drugs once a week by the patient) and DOT (supervised intake of drugs five times a week for 8 weeks and then three times a week for 4 months), while the Thai trial showed a benefit from DOT ensured daily by a family member and reinforced by a weekly motivating visit by health workers. The trial conducted in Pakistan showed no difference between self-supervised treatment (fortnightly collection of drugs by the patients), DOT ensured by a health worker, and DOT ensured by a family member.

There are multiple reports of TB control programmes worldwide using various types of intervention to promote adherence and enhance case-holding, including incentives, tracing of defaulters, legal sanctions and forced detention, patient-centred approaches, staff motivation and supervision.[22] Most of these interventions, however, depend heavily on additional external funding, and their sustainability is questionable. As reported by Klaus Jochem and John Walley of the Nuffield Institute for International Health, University of Leeds, there has been 'considerable debate on the relative importance of provider versus patient factors contributing to non-adherence, on the appropriateness of a universal policy of DOT, on the feasibility and acceptability of DOT in different settings, and on the provider and patients' costs of different DOT options'.[23] There are, indeed, a few studies on the direct and indirect costs incurred by the patients in attending a clinic or health centre daily or thrice-weekly for at least two months. A study in Pakistan found that the additional cost of attending the nearest health facility for two months was equivalent to six days' wages.[24] Other studies have demonstrated that the social stigma associated with the disease is an obstacle to its treatment, and that DOT may aggravate this stigma.[25] Further trials are thus clearly needed in order to assess the efficacy of interventions incorporated in TB control programmes, their cost-effectiveness and their acceptability to the patients and the health staff in different settings.

During the first five years of its promotion by WHO and uptake by national governments, DOTS did not enjoy the success anticipated. While more and more governments adopted the policy, epidemiological analysis reported in 2000 indicated that control was still far from their grasp.[26] Part of this failure can be attributed to the fact that the strategy does not take into consideration the importance of social support in facilitating access and adherence to treatment. It is telling that in one of the model DOTS programmes, the New York City programme of the early 1990s, it was not the biomedical intervention alone that enabled success, but the fact that

> [DOT] was part of an individualized patient treatment plan that also provided accessible services, a reliable source of medication, treatment in a variety of settings, social services, and an integrated system of follow-up. . . . Such an array of services provides an operational definition of *compassion* in health care and shows how supervised therapy can be used as a *positive* rather than a punitive intervention for patients. It will be important to identify the most effective set of comprehensive services that contribute to a successful DOT programme.[27]

Despite the recognition of these enabling factors, however, they were not subsequently included in the international guidelines, leaving policy makers at national level without directions to include these important inputs in their programmes.

The promotion of a universal strategy is thus challenged on operational, epidemiological, economic and sociological grounds. The question posed is whether TB control should remain a biomedical intervention only, focusing on treatment, without efforts to understand and fulfil patients' needs. Volmink and colleagues, conducting a systematic review of published reports on direct observation for TB control, conclude that 'health care delivery oriented towards the needs and preferences of patients seems to lead to more satisfied patients'.[28] They thus point the way to a shift in perspective: considering the well-being of TB patients, taking account of their social and economic environment as well as the presence of TB infection. There is evidence that this shift is now taking place in the international policy arena. In response to critiques of DOTS, and to the 'slow progress of DOTS implementation in countries with a high burden of TB', the strategy is currently being revised and expanded by the WHO. In its new form DOTS is being promoted as 'a comprehensive and multi-sectoral approach'.[29] In support of this effort, and to enable policy makers and programmers to identify ways to develop such an approach, there is a need for more contextualized knowledge about TB treatment and care.

Assessing the patient's perspective in TB control: the qualitative approach

The principle underlying the qualitative approach to infectious diseases is this: because lay people manage and make sense of illness in the context of everyday life, infectious disease interventions must also 'make sense' to people in those terms.[30] While for some aspects of infectious disease control a biomedical focus and orientation may be appropriate, interventions against diseases that require long-term treatment and care, and that have far-reaching social implications, need to take fuller account of social context in their inception and delivery. If patients are being relied on to break the cycle of transmission and to complete a full six-month course of anti-TB treatment, they need programmes that enable them to carry this mandate out.

The various aspects of real life that face patients when trying to get well are influenced by social structures within the household, the community and the wider political economy. These structures will affect the extent to which, and at what point in time, the ill person can adopt the sick role, the range of treatment options available to him or her in seeking care for symptoms, and the extent to which the patient is able to obtain, maintain and complete treatment. These are aspects to which research and policy can respond. The objective of qualitative research is to render people's responses to disease intelligible.[31] If we understand existing structures and responses to ill health we can build on these rather than creating new ones, which may or may not make sense locally. Because the 'all-at-onceness' of social context can make it difficult to grasp in applied research, it is important to identify and map those domains of particular relevance to the problem in question.

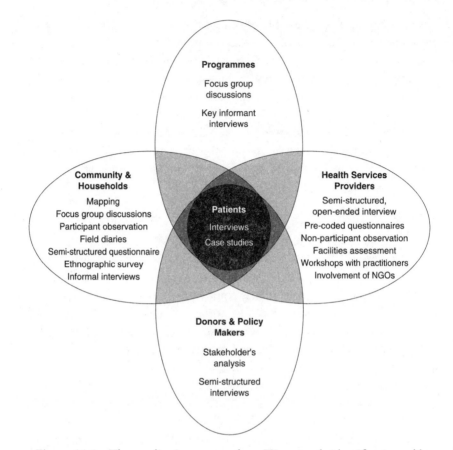

Programmes

Focus group
discussions

Key informant
interviews

**Community &
Households**

Mapping
Focus group discussions
Participant observation
Field diaries
Semi-structured questionnaire
Ethnographic survey
Informal interviews

Patients

Interviews
Case studies

**Health Services
Providers**

Semi-structured,
open-ended interview

Pre-coded questionnaires
Non-participant observation
Facilities assessment
Workshops with practitioners
Involvement of NGOs

**Donors & Policy
Makers**

Stakeholder's
analysis

Semi-structured
interviews

Figure 11.1   The qualitative approach to TB control: identification of key
domains for investigation of adherence to treatment.

A central aspect of this effort is to see what structures of care and
support exist for patients, what structures are missing (and for whom),
and how the programme or health services, maybe in alliance with
other social services, can fill this gap.

The conceptual model developed to illustrate this approach is reproduced as Figure 11.1.[32] This model places the patient at the centre of
four overlapping domains: the community, the health services, the TB
programme and the policy environment. Using a combination of
qualitative and quantitative methods, research can be carried out in
each of these domains in order to understand how the TB patient
experiences this particular illness and how this experience is influenced
by the household and community in which that individual lives. A

patient's choices will be framed and constrained, not only by the physiological impact of the disease but also, and crucially, by the way that person and that disease fit into broader social and cultural structures. Of equal importance is to bring in issues relating to provision of care and support within the health and social services: it is important to understand the range of services available, how they are used and why. Widening the scope still further, these services are themselves resourced and constrained by features in the national and international policy landscape, which may also need to be addressed. This approach has been used in various studies intending to evaluate the relationship between the TB control programme, the general health services, the patient and the community in order to improve access to care and delivery of services.

One such interdisciplinary study is currently under way in West Africa, where five local countries have brought together TB control programme supervisors, medical and social scientists, with the aim of improving TB control policies and practice across the region. After investigating the magnitude of the TB problem and the means to control it in each country, the West African TB Research Initiative intends to explore the perception of the disease and its treatment by all persons concerned: information is sought from key players in the TB control programmes, policy makers and donors as well as the health staff providing treatment, the patients and the community members. On the basis of these findings, the project will develop and test innovative methods to improve case detection and patient adherence.

This type of operational research is an example of how social sciences can be usefully called upon to collaborate with medical sciences, in an effort to improve the treatment and care of people with TB, and the control of the disease in the population. While the strength of the medical approach is in its ability to identify and deliver appropriate drugs for TB treatment, the social science approach outlined here, by investigating and taking account of the key domains of social context relevant to TB care, can enable TB control programmes to develop the most appropriate means of ensuring these drugs get to the people who need them in a timely and appropriate manner. This is a type of partnership that can result in new developments in research and the design of new solutions for disease control.

Prospects for improvement

So long as we consider TB control as a biomedical intervention only, focusing on achieving cure by trying to control patient drug intake, we will be bound to fail. The qualitative approach aims to understand the complex relationship between socio-economic forces and TB infection/ disease, so as to bridge the gap between the individual (as the recipient of care) and society (as a group of individuals deserving well-being) by investigating each level and understanding their interactions.

We have seen above how important it is that health care services ask, 'How can we best enable patients to get well?' and not, 'How can we best control the drug intake of patients?' Results of trials conducted so far question whether, in areas where cure rates are still low, a change to self-administered treatment once a week instead of directly observed therapy three times a week would have a marked impact on cure rates. Studies examining the health care choices of TB patients and reasons for leaving treatment are clearly needed, in order to identify which factors contribute to the success or the failure of treatment in given populations, whatever method is used. Further intervention trials are also needed comparing different approaches for delivery of treatment in various populations. Innovative strategies for TB prevention and treatment must also be developed. Although new areas are being explored to develop new vaccines and improve BCG, there is an urgent need to design new interventions against TB, integrating epidemiological and qualitative approaches.[33] Better understanding of the pathways through which socioeconomic background is associated with specific situations of risk will help in designing new interventions aimed at modifying the environment, so as to minimize the risk of disease at both individual and population level. While waiting for the new vaccines and shorter drug regimens to be developed and tested, the interdisciplinary approach represents a way forward to improve TB control through better prevention and care adapted to local situations and centred on the TB patients and the community.[34]

12

Reflections on the Role of Science in Tuberculosis Control

T. Mark Doherty, Martin E. Munk
and Peter Andersen

The history of scientific attempts to control tuberculosis is very nearly a history of scientific efforts to control infectious disease in general. The identification, over a century ago, of the causative agent of TB was greeted with great rejoicing, as it was assumed that the rapidly evolving microbiology of the time would soon provide a cure. Robert Koch (the discoverer of *Mycobacterium tuberculosis*) and Louis Pasteur, two of the contemporary giants of microbiology, devoted much effort to this cause, and although their efforts were ultimately unsuccessful, their work did lay the foundation of research on TB control. Koch attempted to make a vaccine using a sterile filtrate (tuberculin) from cultures of *M. tuberculin* but this was unsuccessful. Not only did it fail to provide good protection against the virulent organism, but the doubled-edged nature of inflammatory immune responses was revealed by the adverse reactions some recipients experienced. Later known as the Koch phenomenon, this necrotic (tissue-killing) reaction appears to be due to overproduction of the pro-inflammatory cytokine Tumor Necrosis Factor (TNF-α).[1] The failure of tuberculin led Koch to pronounce that only a living vaccine could be efficacious against TB, a doctrine that went largely unchallenged for many decades. Ironically, tuberculin – more carefully administered – became the basis of the first diagnostic reagent for TB, the tuberculin skin test (TST). The skin test has been used for diagnosis of TB for decades, even though its low specificity has restricted it largely to Western settings, where exposure to myco-bacterial other than *M. tuberculosis* infection is uncommon.

Meanwhile, Pasteur's 'principles of attenuation' were enthusiastically put to work by his colleagues.[2] A strain of mycobacteria isolated from the milk of a cow with mastitis was used by Albert Calmette and Camille Guérin of the Pasteur Institute in Lille as a subject for attenuation. It is unknown why this strain was chosen. It may have been because Koch had espoused the opinion that bovine TB was relatively benign in humans, or because of the prevalent belief that consumption of milk from cows with tuberculous mastitis offered some protection from TB. Whatever the reason, this strain of bacteria (Bacillus Calmette Guérin, or BCG) was grown in glass flasks for thirteen years, and continuously tested for reduced virulence in animals. It was soon found that the original bacterium was far from benign *in vivo*, and the degree and stability of the reduction in virulence was a subject for debate for many years. It is still unclear whether the original isolate (now lost) was in fact *M. bovis* or a closely related strain,[3] and there is evidence to suggest that the original vaccine (maintained for approximately a decade after its introduction as three parallel lines all grown from the original isolate) was not entirely homogenous. There is evidence to suggest that the original vaccine may have contained a minority population which was more virulent and that necrotic lesions at the site of subcutaneous vaccination (which are now rare) were more common in the early decades of BCG vaccination.[4]

Despite these concerns, in 1921, the BCG vaccine was administered orally to infants considered at high risk of developing TB, where it proved a resounding success, reducing mortality in vaccinated children by approximately 90 per cent. After testing by various national authorities, the BCG vaccine strain was distributed to various institutions around the globe to establish daughter lines or strains, rapidly becoming one of the most widely used of all vaccines. The administration of BCG increased drastically after the Second World War, and hundreds of millions of people are known to have been immunized with this vaccine.[5] It is known that the vaccine is very safe and the risk of sequelae (side-effects occurring subsequent to the vaccination, such as widespread inflammation) is extremely low, although BCG vaccination can lead to adverse effects at the vaccination site, such as regional suppurative adenitis.[6] However, it is slightly misleading to refer to BCG as a single vaccine. While the loss of the parent strain prevents us from knowing exactly which genes were deleted during the initial period of *in vitro* attenuation, the dissemination of the bacteria to different laboratories at well-defined time points has confirmed that the bacteria continued to lose genes during its initial years of culture, and that it may initially have been much more virulent.[7] The significance of this finding, and its relationship to the current problems with the BCG vaccine, can only be speculative at this point. However, BCG has been a controversial vaccine since its very inception, and the reason this has remained the case may reflect, in part, the changing nature of the vaccine itself over time.

BCG: a controversial past, a contentious present

Despite the widespread use of BCG vaccination, the incidence of TB remained unacceptably high worldwide, and the vaccine's effectiveness was closely studied. Various studies in different locales and populations have found that the efficacy of BCG varies remarkably.[8] The immuno-logical mechanisms, induced by the vaccine, which control infection are still poorly understood. While the BCG vaccine prevents death from disseminated infection in children by impairing the spread of infectious organisms in the blood, it shows less effect against pulmo-nary TB in adults. A trial in the UK demonstrated that the incidence of TB fifteen years after BCG vaccination was equivalent in both vacci-nated and unvaccinated donors.[9] Thus, the protection induced by BCG appears to wane with time. It has been suggested that the practice in developing countries of giving BCG vaccination at birth (which pre-vents most childhood deaths) may account for its limited impact on the development of pulmonary disease in adults. This is consistent with recent research which has shown that, over long periods of time, not even natural infection with *M. tuberculosis* confers full protection against later reinfection.[10] Moreover, BCG efficacy studies are based on protection against primary infection and (endogenous) reactivation of existing TB infection, but not against exogenous reinfection, which further complicates estimation of the true level of protection induced by vaccination. Many reasons have been suggested for the variability in efficacy of BCG vaccination, involving both vaccine- and host-related factors, although no single hypothesis has proved entirely satisfactory, and the major hypotheses are discussed below.

Why has BCG failed in some instances – but not in others?

Hypothesis One: BCG itself has altered from its earlier (successful) incarnations

As described above, BCG strains have been grown in many laboratories under different conditions leading to variations in bacterial morphology, antigen expression or viability.[11] In addition, the different methods used for homogenization and storage of bacilli by vaccine producers may play an important role in controlling microbial dispersion, viability and infectivity of the vaccine itself. The potency of BCG vaccination depends on the proliferation of organisms after the vaccine is given, and different preparations can show great variability in the amount of viable bacilli (thus altering the effective dose). Viability may decline even further in freeze-dried batches not correctly prepared, stored or administered.[12] However, attempts to correlate BCG efficacy with microbial characteristics of the vaccine in animal protection studies have not yet provided convincing evidence that this explains the variation seen in human trials. Initially, the BCG vaccine was administered orally. Due to fears of possibly killing the vaccine in the acid environment of the stomach, and difficulty in quantifying the dose, the route of administration was soon changed to the skin, either by needle, multiple-puncture or jet injection. However, no specific comparison of protection induced by these two routes of administration was ever made, and therefore evidence that this change affected the later course of vaccination is still lacking.

Hypothesis Two: the recipients of successful vaccinations are in some way different from those who were not protected

It is a well-known observation that malnutrition can have a deleterious effect on that part of the immune system responsible for protection against TB.[13] About 95 per cent of all TB cases occur in the poorest countries, such as in sub-Saharan Africa and Southeast Asia, where malnourishment is common; even in the developed world, TB is primarily associated with the most deprived strata of society. Experiments show that guinea pigs (which are highly susceptible to TB) can be effectively protected by BCG vaccination, while animals placed on a diet low in protein and Vitamin D become to some extent immuno-compromised, leading to greatly decreased protective efficacy of sub-sequent BCG vaccination.[14] The implications of this are clear, although no direct evidence exists that responses to BCG are in fact compro-mised in malnourished humans.

It is something of a truism that different people respond to disease differently. More and more of the underlying genes that affect immune responses to TB are now being identified. In mouse experiments, a gene involved in the delivery of toxic molecules inside the cells where the bacteria such as *M. tuberculosis* persist was discovered and the human homologue was soon also identified.[15] Other genes apparently affecting susceptibility to TB continue to be found.[16] However, while a role for genetic factors has been demonstrated,[17] the relatively subtle effects so far described do not appear to explain the enormous variation in BCG vaccine efficacy.

Hypothesis Three: The disease has changed

The virulence of *M. tuberculosis* isolates varies and this has also been suggested as a reason for variation in BCG efficacy. However, BCG has been shown to have similar protective efficacy in guinea pigs challenged with either high- or low-virulence strains of *M. tuberculo-sis*,[18] indicating that this hypothesis is unlikely. However, in the absence of definitive molecular studies in human populations, such an effect cannot be completely ruled out.

Immunity to TB

M. tuberculosis persists inside host cells, and consequently components of the bacilli are potentially always present to stimulate the host's immune response. If a protective immune response is triggered, the infected host cells are capable of killing the pathogen. But what is a protective immune response? Any immune response comprises the activity of a large variety of highly specialized cell populations, which play very different roles in protection against infection. A paradigm shift over the last fifteen years has been the realization that most immune responses fall into two very broad categories often referred to as Type 1 and Type 2. Type 1 immunity involves the activation of inflammatory pathways. This can lead to fever, tissue damage (typically bleeding, swelling, etc.) or (in extreme cases) even death in the infected individual. This kind of immune response is most appropriate to infections such as viruses or bacteria like M. *tuberculosis* that invade host cells. Type 2 immune responses are generally directed against pathogens that live part of their life cycle outside host cells, such as helminths (worms). While these responses can also lead to inflammation, generally it is milder for the host.[19]

Most crucially, however, these two types of immune response are mutually antagonistic – a strong response of one type decreases the ability to make the other. It is known, from both animal studies and analysis of genetic deficiencies in patients, that the Type 1 immune response is crucial for protection against TB, while a Type 2 response may have the opposite effect. It has thus been suggested that other infections may decrease the protection from BCG vaccination, or increase susceptibility to TB. Helminthic infections, which are widespread in many developing countries, are excellent inducers of Type 2 responses and may therefore decrease the effectiveness of BCG vaccination (which aims to induce a Type 1 response) or the immune response against M. *tuberculosis* infection (which relies on a Type 1 response).[20]

Even if the immune response evoked is not antagonistic, it could still interfere with vaccination. Many atypical mycobacteria, which do not normally cause human disease, are common in water and soil (the so-called non-tuberculous mycobacteria). While not closely related to M. *tuberculosis* or BCG, the non-tuberculous mycobacteria can none the less induce some similar immune responses, suggesting that they could interfere with the ability of BCG to survive in the recipient long enough to induce protective immunity. A strong correlation between the degree of protection induced by BCG and the latitude where the vaccinations were carried out has led to the suggestion that local soil and water bacteria might affect immune responses in populations exposed to them.[21] Of course, exposure to soil and untreated water is greater precisely in those countries where the incidence of TB is also high. In support of this idea, infection of experimental animals with atypical mycobacteria can induce cross-reactive immune responses which decrease the relative efficacy of later BCG vaccination and restrict the *in vivo* growth of the vaccine strain.[22]

Prospects for tuberculosis diagnosis and control

In many fields of medicine, there has always been a competition for resources between field workers who see the utility of simple approaches to help control disease spread and those developing new treatments, which promise to cure it completely. However, this dynamic is less evident in TB, because of the nature of the disease. Since casual contact – even for a few minutes – can potentially transmit TB, useful behavioural modifications to limit the spread of TB are very restricted. Moreover, since infection may not be obvious for years, tracing and treating the original source of infection can be very difficult, particularly since someone can be infected (and infectious) for some time without realizing it. One of the major factors influencing the spread of TB is population density, a factor that cannot easily be controlled. Therefore, the mainstays of TB control for the past half-century have been vaccination and chemotherapy. While the cause or causes of BCG failure continue to be debated, research directed towards the control of TB is proceeding along two paths: improving diagnosis and chemotherapy, and the development of new, more reliable vaccines.

In the developed world, TB remains relatively infrequent and management of disease by identifying infected individuals, contact tracing and providing chemotherapy has proved to be a cost-efficient approach. While few new drugs active against TB have reached the market in recent decades, current chemotherapy regimes have remained largely efficacious.[23] This is fortunate since the cost of developing new drugs is enormous and not particularly attractive to pharmaceutical companies, given that most potential customers live in the least economically developed populations in the world. This is changing, however, as private–public partnerships and new technology are beginning to lift the profile and decrease the cost of developing new drugs.

Recommended chemotherapy regimens normally include three or four different drugs to ensure that even drug-resistant strains of TB can be successfully treated. However, a growing concern is the gradual increase in multi-drug-resistant TB strains, which can tolerate many of the common TB drugs and which are therefore very difficult to manage. Even where drugs can be found that are effective, these are often newer, more expensive drugs. The mainstays of current chemotherapy are older drugs, which are now off-patent, greatly reducing their cost. This means that the costs of treatment of MDR-TB strains can be as much as 100 times greater than that of susceptible strains. MDR-TB strains are becoming most common in areas where chemotherapy has been poorly implemented (such as countries of the former Soviet Union) and pose a sufficient threat that ensuring better use of the drugs we have available has become a top priority.

Moreover, increases in both ease of travel and in population movement, whether by refugees or migrants, spreads both normal and MDR-TB, in particular because of the difficulty in detecting the early stages of the disease. Improved diagnosis has therefore also become a priority. Currently, diagnosis relies on the detection of M. *tuberculosis* bacilli in the sputum of infected individuals, directly or by molecular biological methods such as polymerase chain reaction (PCR) testing. However direct examination of sputum by microscopy is difficult and while culture of sputum is more reliable, it can take up to two months to get a result, and neither method is foolproof.[24] PCR of sputum for microbial DNA is sensitive and rapid,[25] and may soon largely replace microscopy in the developed world, but it is expensive and technically demanding. Moreover, all three techniques are limited to detection of active TB where bacteria are present in sputum (by which time the patient is already infectious) and are thus unsuitable for the detection of latent or early disease.

These techniques have therefore been supported by the venerable skin test. This relies on the fact that people previously exposed to mycobacteria will make a measurable immune response to mycobacterial antigens injected under the skin. This kind of immunodiagnosis has the advantage that it can (in theory) detect infection before it reaches the state of overt disease, and is relatively simple to perform, making it ideal for screening. Unfortunately, the only reagent currently available, Purified Protein Derivative (PPD), was derived from Koch's tuberculin and has not been improved in half a century. It is a poorly defined mixture of proteins precipitated from heat-killed cultures of M. *tuberculosis*, many of which are shared with other species of mycobacteria. Individuals sensitized by prior exposure to non-tuberculous mycobacteria, or vaccinated with BCG (both common in developing countries), often respond to PPD as strongly or even more strongly than individuals infected with M. *tuberculosis*. The goal of current research is therefore a more specific test.

While many proteins derived from M. *tuberculosis* are shared with non-tuberculous mycobacteria, it has long been known that others are largely restricted to M. *tuberculosis* or its near relatives. It is recognized that these antigens are the key to genuinely specific immunodiagnosis.[26] Initial attempts to isolate such antigens from complex mixtures of mycobacterial proteins using conventional purification methods met with only limited success.[27] However, identification of targets for immunodiagnosis is advancing dramatically as molecular biology reveals the genomes of different mycobacteria.[28] Comparisons of the genome of BCG with its supposed parent strain M. *bovis* identified stretches of genetic material that were deleted during its long period of *in vitro* attenuation.[29] Today, nearly 100 genes are known that have been deleted in some or all strains of BCG but that are present in disease-causing mycobacteria.[30] While immune responses to any protein encoded by such a gene could in theory discriminate between BCG vaccination and infection with M. *tuberculosis*, a useful immunodiagnostic agent also needs to be strongly immunogenic and not cross-reactive to unrelated proteins.

These are fairly stringent requirements, but several proteins have already been discovered that fulfil them. In particular, two proteins designated ESAT-6 and CFP-10 have shown potential for the immunodiagnosis of M. *tuberculosis* infection. Both are strongly immunogenic in M. *tuberculosis*-infected animals, and the genes are essentially restricted to the TB-causing mycobacteria, being absent in all strains of BCG as well as in most environmental species.[31] Neither of them are recognized by the immune systems of animals successfully vaccinated against TB, or sensitized by environmental exposure.[32] Finally, ESAT-6 has been reported to be strongly recognized by cells from human TB patients and a significant proportion of their contacts, who appear to be subclinically infected, but not by BCG-vaccinated donors or patients with other infections.[33] Tests of these (and other newly identified molecules from the deleted regions of the BCG genome) are continuing and will progress to clinical trials in the very near future. The use of such genuinely specific immunodiagnostic reagents promises to improve greatly our ability to identify and treat TB-infected individuals. Moreover, by identifying infected individuals earlier than is possible with current methods, effective immunodiagnosis may decrease the number of new infections arising from each TB case.

The future of vaccination

While diagnosis may improve management of TB in the developed world, the fact remains that the vast majority of TB cases are found in countries without the budgets or infrastructure for large-scale screening and chemotherapy. Moreover, the slow increase in MDR TB means that even in the developed world, screening and chemotherapy can only ever be a partial answer. To make lasting progress against a disease as widespread as TB, a vaccine is the only realistic solution. Although there is little doubt that BCG has failed to halt the TB epidemic, there is also a consensus that in some cases it has beneficial effects, particularly against childhood TB and leprosy, meaning its use will continue for the foreseeable future.[34]

It is known from animal studies and human disease that the so-called Type 1 immune response is essential for protection against TB. A Type 1 immune response is characterized by large numbers of CD4 cells (a kind of immune cell which responds quickly to a pathogen the body has encountered before) that produce Interferon-gamma (called IFN-g for short, it is a molecule which activates other immune cells to kill foreign organisms). A Type 1 immune response therefore quickly generates an inflammation that can cause fever or organ damage if it is too strong but which is necessary to kill *M. tuberculosis*.[35] Stimulation of this response has therefore been a major goal of vaccine development. However, there is growing agreement that this picture is something of a simplification, particularly with regard to long-term control of infection. While emphasis remains on stimulating strong Type 1 responses, vaccine researchers are therefore beginning to look at augmenting this by stimulating other immune functions as well.[36] The various vaccine strategies are discussed in detail below.

Whole-cell and live vaccines: making a better BCG

There is evidence that current BCG vaccine strains differ significantly from those originally derived. It is possible that the immunogenicity and/or virulence of BCG has been further reduced during this time.[37] Some researchers have therefore attempted to augment BCG by adding human genes to the bacteria that promote the development of the Type 1 immune response.[38] Another approach has been the identification of strongly immunogenic proteins that are lacking in BCG and the use of genetic engineering to add these back to BCG. Reintroduction of genes from the deleted regions into BCG may lead to a more effective vaccine. However, it is possible that these genes may also contribute to the virulence of the parent strain, effectively reversing the attenuation process. Thus, to determine exactly what genes lead to the desired effects will take a great deal of work, and extended safety testing of such a vaccine will be required to ensure that the introduction of genes from virulent mycobacteria does not lead to a reversion to virulence in BCG.

To address these concerns, some researchers have approached this problem from the opposite direction. Instead of attempting to undo some of the attenuation of BCG, they hope to attenuate M. tuberculosis or M. bovis, on the grounds that this would be the closest mimic of a natural infection. Mutant strains with reduced virulence have already been produced and have been shown to induce significant levels of protection against virulent M. tuberculosis in animal models.[39] At the same time, these mutants have proved to be safe even in completely immunodeficient mice, suggesting that they could be given safely to HIV-positive individuals.[40] This last point is important, given the high incidence of HIV in countries with the most severe TB epidemics.[41]

M. tuberculosis, M. bovis and BCG are not the only species being considered for live or whole-cell vaccines. The interesting observation that BCG vaccination appears to reduce the incidence of leprosy (caused by the distantly related M. leprae) suggests that priming the immune system against common mycobacterial antigens can also provide protection against M. tuberculosis.[42] This hypothesis is supported by studies in animals.[43] Other mycobacterial species – in particular M. vaccae – have been tested as vaccines in humans. Live vaccines have the advantages of being cheap to produce and simple to manufacture. However, the same problems of sensitization or risk of severe infection in immunocompromised individuals that apply to BCG could also affect these vaccines. To circumvent these problems, 'booster' or therapeutic vaccines employing high doses of heat-killed bacteria have been tried. While results so far have been disappointing, further trials continue.[44]

Other infective agents, such as recombinant vaccinia virus or Salmonella enterica which have the advantage of being more tractable for genetic manipulation, have also been employed.[45] Both invade host cells like *M. tuberculosis*, but do not establish chronic infections or cause significant disease. Recombinant vaccinia viruses producing different mycobacterial antigens have already been shown to induce protection against experimental infection in animals.

Protein vaccines: the minimalist approach

Koch's opinion was so respected that his assertion that only living vaccines could be efficacious against *M. tuberculosis* influenced vaccine development for almost a century. This was despite evidence that with the proper adjuvants, fractions derived from killed mycobacteria could both prolong survival and reduce infection in infected animals.[46] This work was not followed up, at least partially because of the strong inflammatory responses invoked in some recipients – the same immune response that had alarmed detractors of the early BCG vaccine. More important, these vaccines were believed to evoke predominantly short-lived immune responses.[47] However, the demonstration that purified, soluble proteins derived from *M. tuberculosis* could also induce long-lived protective immune responses revived interest in non-living vaccines.[48] Such vaccines have the advantage of being clearly defined so that they may be subject to rigid quality control and are safe even in immunodeficient recipients. They also appear to be unaffected by presensitization to other mycobacterial strains.

Initial experiments in this field were carried out with material derived from live bacteria, based on the assumption that antigens produced by actively metabolizing bacteria might account for the demonstrated efficacy of live vaccines.[49] However, we now know that with the correct route of delivery and correct choice of adjuvant, many proteins derived from *M. tuberculosis* can also induce protective immunity. Of all the TB vaccines currently under development, protein vaccines are the closest to initial testing in humans.

New adjuvants

It is known that early events can determine the subsequent development of the immune response, and in some cases, the ultimate outcome of infection. Much attention has therefore been devoted to exploring the circumstances under which the immune system first recognizes antigens, and how this response can be manipulated. The ability (or inability) of different adjuvants to prime the immune system for an effective response to M. *tuberculosis* infection has been well demonstrated.[50] While the data caution against a simplistic correlation of magnitude of the immune response induced, with the degree of protection subsequently achieved, none the less it appears to be true that in order to prime an effective immune response against M. *tuberculosis*, a strong Type 1 response is required. In light of this, it is disappointing that the only adjuvant currently approved for use in humans (Alum) generally promotes Type 2 immune responses.[51] As noted above, these do not appear to help towards immunity against TB and may even retard the development of a protective Type 1 immune response. Thus, a number of new adjuvants designed to promote immunity are currently being tested, which aim to enhance Type 1 immune responses. The promise of better delivery systems is exemplified by the recent demonstration in animals that a novel adjuvant could convert a non-protective vaccination into one giving very high levels of protection while at the same time being potentially suitable for use in humans.[52] The implication of these new technologies reaches beyond TB to vaccination in general.

DNA vaccines: a novel approach

All the new vaccine projects discussed above use more advanced technology, but tried and tested concepts. Recently, however, a novel approach has been suggested which holds significant promise. This is the direct delivery of DNA encoding the gene(s) of interest – the so-called 'naked DNA' approach. DNA delivered in this fashion is taken up by the recipient's cells and the proteins(s) it codes for are expressed. This is thought partially to mimic the release of antigens from an infected cell, and has been shown to work successfully in a number of animal models, including TB infection.[53] Moreover, DNA vaccination may stimulate a broader range of immune cells than conventional protein vaccination.[54] Perhaps most intriguing is a recent report that multiple DNA vaccinations using DNA carrying a single mycobacterial gene could prevent reactivation of latent disease in already infected mice. This suggests that appropriate vaccination may offer some benefit to the millions of people who are already infected.[55]

Moving research out of the laboratory

There are, then, multiple paths to a potential new vaccine against TB, and each of these is being vigorously pursued, driven by the awareness that a broadly effective vaccine is urgently needed. There is a growing willingness among both academic and industrial research groups to test promising vaccine candidates against each other, with the goal of settling on the best possible candidate for human trials as soon as possible. This approach has been encouraged by the most influential funding sources. There is also a new emphasis (by both the US government and the European Commission) on the large, cross-disciplinary coalitions needed to conduct large-scale human trials. That the description of TB control as a priority is not mere oratory is shown by the significant increase in annual funds available for TB research and control programmes. This new commitment from the industrialized countries has been matched by efforts in endemic countries where the acceptance of TB as a disease of poverty has been accompanied by a new emphasis on TB as a disease that *causes* poverty, both by striking primarily at young adults and by the consumption of vitally needed national resources in the effort to control it.

The mood in TB research today is more optimistic than at any time since the introduction of effective chemotherapy fifty years ago (though guardedly so, given previous failures to contain TB). It is clear that new tools for TB control will shortly become available, and plans are being made to test them where it matters – in the field – as soon as possible. However, there are still obstacles to be overcome before this can be achieved. Primary to this is a better understanding of why BCG – which functions so well in the laboratory – has not stemmed the TB epidemic in real life. To address this, new animal models that more closely parallel real-life conditions such as latent disease and reactivation, sensitization or post-infection vaccination, have become a priority.[56] The breadth of research has increased also, with detailed examination of the interplay of multiple factors such as the generation of pathology, immune responses and long-term survival after infection.[57] More detailed analysis of these factors may shed light on the still-unresolved question of what a new vaccine should be to contain TB successfully.

Answering this question will be key to the deployment of new vaccines. Any new candidate vaccine would have to provide enormously compelling data before it could be considered as a substitute for BCG. Despite the fact that BCG vaccination has not controlled the TB epidemic, the evidence is good that it has significant beneficial effects. Thus, it is difficult to suggest that it should be withdrawn until we have convincing evidence that any proposed replacement could at least meet the same standard. This means that the most likely scenario – at least in the near future – is that a new vaccine would be used after or together with BCG vaccination.

In addition, the design of vaccine trials in humans is undergoing further consideration. Typically, TB vaccine trials have enrolled huge numbers of people to ensure adequate data, given the rate of the disease in the population as a whole and the extended period during which an infected individual may progress to disease. Other options now being considered are the identification of high-risk groups for smaller vaccine trials. Such individuals have the greatest need for vaccination, while at the same time providing clinically relevant data over a shorter time period. The development of improved diagnostics is relevant in this regard, as it may allow testing in the field, with correspondingly faster assessment of rates of transmission. The rapid progress of TB research in multiple fields – genetics, immunology, molecular biology, protein chemistry and clinical sciences – combined with increased dialogue between these fields, ensures that new vaccine candidates will be introduced and tested in the next few years.

13

Global Poverty and Tuberculosis: Implications for Ethics and Human Rights

Solomon R. Benatar

The magnitude of the problem of tuberculosis in the world presents a paradox that provides insights into the gap between scientific knowledge and its effective application for the promotion of health and human well being. This paradox also serves to remind us that while scientific progress is necessary in the quest for improving health, such knowledge is not sufficient in itself. Deficiencies in our ability to apply knowledge effectively make it clear that new ways of thinking about health and disease are required to promote the use of scientific knowledge to achieve improved global health in the future.[1]

Since Robert Koch discovered the causative organism *Mycobacterium tuberculosis* in 1882, spectacular scientific advances have been made in our understanding of TB and in our ability to treat effectively and cure any individual patient. These advances include major insights into the basic pathobiological processes associated with TB infection and progression to disease, the development of new diagnostic tests and many effective drugs, the evaluation of different drug combinations in a series of well-designed trials, and the implementation of highly cost-effective treatment regimes. These advances gave rise to optimism in the 1970s that it might be possible to eradicate TB from the world.

Sadly this noble aspiration has not been achieved. Indeed quite the opposite has come about. TB is on the increase globally and, as a result of inadequate treatment programmes, multi-drug-resistant TB, for which few new drugs are being developed, is emerging. The cost of treating a single patient with MDR-TB can be up to one hundred times as much as is required to treat a patient with a drug-sensitive organism, and treatment is thus becoming unaffordable in many parts of the world. In the United States, Europe and Latin America, highly resistant strains of *Mycobacterium tuberculosis* have caused numerous explosive institutional outbreaks (in hospitals, prisons and shelters), with high case-fatality rates in immunosuppressed patients and high rates of transmission to immunocompetent caregivers.[2] The World Health Organisation/International Union Against Tuberculosis and Lung Diseases (WHO/IUATLD) global survey of resistance to anti-TB drugs reveals that MDR-TB has become established in almost all participating countries.[3] Prisons in Russia have been described as the 'epicentre of a world-wide epidemic of multidrug resistance'.[4]

This paradox between the extent of our scientific knowledge and the spectre of TB becoming untreatable in the future is frightening – not only in relation to the treatment of TB but also with regard to treatment of other infectious diseases such as HIV/AIDS. The customary explanation given for the failure to achieve global control of TB is the existence of poverty. It is also conventional to express poverty in terms of insufficient economic resources in developing countries to implement effective TB treatment programmes. This is indeed true in part, but the real explanation is much more complex, extending to considerations of the less obvious causes of economic poverty in many developing countries and to other, even more serious, forms of 'non-economic poverty' that afflict privileged societies.

Poverty and health

Poverty means being deficient and deprived materially, socially and emotionally. It includes lack of economic resources, lack of education, lack of access to basic life resources such as food, water and sanitation, and lack of control over one's life and reproductive company. Absolute poverty is defined as a condition of life severely limited by malnutrition, illiteracy, disease, squalid surroundings, high infant mortality and low life expectancy. Poverty brings not only material disadvantage but also social exclusion, which in turn is associated with discrimination across a wide range of social activities that adversely affect health and well-being.[5]

Relative and absolute poverty have been constant characteristics of the human condition. With rapid increases in the wealth of the elite in the past fifty years, relative poverty has become more pronounced. At the beginning of the twentieth century the wealthiest 20 per cent of the world's population were nine times richer than the poorest 20 per cent. This ratio has grown progressively – to thirty times by 1960, sixty times by 1990 and to over eighty times by 1995. One billion people live well, some in great luxury, and three billion live in poverty.

Absolute poverty remains a problem and its extent has increased. The number of extremely poor people in the world more than doubled between 1975 and 1995. Over half of the world's population live on less than $900 a year, and more than a quarter of the world's population live (on less than $1 a day) under conditions of absolute poverty. Of the 4.4 billion people in developing countries, over half lack access to sanitation, over 30 per cent lack access to clean water and essential drugs, and almost a quarter are inadequately nourished.[6]

World debt grew from $0.5 million million in 1980 to $1.9 million million in 1994 and to over $2.2 million million by 1997. The 'debt trade' has been a major factor in perpetuating and intensifying poverty and ill health. Most countries that were forced by the World Bank to pursue structural adjustment programmes during the second half of the twentieth century are in greater debt than ever before. Cuts and underfinancing of public health spending associated with such structural adjustment programmes have led to severe deterioration in health-care delivery systems, especially in Africa. The whole public health agenda (information surveillance, epidemiology, research and behavioural surveillance) has been reduced to a skeleton while the World Bank has continuously promoted cost-recovery for health care. As a result HIV testing, condoms, treatment for sexually transmitted diseases, antituberculosis therapy, and treatments for co-infections of HIV are subject to user charges and therefore unaffordable to many. In Zambia, with an HIV prevalence of over 19 per cent, half the children are now malnourished, a state which reduces resistance to all diseases. Structural adjustment programmes, debt repayments, cuts in aid budgets (especially by the USA), discrimination against African trade, increasing malnutrition and the legacy of the Cold War have all played a significant part in fanning the AIDS pandemic.[7]

Third World debt, although accounting for a small proportion of total world debt, has reached obscene levels in relation to income levels in the Third World and is unpayable. The ways in which such debt has been created and its relationship to the arms trade are indictments against so-called developed nations.[8] It is now abundantly clear that debt relief is an essential first step in the process of achieving improvements in health at a global level. In making a case for debt relief for poor countries, it is reasonable to point out that the extraordinarily high consumption patterns of industrialized nations make these rich nations deeply indebted to us all, and especially to those living in poverty.[9]

Globalization and poverty

The term 'globalization' refers to a process of global integration in which diverse peoples, economies and political processes are increasingly subject to international influences. It is both a complex and an ambiguous concept with social, cultural and economic dimensions. It is generally viewed as the development of an emerging world order characterized both by gradual acceptance and implementation of liberal democracy in many countries, and by the growing impact of a neo-liberal economic system featuring the growing integration of markets in goods, capital and services on a global basis. The driving forces of globalization include advances in information and transport technology and the development of a dense network of international and transnational agreements that facilitate free trade and promote the concept of universal human rights.

Globalization is not a new phenomenon, and the globalization process reflects a long economic and political history, involving a wide range of actors, and resulting in both beneficial and adverse effects. While economic growth has been enhanced, and freedom and prosperity have increased for many, the economic disparities between rich and poor (both within and between nations) have widened in association with the development of a complex web of material, institutional and ideological forces and massive multinational corporations. The influence of the latter on the balance of power in the world effectively blurs boundaries between states, undermines state control (especially that of small states) over their own economies and threatens the ability of states to provide for their citizens.

In addition to the progressive widening of the economic divide between nations and the growing external control over the economies of small countries through the 'debt trade' and markets that are increasingly global, other powerful forces are at work. Evidence is accumulating that, associated with globalization, there has developed a large (but little-discussed) illicit global economy comprising an illicit drugs trade (now an industry worth over $500 billion annually), massive migration and smuggling of people, trafficking in endangered species, toxic waste dumping, prostitution, unprecedented levels of sexual exploitation and child labour, an uncontrolled illicit arms trade, and money laundering. Some scholars claim that globalization aggravates ethnic and cultural violence.[10]

Wealth and disease

It is now well established that there is a definite relationship between wealth/poverty and health/disease, although this relationship is complex and only linear up to annual per capita incomes of $5,000.[11] Anomalies are evident at the poles of wealth and poverty. One of the wealthiest nations in the world, the USA, with per capita annual healthcare expenditure of over $4,000 (amounting to 50 per cent of annual global expenditure on 5 per cent of the world's population) has worse health statistics than some other highly industrialized countries with lower incomes.[12] Some poor provinces (Kerala in India, for example) and poor countries (such as Cuba and Costa Rica) have achieved lower infant mortality rates and greater longevity than many wealthier nations.[13]

Both absolute and relative wealth affect health. Among the developed countries it is not the richest societies that have the best health but rather those with the smallest income differentials between rich and poor.[14] Despite the non-linearity of the relationship between wealth and health above annual per capita gross national products (GNPs) of $5,000, the existence of this relationship and the effect of wide income differentials underscores the need to see health and disease as intimately linked to social and economic conditions.

Poverty directly accounts for almost one third of the global burden of disease. Poverty leads to poor health, which in turn aggravates poverty and reduces human productivity. Of the forty poorest countries in the world, eleven have annual per capita GNPs ranging from US$80 (Mozambique) to US$210 (Sierra Leone), ten from US$220 (Bangladesh) to US$340 (Nigeria), nine from US$370 (China) to US$450

Table 13.1 Health statistics in the forty poorest countries in the world.[13]

Annual per capita GNP (US$)*	168	282	404	570
Life expectancy at birth (years)*	47	51	56	60
Infant mortality rate per 1,000 live births	126	112	90	70
Under 5 years mortality rate	158	169	132	109
Population access to safe water (%)*	37%	53%	53%	63%
Population access to sanitation (%)*	29%	26%	39%	48%
Population per physician (1970)	33,925	39,381	23,009	15,956
Adult literacy rate (1992– %)	42%	44%	46%	63%
Average annual population growth (%)*	2.7%	2.8%	2.6%	2.3%

* 1991 data

Source: G. Gunatilleke, *Poverty and Health in Developing Countries*. WHO/CO/
MESD.16. Geneva: World Health Organization, 1995.

(Nicaragua), and ten from US$500 (Sri Lanka) to US$600 (Zim-babwe).[15] Despite the difficulty in making accurate comparisons it is clear (see Table 13.1) that increments in economic status are associated with better health statistics, and that economic growth is necessary to improve the living conditions conducive to good health, independent of benefits that may arise directly from health care.[16] Ninety-five per cent of TB cases and 98 per cent of TB deaths are in developing countries.[17] TB has a direct bearing on the economies of poor countries as 17 per cent of those who die from this disease are in the economi-cally productive age group of 15–49 years.[18]

'Human rights' and alternative ways of thinking about poverty

It is not only economic or material poverty that prevents the effective treatment of TB. We should consider how we are impoverished by the inadequacy of our ability to feel empathy and to express it in practice. With regard to TB it can be claimed that if those in resource-rich countries find it so impossible to empathize with those suffering from a potentially fatal disease that they cannot sacrifice/donate the US$1 required for each year of life that could be saved by treating TB, there must surely be a deficiency in the ability to reflect on their own potential to suffer and on the misery of being neglected. Of relevance here is the USA's failure to pay its dues to the World Health Organization (WHO): the $35 million that the USA owes to the WHO could do much to promote a global agenda against TB.[19] Minimal respect for the lives of TB victims can be interpreted as an impoverished sense of sincerity regarding the widely acclaimed aspirations expressed in the Universal Declaration of Human Rights (UDHR).

The recent thrust to bring the work of bioethicists and human rights activists closer together in the quest for better global health provides an opportunity to reflect both on the content of the Universal Declaration of Human Rights (and of subsequent supportive covenants and declarations) and on the extent to which these aspirations have not yet been met. Both pessimism and optimism have been expressed regarding the fulfilment of these declarations to date, and what may be achieved in the future. The despair of some at the extent of continuing and even escalating human rights abuses and violations throughout the world – even in highly privileged societies – is countered by the hope of others that with the development of international law and other human rights instruments coupled to intensified educational efforts, the impact of the UDHR will spread more widely. The recent General Comment on the Right to Health by the United Nations Committee on Economic, Social and Cultural Rights is viewed as a significant milestone.[20]

Explanations for the relative lack of success of the UDHR in achieving its noble goals may include: (i) the utopianism expressed in a multiplicity of laws and conventions, (ii) widespread differences in their interpretation and acceptance by various countries, (iii) unrealistic expectations, and (iv) lack of enforcement mechanisms. For example, the USA does not accept, and has not ratified, either the widely accepted Covenant on Social, Economic and Cultural Rights or the more recently agreed to Convention on the Rights of the Child. The appeal to laws that are not uniformly accepted and cannot be enforced weakens the use of a human rights approach to global ideals. The recent description of how the UDHR was crafted is illuminating. Its insight into the discussions central to achieving the promulgation of the UDHR, revealing that signatory countries agreed to differ on the fundamental issues underpinning the declaration, helps to explain its limitations.[21] Another example of lack of integrity is the setting by bodies in rich countries of utopian human rights standards for health-care professionals in other countries, while expecting less in their own country. For example human rights activists in the USA, in making recommendations for the protection of human rights by healthcare professionals in South Africa, have set standards that go well beyond those expected of healthcare professionals in their own country.[22]

The human rights approach to human well-being has potential strengths and weaknesses. In general there is a tendency to celebrate its strengths – and many describe how human rights are more widely acknowledged and honoured around the world today than ever before. However, it is also important to ask why the world at the beginning of the twenty-first century is characterized by widening disparities between rich and poor, by growing injustice within and between nations, by power struggles reflected in wars, torture, human rights violations, and refugeeism on a massive scale, and by escalating ecological deterioration.[23] The spectre of human rights abuses world-wide is a terrible one, and the world now has an estimated 18 million refugees and 25 million displaced persons. Wars, torture and repression continue, and medical personnel are involved. We need to ask why these crises continue to proliferate fifty years after the acceptance of the UDHR and why, despite the efforts of many organizations, abuses are merely being documented instead of being prevented.

It would seem that there is a need to look beyond the obvious violations of human rights to perceive the root causes of such behaviour: to see human rights abuses on a wide scale as a means to restrict access to the basic subsistence rights required for survival. In apartheid South Africa, for example, 20 per cent of the population owned 80 per cent of the wealth – a discrepancy that arose through oppression and domination. The world was correctly critical of the indignities and disparities imposed by legally enforced racial discrimination and exploitation, and justifiably fought to displace the apartheid regime. Now we need to ask why we are not equally critical that in the world as a whole, 20 per cent of the world's people own more than 80 per cent of wealth – and the economic divide continues to widen between and within many countries. While this is not the result of apartheid-like laws that overtly promote racial discrimination and exploitation, it does reflect other forms of covert exploitation and discrimination that have equally offensive results. It is clear, against this background, that human rights abuses are propagated under adverse social and economic circumstances that create divisions and conflict between people. This can be viewed as a form of global apartheid based on the abuse of power, which, given its effects, should surely be contested as vigorously as racial apartheid.[24]

With regard to poverty and racism in the USA, the public health physician Jack Geiger has argued thus:

> ... my country is now embarked on a massive attack on the poor and on people of color. In the US Congress, there are serious attempts to destroy the social welfare system ... to end affirmative action for minorities and women, to deny women's rights to reproductive choice, to slash the funding for health care and public education, to increase taxes for the poor and reduce them for the rich, to reduce food subsidies and heating assistance for the poor and elderly, and even to end the program of free school lunches for low income children. This campaign is driven by a thinly disguised racism.[25]

But this lack of respect within a wealthy nation for the dignity of its own citizens is also only part of the problem. In the USA, prominent economists have also casually dismissed two thirds of the world's population as: 'superfluous from the standpoint of the market. By and large, we do not need what they have; they can't buy what we sell.'[26] 'In the perspective of world capitalism as we know it these people just don't count. . . . Unless that part of the world develops the capacity for terrorist blackmail they will be in the charity ward for a long time.'[27]

The ugly roots of human rights abuses thus seem to lie in the distorted human relationships that arise from exploitation, domination and discrimination. The issues that need to be addressed lie at the core of our humanity. Regrettably, as noted by the Canadian sociologist Rhoda Howard, 'The Western human rights discourse of the late twentieth century has become a discourse of the privileged – of relatively well-off members of social categories who claim the right to equal treatment in law and society, while the poor have little chance of using that discourse to claim their fundamental rights in the economic sphere.'[28] Howard identifies the social minimalism and reactionary conservative ideologies of the USA as permitting social closure against the poor, including blacks and single mothers, and she advocates social democracy as the best means for promoting the whole range of human rights with both respect for individuals and concern for community.[29]

Finally, we need to consider the lack of political will to embark on a global TB programme that has such profound implications for sustainable human well-being.[30] This reflects yet another form of poverty, moral insensitivity and corrosion of character afflicting those who increasingly live self-centred lives, and the extent to which such lives are pervasively diminished by a lack of concern for their fellow human beings.[31] It is not unreasonable to suggest that these various expressions of the 'non-economic poverty' of the wealthy and privileged, who feel entitled to ever-increasing economic resources with little regard for the impact of their way of life on the environment and on the lives of others, diminish our ability to control TB and threaten future peaceful life on our planet.

TB and the ethics of health care

Ethical considerations have long been central concerns in medicine. To a remarkable degree medical ethics was continuous, consistent and largely confined within the profession until the middle of the twentieth century. Medical ethics was centred on the Hippocratic oath, and various declarations (Geneva, Helsinki, Tokyo and others) to which individual practitioners and medical organizations claimed allegiance. Exhortation, apprenticeship and role modelling were the instructional processes. In the latter half of the twentieth century a major change took place. Traditional medical ethics was challenged and the discourse on ethics became multidisciplinary. The rich history of the rebirth and growth of medical ethics has been partially documented and remains the subject of considerable study.[32]

In brief, ethics at the *micro* level of interpersonal relationships is seen today as inclusive of respect for human dignity, for individual self-determination and for access to the resources required to sustain the very basic physical and mental health of individuals conceived of as rational and autonomous. In this context the physician is viewed as committed to the care of each individual patient within a relationship that embraces the concepts of an unwritten but binding contract, respect for patient autonomy, and trust in the physician's concern for the best interest of patients. Such a relationship, in which a physician of good character treats patients as ends in their own right, is rooted in ethical theories concerned primarily either with the inherent 'rightness or goodness' of actions or with theories of virtue. The ethics of the relationship between the doctor and the patient has been extensively debated and written about and will not be further discussed here. Appropriate application of such ethics has the potential to care for and cure any individual patient suffering from TB.

There is also increasing interest in extending the debate on ethics to the *meso* level where such considerations as order and justice within the communities in which individuals are socially embedded come into focus. Here a broader view of the responsibility of health professionals includes concern for public health, and requires participation in the healthcare system of their country for the common good. Considerations of justice require the development of explicit rationing processes, based on well-reasoned notions of distributive justice, and promoted through publicly made policies for equitable access to health care. Such ethics, embracing the idea of a social contract and of utility value at institutional and national levels, are less extensively articulated but are exemplified by the public health policies of countries with a political philosophy of welfare liberalism. Here, interpersonal relationships are broadened to encompass the concept of civic citizenship. The application of good meso-level ethics to TB would result in the creation of an effective public health programme for dealing with this disease at the national level.

In an interdependent global world it is increasingly being appreciated that ethical considerations must extend to the *macro* level to include consideration of ecological security, international relations and the interdependence of all forms of life.[33] The desired conception of the individual here becomes that of an autonomous individual sharing equal rights with all other citizens in the world, in a relationship of interdependence in which the rights of some should not be acquired at the expense of the rights of even distant others. The level of complexity here is much greater because of the way in which the foreign policies of some countries may covertly enhance the lives of their own citizens through the exploitation of unseen persons elsewhere. The role of the physician at this level of ethics includes a commitment to global professional ideals, to the continuing advancement of knowledge, and to concern for health at a global level for present and future generations. Promoting ethics at this level would enable the WHO to implement a global TB control programme.

Some consider the meso and macro levels as widening concentric circles with the degree of moral obligation to others being determined by the closeness to oneself of the people to whom one owes moral obligations. The question that can be asked, with at least some plausibility, is, Why should we bother to go beyond the micro level of ethics? Why should we have moral responsibilities to those who live far from us and whose lives seem to be independent from ours? It can be answered that modern communications, transport, methods of money exchange and the creation of nuclear and other weapons of mass destruction have shrunk distances and differences in many senses, and created common risks and a degree of interdependence between all people worldwide that must be addressed.

The ethical and human rights challenges that must be faced at a global level are the promotion of respect for the dignity of all people, and the reduction of inequity. These goals are required for several reasons. First, there is the ethical imperative to achieve visible respect for individual dignity. Second, there is a need to promote the social stability necessary for human flourishing in a complex world. Hunger, miserable living conditions, lack of education, illiteracy and lack of control over one's own destiny breed anger, violence and crime, and promote the narcotic drug trade and abuse of vulnerable humans – all of which destroy the fabric of society.[34] Third, and not least, is the need to be aware of the adverse ecological effects of modern life and to develop the processes necessary for protecting the environment for the well-being of future generations.[35]

It is clear that too much should not be expected of a single-minded, rights-based approach to improving human life. Whatever might be the present or future anticipated achievements of the human rights approach, the desired goal could hopefully be assisted and even amplified by widespread acceptance and promotion of complementary moral approaches, of which the recently proposed Trieste Declaration of Human Duties is one (Table 13.2). The achievement of a global civil society will require acknowledging and promoting the idea of human duties as an essential component of human rights. The International Council of Human Duties (ICHD), a non-governmental and non-profitmaking organization, has among its objectives to promote international understanding of the concepts of human duties, and to encourage the adoption by the United Nations of a 'Universal Declaration of Human Duties' with comparable stature to the UDHR. Stimulated by the success of the Helsinki Declaration, first issued in

Table 13.2   Trieste Declaration of Human Duties.

Whereas the Declaration of Human Rights represents one of the great advances of the twentieth century, it fails to address Human Duties and Responsibilities as necessary counterparts of these Rights. . . . Recognition of and respect for human rights demand the acceptance of specific duties, in order to assure an adequate quality of life for all people and the persistence of a favourable environment for future generations.

It is the duty of every human being to:

- Respect human dignity as well as ethnic, cultural and religious diversity.
- Work against racial injustice and all discrimination of women and the abuse and exploitation of children.
- Work for the improvement in the quality of life of aged and disabled persons.
- Respect human life and condemn sale of human beings or parts of the living body.
- Support efforts to improve the life of people suffering from hunger, misery, disease or unemployment.
- Promote effective voluntary family planning in order to regulate world population growth.
- Support actions for an equitable distribution of world resources.
- Avoid energy waste and work for reduction of the use of fossil fuels. Promote the use of inexhaustible energy sources, representing a minimum of environmental and health risks.
- Protect nature from pollution and abuse, promote conservation of natural resources and the restoration of degraded environments.
- Respect and preserve the genetic diversity of living organisms and promote constant scrutiny of the application of genetic technologies.
- Promote improvement of urban and rural regions and support endeavours to eliminate the causes of environmental destruction and impoverishment which can lead to massive migrations of people and overpopulation in urban areas.
- Work for maintenance of world peace, condemn war, terrorism and all other hostile activities by calling for decreased military spending in all countries and restriction of the proliferation and dissemination of arms, in particular, weapons of mass destruction.

Source: *Trieste Declaration of Human Duties: a Code of Ethics of Shared Responsibilities*, Trieste University Press, 1997.

1963, the World Medical Association has encouraged several other ambitious ethics statements in recent decades.[36] However, the challenge to the World Medical Association to promote the provocative statement reproduced in Table 13.3 has not been followed up.

The failure to control TB at a global level, and its resurgence with increasing multi-drug resistance in recent decades represent a failure of public health at national and global levels. In the face of such failure despite the clarity of the issues at stake, it is appropriate to ask whether the negotiated political transformation in South Africa in the 1990s will impart a message that can be heard by those interested in the global control of TB. A decade ago a text on TB in South Africa noted that:

> South Africa is embarking on a political journey that offers hope for progress out of the wilderness created by its apartheid policies into a relationship with the world which could make it a catalyst for sub-Saharan development. South Africa reflects the cross-roads in human progress in relation to many conflicts in the modern world – between capitalism and socialism, between individualism and collectivism, between Eurocentric and Afrocentric ideologies, between wealth and poverty, between progress and retrogression, between intercultural belligerence and mutual understanding, and between destruction and conservation of a precious ecology.[37]

It also suggested that the extent to which the conquest of TB in South Africa became a reality would be one of the indicators of progress towards social justice in the new order. It is arguable that these considerations apply to the global control of TB today. The HIV/AIDS epidemic has added to the complexity of the task, but the implications are unchanged. The prospects for dealing with TB (and HIV/AIDS) at a global level will reflect our ability to move beyond global economic apartheid. If ridding South Africa of legalized racial apartheid, and its consequent dehumanizing disparities was a global priority, and I know of no one who disputes this, it would require a powerful argument to refute the similar need to narrow the equally grotesque disparities created by global economic apartheid. The peaceful political transition in South Africa, when most expected that only a civil war could result in change, is an example of the power of the idea that 'might is right' can be replaced by the idea that 'right is might'. The burden of TB at a global level will be a marker of whether the widely acclaimed political shift made by South Africa is being emulated at a global level.

Table 13.3   Proposed World Medical Association Code.

Whereas the World Medical Association:

A. Recognizes that:
- We live in a divided world, a world in which 23 per cent of the world's population lives in affluence on 85 per cent of the annual global economic output, while 77 per cent live poorly, often in misery, on 15 per cent;
- These disparities have deep roots in centuries of complex human development and progress that has regrettably been associated with military and economic conflict and exploitation;
- The gap continues to widen as human and material resources flow from poor countries into the rich;
- These disparities and their causes aggravate population growth, human misery and ecological degradation in all countries;
- Vast resources are wastefully expended year after year on militarization worldwide;

B. Notes that health care professionals have:
- Traditionally seen themselves as part of a global moral community with shared goals for the promotion of life and health;
- Formulated codes of ethics that reflect the universal nature of these professional obligations;
- Committed themselves through their nations to support universal human rights, including health for all;
- Responsibility towards the common good as well as individual patients;

C. Acknowledges that:
- The principle of justice requires access to health care in all countries as a basic human right without which people will suffer individually and communities collectively;
- We live in an interdependent world in which modern communication and transport systems inform us about and expose us all to individual and collective threats to human health and survival;

The World Medical Association urges all health care professionals and their professional associations to:

- Acknowledge that their responsibility for individual and population health should not be subverted by political and other ideologies either in wealthy or in poor countries;
- Expose and contest actions taken by their respective governments that may adversely affect the health of individuals or populations, at home or abroad;
- Assist professional organizations to work toward creating national and international concepts of the practice of medicine that will contribute to the health of populations as well as to the health of individuals.

EPILOGUE
Politics, Science and the 'New' Tuberculosis

Alimuddin Zumla and Matthew Gandy

The history of TB is a story of medical failure. This seemingly harsh indictment reflects the paradox that modern treatment for TB is among the most effective and inexpensive of all therapies for life-threatening diseases yet TB remains the leading infectious cause of morbidity and mortality worldwide. The fact that TB was declared a global emergency by the World Health Organization (WHO) in 1993 raises the question of whether control strategies have failed because they have been used incorrectly or because they are intrinsically flawed. Above all, it is the sense of surprise that has surrounded this public health crisis which suggests that the international community has overlooked the significance of TB until it has been faced with a threat to some of the wealthiest cities and regions in the world, exemplified by the New York City outbreak of the 1980s. No longer a 'tropical disease' of merely historical or scientific curiosity, TB has had a resurgence that has become global in scope, ranging from schools in the UK to prisons in Russia, from refugee camps in central Africa to North American suburbs. Like the cholera epidemics of the nineteenth century, which threatened all of urban society, the global scale of the TB epidemic has forced the international community to act.

The scientific response to the crisis has fostered a new wave of research into what had until recently been a relatively neglected field of study in relation to its human impact. The development of improved tools for diagnosis, treatment and prevention of TB through the use of vaccines appear attractive options for continued emphasis but there are doubts about whether these could ever be effective by themselves in eradicating the disease.[1] The basic biomedical approach to TB cannot *per se* be deemed a failure; indeed, the development of modern short-course anti-TB therapy can be hailed as one of the greatest triumphs of medical science. The key question facing us today is why the available means of treatment and control have not been more widely applied. Since the problem lies with delivery of care, a shift of emphasis is required away from the TB bacillus as the 'cause' of the pandemic towards the social and political factors underlying the epidemiology of disease.[2] A concerted effort from the medical sciences is required to work closely with other disciplines such as anthropology, geography and social policy. These efforts must be linked with those of governments and donor agencies in order to maximize the availability of much-needed resources for TB control.

The chapters in this book illustrate the fact that immense forces are counteracting efforts to tackle the spread of TB. Political and demographic factors, the HIV/AIDS epidemic, poverty and social marginalization, mass displacements of people and the growth of drug resistance have all been important in impeding control measures and creating the current pandemic. The debates generated in this book highlight a series of dilemmas regarding which aspects of control should be emphasized. Better tools for diagnosis and treatment or the strengthening of existing TB control programmes? The development of newer vaccines or more effective campaigns to combat poverty? In practice, of course, there are likely to be a combination of different strategies involved in any successful attempt to control the disease, but a reliance on biomedical innovations alone cannot hope to have any lasting impact.

Renewed recognition of the link between TB and poverty led to the creation in 2000, and under the auspices of the WHO and UNAIDS, of the Advocacy Forum for Massive Effort Against Diseases of Poverty. The international community clearly has the financial means, the medications and the know-how to take a stand against a small number of diseases that cause tremendous suffering and economic loss. This 'Massive Effort' initiative against diseases of poverty is forcing the international community from words to action – action that can facilitate more equitable forms of development, stimulate economic growth, ensure greater global public health security and, most important, save human lives. Yet other organizations such as Médecins sans Frontières have openly questioned whether the WHO's 'Massive Effort' initiative has any real prospect of success without better access to available drugs for the world's poor of whom only about 20 per cent receive adequate treatment.[3]

The launch of the Stop TB initiative by the WHO in March 2000 involved setting up a new organization called the Global TB Drug Facility which will purchase quality anti-TB drugs for countries with a high burden of the disease. The aim of the Global TB Drug Facility is to provide drugs for 10 million TB patients over the next five years and for 45 million patients over a ten-year period. Also in 2000, the health ministers from the twenty countries with the greatest burden of TB, in what has been termed the Amsterdam Declaration, pledged support for the WHO's Stop TB initiative. Yet the WHO's most recent research into the prevalence of drug-resistant strains of TB shows that the problem has significantly worsened since their first survey in 1997. In Estonia some 14 per cent of new cases of TB are resistant to both isoniazid and rifampicin, and in Latvia, Iran and parts of Russia and China rates of MDR-TB now exceed 5 per cent, presenting a steadily worsening outlook for the control of the disease. Furthermore, the rapid spread of the HIV pandemic beyond its current epicentre in sub-Saharan Africa to South Asia and elsewhere now threatens to undermine global efforts to control TB.[4]

In October 2000 the Global Alliance for TB Drug Development was launched at the International Conference on Health Research for Development in Bangkok. The members of this new alliance, including governments, non-governmental organizations, pharmaceutical companies and funding agencies, made a pledge to apply recent scientific breakthroughs to the development of new cost-effective anti-TB drugs that will shorten the duration of treatment, simplify the use of drugs, improve the elimination of latent infection and be effective against multi-drug-resistant tuberculosis (MDR-TB). This marks the first attempt to systematically develop a new TB drug in thirty years but is little more than a belated response of biotechnology and pharmaceutical companies to the widespread condemnation of their failure to make drugs more widely available for the treatment of infectious diseases in developing countries.[5] Yet even if new drugs are developed, unless there is radical change in the use of drugs away from what the WHO has termed 'therapeutic anarchy', then any new antibacterial agents will be countered by renewed forms of drug resistance. There is, therefore, a need for new vaccines to supplement any advances in the development of drugs. Much effort is currently being put into unravelling the complexities of human immune responses to TB, but the difficulties in evaluating any new vaccine, and the time required for its full development, should not be underestimated. Vaccines account for a very small share of the global pharmaceuticals market – just 1.5 per cent – a figure that underlines the complexity of any fundamental shift in the research and development of new medicines towards the needs of preventive health care. New initiatives such as the Global Alliance on Vaccines and Immunization supported by the World Bank, the WHO and the vaccine industry reflect a change in priorities driven at least in part by Western fears that diseases such as HIV and MDR-TB cannot be contained by conventional means.[6] The danger, however, is that vaccines will become the new 'magic bullet', deflecting attention yet again away from the structural causes and devastating impacts of ill health. Although the pharmaceutical industry has begun to respond to global demands for affordable medicine – most notably in the wake of the rancorous international AIDS summit hosted by South Africa in July 2000 – there remains an immense gulf between the commercial interests of drug companies and ethical demands for affordable health care. Indeed, the offer to reduce the cost of antiretroviral drugs in selected developing countries to one eighth of their price in the USA has raised a host of further issues. Why should HIV be afforded a different priority to other killer diseases such as malaria and TB? How should different 'cheap' markets be selected in the face of global poverty and inequality? And what kind of profit margins are being sustained anyway by the pharmaceutical industry if they are able to make such drastic price cuts without threatening their financial viability?[7]

At the 2000 G8 summit at Okinawa, Japan, an ambitious commitment was made by the world's richest countries to achieve substantial reductions in the global burden of disease and death due to HIV/AIDS, TB and malaria by the year 2010.[8] Funds will be additional to existing aid from multilateral and bilateral agencies and will be managed and disbursed by a new entity called the Global Health Fund. The Global Health Fund has the potential to help coordinate ongoing international efforts and reduce potential duplication among the different global public–private partnerships and health initiatives. Yet the precise remit of this fund and its relationship to existing disease control programmes remain uncertain. There is a tension, for example, between renewed emphasis on scientific developments such as vaccine development and wider goals such as better nutrition or the stated aim to halve absolute poverty by the year 2015. Countries receiving the aid will have to build up their healthcare systems in order to deliver new treatment programmes, but this may conflict with the impetus of structural adjustment programmes and pressures on developing countries to reduce social expenditure. The Global Health Fund has, however, sent out a message that rich countries have a moral and political responsibility to do something about TB and other preventable killer diseases. Yet at the same time the inequities of global trade and the burden of Third World debt suggest that the G8 nations remain at the very least Janus-faced towards the plight of the world's poor: the failure of the G8 leaders to implement previous agreements on debt relief is reflective of the contradictory character of any apparent commitment to tackle global health issues.[9]

Notwithstanding these recent developments, it is the responsibility of all those involved in the global campaign against TB to be relentless in their advocacy efforts to ensure that declarations, initiatives and intentions are translated into sustained and effective action. The currently available tools for the control of TB – bacteriological diagnosis, BCG vaccination and standard short-course therapy – have been widely and often successfully deployed against the disease. Nevertheless, TB remains a major cause of illness and death worldwide and, despite the WHO's 1993 declaration of a global emergency, its incidence has continued to rise. There is an increasing awareness that the failure to control TB worldwide is a direct consequence both of poor political leadership and of the burden of poverty borne by the great majority of its sufferers.

Notes

Introduction

1. Friedrich Engels, *The Condition of the Working Class in England*, trans. W. O. Henderson and W. H. Chaloner, Stanford: Stanford University Press, 1958 [1845], p. 111.
2. René Dubos and Jean Dubos, *The White Plague: Tuberculosis, Man, and Society*, Boston: Little, Brown and Company, 1952, p. 220.
3. Gordon L. Snider, 'Tuberculosis then and now: a personal perspective on the last fifty years', *Annals of Internal Medicine*, vol. 126 (3), 1997, p. 237.
4. William D. Johnston, 'Tuberculosis', in Kenneth F. Kiple, ed. *The Cambridge World History of Human Disease*, Cambridge: Cambridge University Press, 1993, pp. 1059–68; Richard Levins *et al.*, 'The emergence of new diseases', *American Scientist*, January 1994, pp. 52–60; World Health Organization, *The World Health Report 1996: Fighting Disease, Fostering Development*, Geneva: World Health Organization, 1996.
5. See L. K. Altman, 'Deadly strain of TB is spreading fast, US finds', *New York Times*, 24 January 1992; L. Belkin, 'Top TB peril: not taking the medicine', *New York Times*, 18 November 1991; Sarah Boseley, 'School at centre of rare TB outbreak', *Guardian*, 5 April 2001.
6. For an overview of the medical aspects of TB see, for example, Arthur M. Dannenberg, 'Pathophysiology: basic aspects', in David Schlossberg, ed., *Tuberculosis and Nontuberculous Mycobacterial Infections*, London: W. B. Saunders, 1999, pp. 17–47, and Philip C. Hopewell, 'Overview of clinical tuberculosis', in Barry R. Bloom, ed., *Tuberculosis: Pathogenesis, Protection and Control*, Washington, DC: American Society for Microbiology, 1994, pp. 25–46.
7. Katherine Mansfield, cited in Lewis J. Moorman, *Tuberculosis and Genius*, Chicago: Chicago University Press, 1940, p. 120.

8. John Keats, cited in Harley Williams, *Requiem for a Great Killer*, London: Health Horizon, 1973.

9. Charles Dickens, *Nicholas Nickleby*, London: Penguin, 1999 [1839], p. 60.

10. Matthew Gandy, 'Science, society and disease: emerging perspectives', *Current Opinion in Pulmonary Medicine*, vol. 7, 2001, pp. 12–19; Matthew Gandy and Alimuddin Zumla, 'The resurgence of disease: social and historical perspectives on the "new" tuberculosis', *Social Science and Medicine*, vol. 55, 2002, pp. 385–96; Matthew Gandy and Alimuddin Zumla, 'Theorizing tuberculosis: a reply to Porter and Ogden', *Social Science and Medicine*, vol. 55, 2002, pp. 399–401.

11. See, for example, Paul Farmer, 'DOTS and DOTS-plus: not the only answer', *Annals of the New York Academy of Science*, vol. 953, 2001, pp. 165–84, and I. Bastian, L. Rigouts, A. Van Deun and F. Portaels, 'Directly observed treatment, short-course strategy and multidrug-resistant tuberculosis: are any modifications required?' *Bulletin of the World Health Organization*, vol. 78, 2000, pp. 238–51.

1 Life without Germs: Contested Episodes in the History of Tuberculosis

Many thanks to Michael Warboys for his helpful comments on an earlier draft of this chapter. Thanks also to Ana Francisca de Alvezedo for assistance with the translation of the article by Diego Armus. The principal data sources used were the British Library, the New-York Historical Society, the London School of Hygiene and Tropical Medicine and the Wellcome Library for the History and Understanding of Medicine, London.

1. Arturo Castiglioni, 'History of tuberculosis', trans. Emilie Recht, *Medical Life* 40, 1933, p. 5.

2. Cited in Robert Koch, 'Epidemiology of tuberculosis', a lecture given before the Academy of Sciences of Berlin at its session of 7 April 1910. Translated from *Zeitschrift für Hygiene* and published in *The Annual Report of the Board of Regents of the Smithsonian Institution, Washington*, 1991, p. 660.

3. Early accounts of the history of TB include Richard M. Burke, *An Historical Chronology of Tuberculosis*, Springfield, IL: Charles C. Thomas 1938; Lyle Cummins, *Tuberculosis in History*, London: Baillière, Tindall and Cox 1949; Robert Koch, *Die Ätiologie und die Bekämpfung der Tuberkulose*, Leipzig: Johann Ambrosius Barth, 1912. Recent archaeological debates are discussed in György Palfi, Olivier Datour, Jufith Deák and Imre Hutás, eds., *Tuberculosis Past and Present*, Szeged: Tuberculosis Foundation, 1999. An excellent anthology of sources is contained in Barbara Gutmann Rosenkrantz, *From Consumption to Tuberculosis: a Documentary History*, London and New York: Garland Publishing, 1994.

4. This very high estimate of TB infection is derived from William D. Johnston, 'Tuberculosis', in Kenneth F. Kiple, ed., *The Cambridge World History of Human Disease*, Cambridge: Cambridge University Press, 1993, pp. 1059–68.

5. Ibid.

6. Sir Richard Blackmore, *Discourses on the Gout, Rheumatism, and the King's Evil*, London: J. Pemberton, 1726, pp. 38, 33.

7. For a classic overview of the disease and its human consequences see René Dubos and Jean Dubos, *The White Plague: Tuberculosis, Man and Society*, London: Victor Gollancz, 1953.

8. Sir James Clark, *A Treatise on Pulmonary Consumption, Comprising an Inquiry into the Causes, Nature, Prevention, and Treatment of Tuberculosis and Scrofulous Diseases*, London: Sherwod, Gilbert and Piper, 1837, p. xi. See also Samuel Sheldon Fitch, *Six Lectures on the Uses of the Lungs*, New York: H. Carlisle, 1847.

9. W. Beach, *A Treatise on Pulmonary Consumption: Phthisis Pulmonalis*, New York: Joseph B. Allee, 1840, pp. 4, 16.

10. See, for example, Castiglioni.

11. Ibid.

12. J. Arthur Myers, *Captain of All These Men of Death: Tuberculosis Historical Highlights*, St Louis, MS: Warren H. Green, 1977.

13. Robert Koch, 'The etiology of tuberculosis', trans. William de Rouville, in *Medical Classics*, vol. 2, 1938 [1882], p. 879.

14. See Barbara Gutmann Rosenkrantz, 'The trouble with bovine tuberculosis', *Bulletin of the History of Medicine*, vol. 59, 1985, pp. 155–75.

15. Susan Sontag, *Illness as Metaphor*, New York: Farrar, Straus and Giroux, 1978, p. 15.

16. Johnston, 'Tuberculosis'.

17. Sontag, p. 73.

18. Castiglioni, p. 80.

19. The Grand Tour undertaken by wealthy northern Europeans of Italy and the Mediterranean was rooted in the Romantic reaction to TB. The presence of these pallid travellers was met with widespread fear and hostility in southern Europe, however, because of the greater emphasis on contagionist conceptions of TB in southern Europe. See J. N. Hays, *The Burdens of Disease: Epidemics and Human Response in Western History*, New Brunswick, NJ: Rutgers University Press, 1998.

20. Gilles Boetsch, 'The white death in black and colour: from romantic phthisis to tuberculosis as a social disaster', in Palfi *et al.*, pp. 63–8.

21. Sontag, pp. 19–20.

22. Clark Lawlor and Akihito Suzuki, 'The disease of the self: representing consumption, 1700–1830', *Bulletin of the History of Medicine*, vol. 74, 2000, pp. 458–94.

23. See H. D. Chalke, 'The impact of tuberculosis on history, literature and art', *Medical History*, vol. 6, 1962, pp. 301–18; René and Jean Dubos,

'Consumption and the Romantic age', in *The White Plague*, pp. 44–66; Dan Latimer, 'Erotic susceptibility and tuberculosis: literary images of a pathology', *Modern Language Notes*, vol. 105, 1990, pp. 1016–31; David Farrell Krell, *Contagion: Sexuality, Disease and Death in German Idealism and Romanticism*, Bloomington: Indiana University Press, 1998; Lewis J. Moorman, *Tuberculosis and Genius*, Chicago: Chicago University Press, 1940.

24. It was implied that writers in good health, such as Victor Hugo, would have been better still had they become ill. Dubos and Dubos, 'Consumption and the Romantic age', p. 64.

25. On the sanatoria movement see, for example, Linda Bryder, 'Papworth village settlement – a unique experiment in the treatment and care of the tuberculous?' *Medical History*, 28, 1984, pp. 372–90; Linda Bryder, *Below the Magic Mountain: a Social History of Tuberculosis in Twentieth-century Britain*, Oxford: Oxford University Press, 1988; Guy Hinsdale, 'Atmospheric air in relation to tuberculosis', *Smithsonian Miscellaneous Collections*, vol. 63, 1914, pp. 1–136; Robert Taylor, *Saranac: America's Magic Mountain*, Boston: Houghton Mifflin, 1986. On the later phase see Michael Warboys, 'The sanatorium treatment for consumption in Britain, 1890–1914', in John V. Pickstone, ed., *Medical Innovations in Historical Perspective*, London: Macmillan, 1992, pp. 47–73.

26. In 1904, for instance, the Adirondack Cottage Sanitorium in up-state New York began publishing its own magazine entitled *Journal of Outdoor Life* which stressed the centrality of fresh air, sunlight and oudoor recreation for the eradication of TB. Even after the bacterial origins of TB had been clearly established, climatic perspectives on the disease continued to a play a powerful role in the medical literature. Articles printed by the Southern California Medical Society in the 1890s, for example, continue to extol the benefits of warm dry climates for conferring immunity against TB. See P. C. Remondino, 'The marine climate of the southern California coast and its relations to phthisis', 1888. Reprint from the *Proceedings of the Southern California Medical Society*, 1888, held in the archives of the New York Historical Society.

27. R. Y. Keers, B. G. Rigden and F. H. Young, *Pulmonary Tuberculosis: A Handbook for Students and Practitioners*, Edinburgh: E & Livingston, 1945, p. 139.

28. The transformation of cities in Europe and North America also had a wider resonance for the processes of urbanization in the colonial and post-colonial centres of Africa and Latin America. In Buenos Aires, for instance, the control of TB became a central element in utopian conceptions of urban planning which varied from the complete eradication of the disease to the scientific ideal of biological containment through vaccination. See Diego Claudio Armus, 'O discurso da regeneração: espaço urbano, utopias e tuberculose em Buenos Aires, 1870–1930', *Estudos Historicos*, vol. 8, 1995, pp. 235–50, and Diego Claudio Armus, 'The years of tuberculosis.

Disease, culture and society: Buenos Aires 1870–1930', unpublished PhD thesis, University of California at Berkeley, 1996.

29. Pierre Hulliger, *A New Treatment of Tuberculosis*, London: H. K. Lewis, 1930, p. 47.

30. Neil McFarlane, 'Hospitals, housing, and tuberculosis in Glasgow, 1911–51', *Social History of Medicine*, vol. 2, 1989, p. 65. McFarlane suggests that institutional treatment 'provided, perhaps unwittingly, a smokescreen behind which the social conditions which predisposed to infection were obscured'. *Ibid.*, p. 85. For a detailed contemporary investigation into the effectiveness of sanatoria see Sir Arthur MacNalty, *Report on Tuberculosis: Including an Examination of the Results of Sanatorium Treatment*, London: HMSO, 1932.

31. Dubos and Dubos, 'Consumption and the Romantic Age', p. 65.

32. Cited in Linda Bryder, ' "Not always one and the same thing": the registration of tuberculosis deaths in Britain, 1900–1950', *Social History of Medicine*, vol. 9, 1996, p. 264.

33. Warboys.

34. See, for example, Thomas McKeown, *The Modern Rise of Population*, London: Edward Arnold, 1976; Thomas McKeown, *The Role of Medicine: Dream, Mirage, or Nemesis?*, Oxford: Blackwell, 1979 [1976]; Thomas McKeown, *The Origins of Human Disease*, Oxford: Blackwell, 1988. For other literature that broadly supports McKeown's interpretation for the decline of TB see, for example, William D. Johnston, *The Modern Epidemic: a History of Tuberculosis in Japan*, Harvard East Asian Monographs, 1995; F. B. Smith, *The Retreat of Tuberculosis, 1850–1950*, New York: Croom Helm, 1988; Heikki S. Vourinen,'The tuberculosis epidemic in Finland from the 18th to the 20th century' in Palfi *et al.*, pp. 107–12.

35. McKeown, *Modern Rise of Population*, pp. 94–5.

36. See, for example, John Duffy, *The Sanitarians: a History of American Public Health*, Urbana: University of Illinois Press, 1990; Richard J. Evans, 'Epidemics and revolutions: cholera in nineteenth-century Europe', in T. Ranger and P. Slack, eds., *Epidemics and Ideas: Essays on the Historical Perception of Pestilence*, Cambridge: Cambridge University Press, 1992, pp. 149–73; Anne Hardy, *The Epidemic Streets: Infectious Disease and the Rise of Preventive Medicine, 1856–1900*, Oxford: Clarendon Press, 1993; Gerry Kearns, 'Biology, class and the urban penalty', in Gerry Kearns and W. J. Withers, eds., *Urbanising Britain: Essays on Class and Community in the Nineteenth Century*, Cambridge: Cambridge University Press, 1991, pp. 12–30; Constance A. Nathanson, 'Disease prevention as social change: toward a theory of public health', *Population and Development Review*, vol. 22, 1996, pp. 609–37; Simon Szreter, 'The importance of social intervention in Britain's mortality decline c. 1850–1914: a reinterpretation of the role of public health', *Social History of Medicine*, vol. 1, 1988, pp. 1–37; Simon Szreter, 'Economic growth, disruption, deprivation, disease and death: on the importance of the politics of public

health for development', *Population and Development Review*, vol. 23, 1997, pp. 693–728.

37. Amy L. Fairchild and Gerald M. Oppenheimer, 'Public health nihilism versus pragmatism: history, politics, and the control of tuberculosis', *American Journal of Public Health*, vol. 88, 1998, pp. 1105–17.

38. Leonard G. Wilson, 'The historical decline of tuberculosis in Europe and America: its causes and significance', *Journal of the History of Medicine and Allied Sciences*, vol. 45, 1990, pp. 366–96.

39. See the exchange between Linda Bryder and Leonard Wilson in the *Journal of the History of Medicine and Allied Sciences*, vol. 46, 1991, pp. 358–68.

40. Koch, 'Epidemiology of tuberculosis', p. 37. See also Jacques Chrétien, 'La contribution française à la lutte contre la tuberculose et sa maîtrise', *Histoire des Sciences Médicales*, vol. 27, 1993, pp. 241–8; R.-H. Guerrand, 'Guerre à la tuberculose', *Histoire*, vol. 74, 1984, pp. 78–81.

41. Allan Mitchell, 'An inexact science: the statistics of tuberculosis in late nineteenth-century France', *Social History of Medicine*, vol. 3, 1990, p. 399.

42. David S. Barnes, 'The rise and fall of tuberculosis in Belle-Epoque France: a reply to Allan Mitchell', *Social History of Medicine*, vol. 5, 1992, pp. 279–90.

43. Koch, 'Epidemiology of tuberculosis'.

44. Fairchild and Oppenheimer.

45. Koch's observations on housing are in his 'Epidemiology of tuberculosis'. On Glasgow, see McFarlane. See also Gillian Cronje, 'Tuberculosis and mortality decline in England and Wales, 1851–1910', in Robert Woods and John Woodward, eds., *Urban Disease and Mortality in Nineteenth-century England*, New York: St Martin's Press, 1984.

46. There has been some degree of evolution between different regional strains of TB marked by varying degrees of virulence but the very limited degree of mutation in the TB bacillus suggests that these genetic variations cannot account for the epidemic of the disease through the nineteenth century and its gradual decline before the introduction of streptomycin in the 1940s. On the contribution of disease resistance to declining mortality see, for example, Silvia Bello, Michel Signoli, Márta Maczel and Olivier Dutour 1999, 'Evolution of mortality due to tuberculosis in France (18–20th centuries)' in Palfi *et al.*, pp. 95–104; R. P. O. Davies *et al.*, 'Historical declines in tuberculosis in England and Wales: improving social conditions or natural selection?' *Vesalius*, vol. 5, 1999, pp. 25–9.

47. Emily K. Abel, 'Taking the cure to the poor: patients' responses to New York City's tuberculosis program, 1894–1918', *American Journal of Public Health*, vol. 87, 1997, pp. 1808–15.

48. Daniel M. Fox, 'Social policy and city politics: tuberculosis reporting in New York, 1889–1900', *Bulletin of the History of Medicine*, vol. 49, 1975, pp. 169–95.

49. Ibid.

50. See, for example, Susan Craddock, *City of Plagues: Disease, Poverty, and Deviance in San Francisco*, Minneapolis: University of Minnesota Press, 2000; Sander L. Gilman, *Difference and Pathology: Stereotypes of Sexuality, Race, and Madness*, Ithaca: Cornell University Press, 1985; Sander L. Gilman, *Disease and Representation: Images of Illness from Madness to AIDS*, Ithaca: Cornell University Press, 1988.

51. Mark Harrison and Michael Warboys, ' "A disease of civilization": tuberculosis in Africa and India', in Lara Marks and Michael Warboys, eds., *Migrants, Minorities and Health: Historical and Contemporary Studies*, London and New York: Routledge, 1997, pp. 93–124; Michael Warboys, 'Tuberculosis and race in Britain and its empire, 1900–50', in Waltraud Ernst and Bernard Harris, eds., *Race, Science and Medicine, 1700–1960*, London and New York: Routledge, 1999, pp. 144–66.

52. Georgina D. Feldberg, *Disease and Class: Tuberculosis and the Shaping of Modern North American Society*, New Jersey: Rutgers University Press, 1995; Barbara Bates, *Bargaining for Life: a Social History of Tuberculosis, 1876–1938*, Philadelphia: University of Pennsylvania Press, 1992. On the surveys, see David McBride, *From TB to AIDS: Epidemics among Urban Blacks since 1900*, Albany: State University of New York Press, 1991.

53. See Harrison and Warboys, p. 102

54. George E. Bushnell, *A Study in the Epidemiology of Tuberculosis with Especial Reference to Tuberculosis of the Tropics and of the Negro Race*, London: John Bale, Sons & Danielsson, 1920, pp. 210, 155, 156.

55. Marion M. Torchia, 'The tuberculosis movement and the race question, 1890–1950', *Bulletin of the History of Medicine*, vol. 49, 1975, p. 161. See also Marion M. Torchia, 'Tuberculosis among American Negroes: medical research on a racial disease, 1830–1950', *Journal of the History of Medicine and Allied Sciences*, vol. 32, 1977, pp. 252–79.

56. Jessica M. Robbins, 'Class struggles in the tubercular world: nurses, patients, and physicians', *Bulletin of the History of Medicine*, vol. 71, 1997, pp. 412–34.

57. Peter Bryce, 'Tuberculosis in Relation to Feeblemindedness', Tuberculosis Monograph No. 3, New York City: Department of Health 1917, p. 5.

58. Harrison and Warboys.

59. Sontag, *Illness as Metaphor*, p. 83. See also Bruno Latour, *The Pasteurization of France*, Cambridge, MA: Harvard University Press, 1988; Allan Mitchell, 'Obsessive questions and faint answers: the French response to tuberculosis in the Belle Epoque', *Bulletin of the History of Medicine*, vol. 62, 1988, pp. 215–35; and P. Weindling, *Health, Race and German Politics between National Unification and Nazism, 1870–1945*, Cambridge: Cambridge University Press, 1989; Aly Götz, Peter Chroust and Christian Pross, *Cleansing the Fatherland: Nazi Medicine and Racial Hygiene*, Baltimore: Johns Hopkins University Press, 1994.

60. Johnston, 'Tuberculosis'.

61. Hinsdale, 'Atmospheric air in relation to tuberculosis'. On the develop-

ment of a vaccine, see Simon Flexner, 'Immunity in tuberculosis', *Annual Report of the Board of Regents of the Smithsonian Institution*, 1907, pp. 627–45; Hays, *The Burdens of Disease*.

62. Feldberg, *Disease and Class*.

63. Anne Marie Moulin, 'The impact of BCG on the history of tuberculosis', in Palfi *et al.*, pp. 77–86.

64. See, for example, Barron H. Lerner, 'From careless consumptives to recalcitrant patients: the historical construction of noncompliance', *Social Science and Medicine*, vol. 45, 1997, pp. 1423–31.

65. Typical examples of cultural explanations for high black rates of TB in the apartheid era include A. Barker, 'New doctors for an altered society', *South African Medical Journal*, vol. 45, 1971, pp. 558–61 and H. Dubovsky, 'Tuberculosis and art', *South African Medical Journal*, 64, 1983, pp. 823–6. For a detailed indictment of TB disparities in modern South Africa see Neil Andersson, 'Tuberculosis and social stratification in South Africa', *International Journal of Health Services* 20, 1990, pp. 141–65; Randall M. Packard, *White Plague, Black Labor: Tuberculosis and the Political Economy of Health and Disease in South Africa*, Berkeley, CA: University of California Press, 1989.

66. Mahfouz H. Zaki and Mary E. Hibberd, 'The tuberculosis story: from Koch to the year 2000', *Caduceus*, vol. 12, 1996, pp. 43–60.

67. F. J. C. Millard, 'The rising incidence of tuberculosis', *Journal of the Royal Society of Medicine*, vol. 89, 1996, p. 497.

68. J. Arthur Myers, *Tuberculosis: a Half Century of Study and Conquest*, St Louis, Missouri: Warren H. Green, 1970, p. 309.

69. See Karen Brudney and Jay Dobkin, 'Resurgent tuberculosis in New York City: human immunodeficiency virus, homelessness, and the decline of tuberculosis control programs', *American Review of Respiratory Disease*, vol. 144, 1991, pp. 745–9; E. Drucker *et al.*, 'Childhood tuberculosis in the Bronx, New York', *Lancet*, vol. 343, 1994, pp. 1482–5; Barron H. Lerner, 'New York City's tuberculosis control efforts: the historical limitations of the "war on consumption"', *American Journal of Public Health*, 83, 1993, pp. 758–67; Dixie E. Snider, Louis Salinas and Gloria D. Kelly, 'Tuberculosis: an increasing problem among minorities in the United States', *Public Health Reports*, vol. 104, 1989, pp. 646–53.

70. K. Neville, A. Bromberg and R. Bromberg, 'The third epidemic – multidrug-resistant tuberculosis', *Chest*, vol. 105, 1994, 45–8; C. M. Nolan, 'Nosocomial multidrug-resistant tuberculosis – global spread of the third epidemic', *Journal of Infectious Diseases*, vol. 76, 1997, pp. 748–51; P. Small and A. Moss, 'Molecular epidemiology and the new tuberculosis', *Infections and Agents of Disease*, vol. 2, 1993; P. Small, R. Shafer and P. Hopewell, 'Exogenous reinfection with multidrug-resistant *Mycobacterium tuberculosis* in patients with advanced HIV infection', *New England Journal of Medicine*, vol. 328, 1993.

71. See I. N. Okeke, A. Lamikanra and R. Edelman, 'Socio-economic and

behavioural factors leading to acquired bacterial resistance to antibiotics in developing countries', *Emerging Infectious Diseases*, vol. 5, 1999, pp. 18–27.

72. Paul Farmer and J. Y. Kim, 'Community based approaches to the control of multidrug resistant tuberculosis: introducing "DOTS-plus"', *British Medical Journal*, 317, 1998, p. 671–4.

73. A. Kochi, B. Vareldzis and K. Styblo, 'Multidrug-resistant tuberculosis and its control', *Res Microbiol*, vol. 144, 1993, pp. 104–10.

74. Farmer and Kim, 'Community based approaches'.

75. Sarah Boseley, 'Warning as TB cases increase', *Guardian*, 14 December 1999.

76. See A. Zumla, M. Johnson and R. F. Miller, eds., *AIDS and Respiratory medicine*, London: Chapman and Hall, 1997.

77. L. K. Altman, 'Parts of Africa showing HIV in 1 in 4 adults', *New York Times*, 24 June 1998. In the absence of immuno-suppression, people who have overcome primary TB have about a 5 per cent chance of developing post-primary tuberculosis at some time during the remainder of their lives. In contrast, HIV-positive persons have an 8 per cent chance annually of developing TB, rising to a total of 50 per cent during the remainder of their shortened life span. Jacques Chrétien, 'Tuberculosis and HIV: the cursed duet', *Bulletin of the International Union against Tuberculosis and Lung Disease*, 65, 1990, pp. 25–8; R. Coker and R. F. Miller, 'HIV associated tuberculosis', *British Medical Journal*, vol. 314, 1997, p. 1847; Frances Elender, Graham Bentham and Ian Langford, 'Tuberculosis mortality in England and Wales during 1982–1992: its association with poverty, ethnicity and AIDS', *Social Science and Medicine*, vol. 46, 1998, pp. 673–81; World Health Organization, *Tuberculosis in the Era of HIV: a Deadly Partnership*, Geneva: World Health Organization, 1996.

78. M. Van Cleef and H. J. Chum, 'The proportion of tuberculosis cases in Tanzania attributable to human immunodeficiency virus', *International Journal of Epidemiology*, vol. 24, 1995, pp. 637–42.

79. See Ronald Bayer, 'Public health policy and tuberculosis', *Journal of Health Politics, Policy and Law*, vol. 19, 1994, pp. 149–54; Ronald Bayer and David Wilkinson, 'Directly observed therapy for tuberculosis: history of an idea', *Lancet*, vol. 345, 1995, pp. 1545–8; R. Bayer, *Private Acts, Social Consequences: AIDS and the Politics of Public Health*, New Brunswick, NJ: Rutgers University Press, 1991; R. Bayer, N. N. Dubler, and S. Landesman, 'The dual epidemics of tuberculosis and AIDS: ethical and policy issues in screening and treatment', *American Journal of Public Health*, vol. 83, 1993, pp. 649–54; Richard J. Coker, *From Chaos to Coercion: Detention and the Control of Tuberculosis*, New York: St Martin's Press, 2000.

80. See, for example, Matthew Smallman-Raynor and Andrew Cliff, 'Civil war and the spread of AIDS in Africa', *Epidemiology and Infection*, vol. 107, 1991, pp. 69–79.

81. See Paul Farmer, 'Social scientists and the new tuberculosis', *Social Science and Medicine*, vol. 44, 1997, pp. 347–58.

82. Eric Naterop and Ivan Wolffers, 'The role of the privatization process on tuberculosis control in Ho Chi Minh City Province, Vietnam', *Social Science and Medicine*, vol. 48, 1999, pp. 1589–98. See also P. Kamolratanakul *et al.*, 'Economic impact of tuberculosis at the household level', *International Journal of Tuberculosis and Lung Disease*, vol. 3, 1999, pp. 596–602.

83. Theodore H. Tulchinsky and Elena A. Varavikova, 'Addressing the epidemiologic transition in the former Soviet Union: strategies for health system and public health reform in Russia', *American Journal of Public Health*, vol. 86, 1996, pp. 313–23; R. Wallace *et al.*, 'The spatiotemporal dynamics of AIDS and TB in the New York metropolitan region from a sociogeographic perspective: understanding the linkages of central city and suburbs', *Environment and Planning A*, vol. 27, 1995, 1085–1108; R. Wallace and D. Wallace, 'The destruction of US minority urban communities and the resurgence of tuberculosis: ecosystem dynamics and the white plague in the de-developing world', *Environment and Planning A*, vol. 29, 1997, 269–91.

84. World Health Organization 1948 cited in Mildred Blaxter, 'Health', in William Outhwaite and Tom Bottomore, eds., *The Blackwell Dictionary of Twentieth-century Social Thought*, Oxford: Blackwell, 1993, p. 254.

85. World Health Organization, *TB – A Global Emergency*, Geneva: WHO, 1994.

86. Laurie Garrett, *Betrayal of Trust: The Collapse of Global Public Health*, New York: Hyperion, 2000; Claire Ainsworth and Debora MacKenzie, 'Coming home', *New Scientist*, vol. 171, 7 July 2001, pp. 28–33.

2 Immigration, Race and Geographies of Difference in the Tuberculosis Pandemic

This chapter contains material from Chapter 4 of my PhD thesis, 'Infectious disease in a world of goods', Harvard University, 2001. I would like to thank Orit Halpern, Allan M. Brandt, Jeremy Greene, David Jones, Julie Livingston, and Abena D. A. Osseo-Asare for helpful comments on earlier drafts of this chapter.

1. Susan Sachs, 'More screening of immigrants for TB sought', *New York Times*, 3 January 2000, p. A1.

2. Bruce Johnston, 'Italians fear new surge of illegal migrants', *Sunday Telegraph*, 19 October 1997.

3. Preecha Srisathan Kanchanaburi, 'New drive to promote regional trade links. Opening checkpoints "may spread diseases" ', *Bangkok Post*, 5 April 1998.

4. S. Jody Heymann et al., 'The need for global action against multidrug-resistant tuberculosis', Journal of the American Medical Association, vol. 281, 9 June 1999, pp. 2138–40; David E. Griffith, 'The United States and worldwide tuberculosis control: a second chance for Prince Prospero', Chest, vol. 113, June 1998, pp. 1434–6; Charles D. Wells, 'A study of tuberculosis among foreign-born Hispanic persons in the US states bordering Mexico', American Journal of Respiratory and Critical Care Medicine, vol. 159, 1999, pp. 834–7. See also Patrick L. F. Zuber, 'Long-term risk of tuberculosis among foreign-born persons in the United States', Journal of the American Medical Association, vol. 278, 23 July 1997, pp. 304–7.

5. For providing a model for the role of historical scholarship in the analysis of contemporary epidemics, I am indebted to Allan M. Brandt's essay, 'AIDS in historical perspective: four lessons from the history of sexually transmitted diseases', American Journal of Public Health, vol. 78, April 1988, pp. 367–71.

6. For the sake of clarity and brevity, this chapter focuses primarily on the United States and, to a lesser extent, Western Europe. Many of the points contained in it are applicable to other parts of the world. However, it is important to note that American and European understandings of race and immigration are rooted in those countries' peculiar histories, and thus do not necessarily reflect the experience of other countries or regions.

7. Paul Farmer, AIDS and Accusation: Haiti and the Geography of Blame, Berkeley: University of California Press, 1992.

8. Roy Porter, The Greatest Benefit to Mankind, New York: W. W. Norton, 1997, p. 166.

9. Judith Walzer Leavitt, Typhoid Mary: Captive to the Public's Health, Boston: Beacon Press, 1996.

10. Paula Treichler, 'AIDS and HIV infection in the Third World: a First World chronicle', in Barbara Kruger, ed., Remaking History, Seattle: Bay Press, 1989; Simon Watney, 'Missionary positions: AIDS, "Africa", and race', in Russell Ferguson et al., eds., Out There: Marginalization and Contemporary Culture, Cambridge: MIT Press, 1990; Sander L. Gilman, 'Plague in Germany, 1939/1989: cultural images of race, space, and disease', in Andrew Parker et al., eds., Nationalisms and Sexualities, New York: Routledge, 1992; Paul Farmer, AIDS and Accusation.

11. This topic is covered in detail in my PhD thesis, 'Infectious disease in a world of goods'. See also: Joshua Lederberg et al., eds., Emerging Infections: Microbial Threats to Health In the United States, Washington: National Academy Press, 1992; Board on International Health, Institute of Medicine, America's Vital Interest in Global Health: Protecting Our People, Enhancing Our Economy, and Advancing Our International Interests, Washington, DC: National Academy Press, 1997.

12. Geoffrey Cowley, 'Outbreak of fear', Newsweek, 22 May 1995, p. 52.

13. Often used inconsistently and without clear or precise definition, the terms 'race', 'ethnicity', and 'immigrant' present any researcher with a number

of problems. Each has long been recognized by scientists and social scientists alike as social constructs rather than essential biological characteristics, and there is considerable debate over whether these terms have any utility in the theory and practice of public health. In this chapter, I assume that – whether or not they are either 'real' or useful – the continued usage of these categories by social actors (including scientists, policymakers and lay people) has important ramifications on both health and health policy. See Nancy Kreiger, 'Refiguring "race": epidemiology, racialized biology, and biological expressions of race relations', *International Journal of Health Services*, vol. 20, no. 1, 2000, pp. 211–16; Lara Marks and Michael Worboys, 'Introduction', in Marks and Worboys, eds., *Migrants, Minorities and Health*, London: Routledge, 1997.

14. Georgina D. Feldberg, *Disease and Class: Tuberculosis and the Shaping of Modern North American Society*, New Brunswick: Rutgers University Press, 1995, pp. 104–9; Alan M. Kraut, *Silent Travelers: Germs, Genes, and the 'Immigrant Menace'*, Baltimore: Johns Hopkins University Press, 1994.

15. On the relationship between tuberculosis and racial and cultural difference, see the following: Mark Harrison and Michael Worboys, 'A disease of civilization: tuberculosis in Britain, Africa and India, 1900–39', in Marks and Worboys, eds., *Migrants, Minorities and Health*; Randall M. Packard, *White Plague, Black Labor: Tuberculosis and the Political Economy of Health and Disease in South Africa*, Berkeley: University of California Press, 1989, pp. 105–8.

16. David McBride calls this 'sociomedical racism'. See Chapter one of his *From Tuberculosis to AIDS: Epidemics Among Urban Blacks Since 1900*, Albany: State University of New York, 1991. See also: Kraut, *Silent Travelers*; Treichler, 'AIDS and HIV infection in the Third World'; Watney, 'Missionary positions'.

17. Quoted in 'Perspectives 1994', *Newsweek*, 26 December 1994, p. 85.

18. The terms 'essentialist' and 'anti-essentialist' are not used by public health researchers themselves. The distinction between strategies that emphasize essential and contingent differences is, of course, itself an oversimplification. The two approaches are not necessarily mutually exclusive, and observers often display a wide range of both responses simultaneously. Nevertheless, I believe that the distinction is useful as a heuristic device in evaluating political and public health responses to health disparities.

19. The classic source for the formulation of tuberculosis as a 'social disease' is Rene Dubos and Jean Dubos, *The White Plague: Tuberculosis, Man, and Society*, New Brunswick: Rutgers University Press, 1987 [1952]; see also Barbara Rosenkrantz's introductory essay to the Dubos volume; Kevin B. Weiss, 'Tuberculosis: poverty's penalty', *American Journal of Respiratory and Critical Care Medicine*, vol. 157, 1998, p. 1011.

20. The exact relationship between these factors and tuberculosis is extremely complicated, and has inspired considerable debate in a number of areas.

For example, a number of historians contend that changes in political economy – including rising standards of living and better sanitation and nutrition – rather than specific therapeutic or preventive efforts were responsible for the massive mortality decline in the nineteenth and early twentieth centuries. This debate has been carried into the present by those who wonder what is the most appropriate strategy to address TB in the future. The classic source is Thomas McKeown, *The Role of Medicine: Dream, Mirage, or Nemesis?* Oxford: Blackwell, 1979 [1976]. See also: Nancy J. Tomes, 'Essay review: the White Plague revisited', *Bulletin of the History of Medicine*, vol. 63, 1989, pp. 467–80; Leonard G. Wilson, 'The historical decline of tuberculosis in Europe and America: its causes and significance', *Journal of the History of Medicine and Allied Sciences*, vol. 45, July 1990, pp. 366–96; David S. Barnes, 'The rise or fall of tuberculosis in Belle-Epoque France', *Social History of Medicine*, vol. 5, 1992, pp. 279–90; Simon Szreter, 'The importance of social intervention in Britain's mortality decline, 1850–1914: a re-interpretation of the role of public health', *Social History of Medicine*, vol. 1, 1988, pp. 1–37; Amy Fairchild and Gerald Oppenheimer, 'Public health nihilism vs. pragmatism: history, politics, and the control of tuberculosis', *American Journal of Public Health*, vol. 88, July 1998, pp. 1105–17; Paul Farmer and Edward Nardell, 'Editorial: nihilism and pragmatism in tuberculosis control', *American Journal of Public Health*, vol. 88, July 1998, pp. 1014–15.

21. S. C. Pang *et al.*, 'Tuberculosis surveillance in immigrants through health undertakings in Western Australia', *International Journal of Tuberculosis and Lung Disease*, vol. 4, no. 3, March 2000, pp. 232–6; R. Bwire, 'Tuberculosis screening among immigrants in the Netherlands: what is its contribution to public health?' *Netherlands Journal of Medicine*, vol. 56, 2000, pp. 63–71.

22. Statistics for the United States from Zuber, 'Long-term risk of tuberculosis'; Nancy J. Binkin, 'Overseas screening for tuberculosis in immigrants and refugees to the United States: current status', *Clinical Infectious Diseases*, vol. 23, 1996, pp. 1226–32; P. L. Zuber *et al.*, 'Tuberculosis among foreign-born persons in Los Angeles County', 1992–1994', *Tuberculosis and Lung Disease*, vol. 77, December 1996, pp. 524–30; Michael F. Cantwell, 'Epidemiology of tuberculosis in the United States, 1985 through 1992', *Journal of the American Medical Association*, vol. 272, 17 August 1994, pp. 535–9.

23. Barbara Sibbald, 'Infected MD calls for tougher medical screening of newcomers to Canada', *Canadian Medical Association Journal*, vol. 160, 20 April 1999, pp. 1201; Michael D. Iseman and Jeffrey Starke, 'Immigration and tuberculosis control', *New England Journal of Medicine*, vol. 332, 20 April 1995, pp. 1094–5.

24. Kevin R. Johnson, 'Fear of an "Alien Nation": race, immigration, and immigrants', *Stanford Law and Policy Review*, vol. 7, 1996, pp. 111–26.

25. Since tuberculosis is not recognized as a medical emergency (unless it is

meningeal, pulmonary with respiratory failure, or involves massive haemoptysis), Proposition 187 effectively prevented tubercular immigrants
from receiving a timely diagnosis and treatment.

26. Kimberly A. Johns and Christos Varkoutas, 'The tuberculosis crisis:
the deadly consequence of immigration policies and welfare reform',
Journal of Contemporary Health Law and Policy, vol. 15, Fall, 1998,
pp. 101–30; Julia A. Martin, 'Proposition 187, tuberculosis, and the
immigration epidemic?' *Stanford Law and Policy Review*, vol. 7, 1996,
pp. 89–109; Guido S. Weber, 'Unresolved issues in controlling the tuberculosis epidemic among the foreign-born in the United States', *American
Journal of Law and Medicine*, vol. 22, 1996, pp. 503–36; Steven Asch,
'Does fear of immigration authorities deter tuberculosis patients from
seeking care?' *Western Journal of Medicine*, vol. 161, October 1994,
pp. 373–6.

27. The following argument also applies to its more palatable but no less
ambiguous cousin, 'foreign-born'.

28. Johnson, 'Fear of an "alien nation"'; Margaret A. Somerville, 'Crossing
boundaries: travel, immigration, human rights and AIDS', *McGill Law
Journal*, vol. 43, 1998, pp. 781–834; Kraut, *Silent Travelers*; David Theo
Goldberg, *Racist Culture: Philosophy and the Politics of Meaning*, Cambridge: Blackwell, 1993.

29. Johnston, 'Italians fear new surge of illegal migrants'.

30. P. M. Small *et al.*, 'The epidemiology of tuberculosis in San Francisco: a
population-based study using conventional and molecular methods', *New
England Journal of Medicine*, vol. 330, 16 June 1994, pp. 1703–9; C. R.
MacIntyre and A. J. Plant, 'Longitudinal incidence of tuberculosis in
South-East Asian refugees after resettlement', *International Journal of
Tuberculosis and Lung Disease*, vol. 3, April 1999, pp. 287–93; Bwire,
'Tuberculosis screening among immigrants in the Netherlands'.

31. N. W. Schluger, 'The impact of drug resistance on the global tuberculosis
epidemic', *International Journal of Tuberculosis and Lung Disease*, vol. 4,
p. S74.

32. MacIntyre and Plant, 'Longitudinal incidence', p. 287.

33. R. M. Jasmer *et al.*, 'Tuberculosis in Mexican-born persons in San
Francisco: reactivation, acquired infection and transmission', *International
Journal of Tuberculosis and Lung Disease*, vol. 1, 1997, pp. 536–41; M.
W. Borgdorff *et al.*, 'Transmission of tuberculosis in San Francisco and its
association with immigration and ethnicity', *International Journal of
Tuberculosis and Lung Disease*, vol. 4, April 2000, pp. 287–94. See also
Matthew T. McKenna, 'The epidemiology of tuberculosis among foreign-
born persons in the United States, 1986 to 1993', *New England Journal
of Medicine*, vol. 332, 20 April 1995, pp. 1071–6.

34. On the US, see Daniel P. Chin *et al.*, 'Differences in contributing factors
to tuberculosis incidence in US-born and foreign-born persons', *American
Journal of Respiratory and Critical Care Medicine*, vol. 158, 1998,

pp. 1797–1803; Kathryn DeRiemer, 'Tuberculosis among immigrants and refugees', *Archives of Internal Medicine*, vol. 158, 13 April 1998, pp. 753–60. On the UK, see Peter Ormerod, 'Screening immigrants at risk of tuberculosis', *British Medical Journal*, vol. 308, 12 March 1994, pp. 720–1.

35. Paul Farmer, Mercedes Becerra and Jim Yong Kim, eds., *The Global Impact of Drug-resistant Tuberculosis*, Boston: Program in Infectious Disease and Social Change, Harvard Medical School, 1999, especially Chapter 2; Jim Yong Kim *et al.*, eds., *Dying For Growth: Global Inequality and the Health of the Poor*, Monroe, ME: Common Courage Press, 2000.

36. David McBride, 'Tuberculosis in African-American and minority populations: historic epidemiology of a nonclassic contagious process', *Journal of the Association for Academic Minority Physicians*, vol. 5, January 1994, pp. 11–15. The figures are from Cantwell, 'Epidemiology of tuberculosis in the United States'.

37. Ormerod, 'Screening immigrants'.

38. Zhiyuan Liu, 'Distinct trends in tuberculosis morbidity among foreign-born and US-born persons in New Jersey, 1986 through 1995', *American Journal of Public Health*, vol. 88, July 1998, pp. 1064–7.

39. See note 11 above.

40. W. W. Stead *et al.*, 'Racial differences in susceptibility to infection by *Mycobacterium tuberculosis*', *New England Journal of Medicine*, vol. 22, 1990, pp. 422–7; R. Bellamy *et al.*, 'Variations in the *NRAMP1* gene and susceptibility to tuberculosis in West Africans', *New England Journal of Medicine*, vol. 338, 1998, pp. 640–4. See also David S. Barnes, 'Historical perspectives on the etiology of tuberculosis', *Microbes and Infection*, vol. 2, 2000, pp. 431–40.

41. This does not mean that *no* health disparities are rooted in physiology or genetics. For example, the higher prevalence of disorders such as sickle-cell disease among African-Americans is likely due to genetic differences.

42. We should note that there is some debate as to the exact linkage between homelessness and health status – that is, are people more likely to be ill because they are homeless, or do those with health problems run a greater risk of becoming homeless? Statistics on homelessness from Kristy Woods, 'Homelessness: a risk factor for poor health', in Annette Dula and Sara Goering, eds., *'It Just Ain't Fair': The Ethics of Health Care for African Americans*, Westport: Praeger, 1994, p. 106.

43. Victor W. Sidel, 'The resurgence of tuberculosis in the United States: societal origins and societal response', *Journal of Law, Medicine and Ethics*, vol. 21, Fall–Winter 1993, pp. 303–16.

44. However, this adjustment had little apparent impact on rates for foreign-born African Americans and Asians. Michael F. Cantwell, 'Tuberculosis and race/ethnicity in the United States', *American Journal of Respiratory and Critical Care Medicine*, vol. 157, 1998, pp. 1016–20.

45. McBride, 'Tuberculosis in African-American and minority populations'.

However, we should note the difficulty inherent in comparing studies conducted according to different methodologies and in different time periods, especially since the definition and understanding of racial difference itself changes over time.

46. George Davey Smith *et al.*, 'Mortality differences between black and white men in the USA: contribution of income and other risk factors among men screened for the MRFIT', *Lancet*, vol. 351, 28 March 1998, pp. 934–9.

47. For a comprehensive review, see Nancy Kreiger, 'Discrimination and health', in Lisa F. Berkman and Ichiro Kawachi, eds., *Social Epidemiology*, New York: Oxford University Press, 2000.

48. Victor W. Sidel, 'The resurgence of tuberculosis in the United States: societal origins and societal response', *Journal of Law, Medicine and Ethics*, vol. 21, Fall–Winter 1993, pp. 303–16; Woods, 'Homelessness: a risk factor for poor health'.

49. The experiment involved pretending to treat African-Americans for syphilis in order to observe the long-term progression of the disease. Allan M. Brandt, 'Racism and research: the case of the Tuskegee syphilis study', in Judith Leavitt and Ronald Numbers, eds., *Sickness and Health in America: Readings in the History of Medicine and Public Health*, Madison: University of Wisconsin Press, 1997, pp. 392–404; Stephen J. Gould, *The Mismeasure of Man*, New York: Norton, 1996.

50. Barron H. Lerner, 'Tuberculosis in Seattle, 1949–1973: balancing public health and civil liberties', *Western Journal of Medicine*, vol. 171, July 1999, pp. 44–9.

51. M. C. Becerra, P. E. Farmer and J. Y. Kim, 'The problem of drug-resistant tuberculosis: an overview', in Farmer *et al.*, eds. *The Global Impact of Drug-Resistant Tuberculosis*, p. 37.

52. Saskia Sassen, 'Immigration and local labor markets', in Alexander Portes, ed., *The Economic Sociology of Immigration: Essays in Networks, Ethnicity, and Entrepreneurship*, New York: Russell Sage Foundation Press, 1994; M. Patricia Fernandez-Kelly, 'Migration, race, and ethnicity in the design of the American city', in Russell Ferguson, ed., *Urban Revisions: Current Projects for the Public Realm*, Cambridge, MA: MIT Press, 1994.

3   Gender and Tuberculosis: A Conceptual Framework for Identifying Gender Inequalities

1. I. Smith, *Women and Tuberculosis: gender issues and tuberculosis control in Nepal*, unpublished MA dissertation, Nuffield Institute for Health, 1994.

2. J. A. Kumaresan *et al.*, eds., *The Global Burden of Disease and Risk Factors in 1990*, Geneva: World Health Organization, 1996.

3. G. Rubin, 'The traffic in Women: notes on the political economy of sex', in R. Reiter, ed., *Toward an Anthropology of Women*, New York: Monthly Review Press, 1975.

4. See, for example, Butler, *Gender Trouble: Feminism and the Subversion of Identity*, New York: Routledge, 1990.

5. World Health Organization, *Global Tuberculosis Report 1999*, Geneva: World Health Organization, 2000.

6. E. M. Rathgeber and C. Vlassoff, 'Gender and tropical diseases: a new research focus', *Social Science and Medicine*, vol. 37, 1993, pp. 513–20.

7. L. Doyal, *What Makes Women Sick: Gender and the Political Economy of Health*, London: Macmillan, 1995.

8. A. G. Tinker *et al.*, *Women's Health and Nutrition: Making a Difference*, Washington, DC: World Bank, 1994.

9. Rathgeber and Vlassoff, 'Gender and tropical diseases'.

10. L. Manderson, J. Jenkins and M. Tanner, 'Women and tropical diseases', *Social Science and Medicine*, vol. 37, 1993, pp. 441–3.

11. S. Rao *et al.*, 'Gender differentials in the social impact of leprosy', Pune, India: Aghakar Research Institute, unpublished report, 1996; P. Boonmongkon, 'Khi thut, *'The Disease of Social Loathing'*: An Anthropological Study of the Stigma in Leprosy in Rural North–North-East Thailand, Washington: UN Development Programme, Social and Economic Research Project Report, no. 17, 1994; J. C. Paz, I. R. Medina and E. R. Ventura, *A Multidisciplinary Study of Stigma in Relation to Hansen's Disease among the Tausug in the Philippines*, (Social and Economic Research Project Report, no. 7), Washington: UN Development Programme, 1994.

12. S. Rao *et al.*, 'Differences in detection patterns between male and female leprosy patients in Maharashtra', Pune, India: Aghakar Research Institute, 1996.

13. M. B. Ettling *et al.*, 'Evaluation of malaria clinics in Maesot, Thailand: use of serology to assess coverage', *Transactions of the Royal Society for Tropical Medicine and Hygiene*, vol. 83, 1989, pp. 325–31.

14. World Health Organization, *Gender and leishmaniasis in Colombia, a Redefinition of Existing Concepts?* (Gender and Tropical Diseases Resource Paper no. 2), Geneva: World Health Organization, 1996.

15. World Health Organization, *Global Tuberculosis Report 1999*.

16. V. Diwan and A. Thorson, 'Sex, gender and tuberculosis', *Lancet*, vol. 353, 1999, pp. 1000–1; V. Diwan, A. Thorson and A. Winkvist, eds., *Gender and Tuberculosis: An International Research Workshop*, Göteborg: Nordic School of Public Health, 1998.

17. N. H. Long, 'Gender specific epidemiology of tuberculosis in Vietnam', unpublished PhD thesis, Stockholm: Karolinska Institute, 2000.

18. C. B. Holmes, H. Hausler and P. Nunn, 'A review of sex differences in the epidemiology of tuberculosis', *International Journal of Tuberculosis and Lung Disease*, vol. 2, 1998, pp. 96–104.

19. K. Kurosawa, 'Tuberculin skin tests of patients with active pulmonary tuberculosis and non-tuberculosis pulmonary disease', *Kekkaku*, vol. 65, 1990, pp. 47–52.

20. M. A. Shaaben *et al*, 'Revaccination with BCG: its effect on skin tests in Kuwaiti senior school children', *European Respiratory Journal*, vol. 3, 1990, pp. 187–91.

21. G. Bothamley, 'Sex and gender in the pathogenesis of infectious tuberculosis: a perspective from immunology, microbiology and human genetics', in Diwan *et al.*, *Gender and Tuberculosis*.

22. T. Olakowski, *Tuberculosis longitudinal survey*, Bangalore, India: National Tuberculosis Institute/WHO Regional Office for South East Asia, 1973.

23. G. W. Comstock, V. T. Livesay and S. F. Woolpert, 'The prognosis of a positive tuberculin reaction in childhood and adolescence', *American Journal of Epidemiology*, vol. 99, 1974, pp. 131–8.

24. Holmes *et al.*, 'A review of sex differences'.

25. J. Grange, A. Ustianowski and A. Zumla, 'Tuberculosis and pregnancy', in Diwan *et al.*, *Gender and Tuberculosis*.

26. M. Espinal, A. L. Reingold and M. Lavandera, 'Effect of pregnancy on the risk of developing active tuberculosis', *Journal of Infectious Disease*, vol. 173, 1996, pp. 488–91.

27. J. Grange, A. Ustianowski and A. Zumla, 'Tuberculosis and pregnancy'.

28. A. Thorson, N. P. Hoa and N. H. Long, 'Health seeking behaviour of men and women with a cough for more than three weeks', *Lancet*, forthcoming.

29. E. Johansson, 'Emerging perspectives on tuberculosis and gender in Vietnam', unpublished thesis, Umeå University, Sweden, 2000.

30. Bi Puranen, 'Tuberkulos: en sjukdoms förekomst och dess orsaker: Sverige, 1750–1980', unpublished PhD thesis, Umeå University, 1984.

31. E. Johansson *et al.*, 'Attitudes to compliance with tuberculosis treatment among men and women in Vietnam', *International Journal of Tuberculosis and Lung Disease*, vol. 3, 1999, pp. 1–7.

32. Long, 'Gender specific epidemiology of tuberculosis in Vietnam'.

33. H. L. Reider, D. E. Snider, G. H. Cauthen, 'Extrapulmonary tuberculosis in the United States', *American Review of Respiratory Disease*, vol. 141, 1990, pp. 347–51.

34. Bothamley, 'Sex and gender'.

35. World Health Organization, *Global Tuberculosis Control*.

36. Holmes *et al.*, 'A review of sex differences'.

37. A. Cassels, E. Heineman and S. Le Clerq, 'Tuberculosis case-finding in Eastern Nepal', *Tubercle*, vol. 63, 1982, pp. 173–85.

38. M. Borgdorff *et al.*, 'Gender and tuberculosis: a comparison of prevalence surveys with notification data to explore sex differences in case detection', *International Journal of Tuberculosis and Lung Disease*, vol. 4, 2000, pp. 123–32.

39. N. H. Long *et al.*, 'Longer delays in tuberculosis diagnosis among women in Vietnam', *International Journal of Tuberculosis and Lung Disease*, vol. 3, 1999, pp. 388–93.

40. Long, 'Gender specific epidemiology'.
41. N. K. Wenger, 'Coronary heart disease in women: gender differences in diagnostic evaluation', *Journal of the American Medical Association*, vol. 49, 1994, pp. 181–5.
42. R. Liefooghe, 'Gender differences in beliefs and attitudes towards tuberculosis and their impact on tuberculosis control: what do we know?' in Diwan *et al.*, eds., *Gender and Tuberculosis*.
43. M. Zwarenstein *et al.*, 'Randomized controlled trial of self-supervised and directly-observed treatment of tuberculosis', *Lancet*, vol. 352, 1998, pp. 1340–3.
44. J. Volmink, P. Matchaba and P. Gamer, 'Directly observed therapy and treatment adherence', *Lancet*, vol. 355, 2000, pp. 1345–50.
45. Johansson, 'Emerging perspectives on tuberculosis and gender'.
46. E. Johansson and A. Winkvist, 'Trust and transparency in human encounters in tuberculosis control: lessons learned from Vietnam', *Qualitative Health Research*, vol. 12, 2002, pp. 473–91.
47. Olakowski, *Tuberculosis longitudinal survey*.
48. Holmes *et al.*, 'A review of sex differences'.
49. J. E. Olle-Goig, 'Patients with tuberculosis in Bolivia: why do they die?' *Revista Panam Salud Publica*, vol. 8, 2000, pp. 151–5.
50. R. F. Grimble, 'Malnutrition and the immune response 2: impact of nutrients on cytokine biology infection', *Transactions of the Royal Society for Tropical Medicine and Hygiene*, vol. 6, pp. 615–19.
51. D. Shimeles and S. Lulseged, 'Clinical profile and pattern of infection in Ethiopian children with severe protein-energy malnutrition', *East Africa Medical Journal*, vol. 71, 1994, pp. 264–7; M. Vijayakumar, M. Bhaskaram, and P. Hemalatha, 'Malnutrition and childhood tuberculosis', *Journal of Tropical Paediatrics*, vol. 36, 1990, pp. 294–8.
52. Johansson, 'Emerging perspectives on tuberculosis'.

4   War and Disease: Some Perspectives on the Spatial and Temporal Occurrence of Tuberculosis in Wartime

The research for this chapter has been undertaken as part of a five-year programme of research entitled 'Disease in War, 1850–1990: Geographical Patterns, Spread and Demographic Impact', funded by the Leverhulme Trust. Its financial support is gratefully acknowledged.

1. Marc Daniels, 'Tuberculosis in post-war Europe: an international problem', *Tubercle*, vol. 28, no. 10, 1947, p. 201.
2. See, for example, Friedrich Prinzing, *Epidemics Resulting from Wars*, Oxford: Clarendon Press, 1916; Ralph Major, *War and Disease*, London: Hutchinson, 1940; Clara E. Councell, 'War and infectious disease', *Public Health Reports*, vol. 56, no. 12, 1941; Barry S. Levy and Victor W. Sidel, eds., *War and Public Health*, Oxford: Oxford University Press, 1997;

Samuel Dumas and K. O. Vedel Petersen, *Losses of Life Caused by War*, Oxford: Clarendon Press, 1923, pp. 49–50.

3. On this influenza pandemic, see Edwin O. Jordan, *Epidemic Influenza: A Survey*, Chicago: American Medical Association, 1927.

4. Councell, 'War and infectious disease'.

5. See, for example: ibid.; Henry O. Lancaster, *Expectations of Life: A Study in the Demography, Statistics, and History of World Mortality*, Berlin: Springer-Verlag, 1990, pp. 314–40.

6. Daniels, 'Tuberculosis in post-war Europe', p. 201.

7. See, for example: Matthew Smallman-Raynor and Andrew D. Cliff, 'The spatial dynamics of epidemic diseases in war and peace: Cuba and the insurrection against Spain, 1895–98', *Transactions of the Institute of British Geographers*, vol. 24, no. 3, 1999; Matthew Smallman-Raynor and Andrew D. Cliff, 'The epidemiological legacy of war: the Philippine-American War and the diffusion of cholera in Batangas and La Laguna, South-West Luzón, 1902–1904', *War in History*, vol. 7, no. 1, 2000.

8. Although the years of the Austro-Prussian War (1866) and the Franco-Prussian War (1870–71) were accompanied by marked increases in mortality from pulmonary TB in England and Wales (Figure 4.1), evidence for a direct epidemiological link with the conflicts is generally lacking. We note, however, that fugitives from the warring states played a pivotal role in the spread of other infectious diseases (most notably, smallpox in 1870–71) to, and within, England and Wales (see, for example: J. D. Rolleston, 'The smallpox pandemic of 1870–1874', *Proceedings of the Royal Society of Medicine, Section of Epidemiology and State Medicine*, vol. 27, no. 1, 1933). Under these circumstances, and by analogy with the international movements of tuberculous refugees in more recent conflicts, the mortality levels associated with the Austro-Prussian and Franco-Prussian wars in Figure 4.1 may have been inflated – to a greater or lesser extent – by continental Europeans in search of refuge from the troubles.

9. For an overview of host-dependent and primary environmental factors in the aetiology of TB, see: William D. Johnston, 'Tuberculosis', in Kenneth F. Kiple, ed., *Cambridge World History of Human Disease*, Cambridge: Cambridge University Press, 1993, pp. 1059–68.

10. For contemporary overviews of the factors that may contribute to the occurrence of TB in wartime, with special reference to Europe during the world wars, see: R. Murray Leslie, 'Tuberculosis and the war', *British Journal of Tuberculosis*, vol. 9, no. 1, 1915; Frederick Heaf, 'Prevention of tuberculosis in war-time', *British Journal of Tuberculosis*, vols. 35–6, nos. 3–4, 1941–42; Daniels, 'Tuberculosis in post-war Europe'; Marc Daniels, 'Tuberculosis in Europe during and after the Second World War', *British Medical Journal*, vol. 2, no. 4636, 1949.

11. Johnston, 'Tuberculosis'.

12. Daniels, 'Tuberculosis in post-war Europe', pp. 202–3.

13. Ibid., pp. 204–7.

14. Myron Allukian and Paul L. Atwood, 'Public health and the Vietnam War', in Levy and Sidel, eds., *War and Public Health*, pp. 215–37; Mam B. Heng and P. J. Key 'Cambodian health in transition', *British Medical Journal*, vol. 311, no. 7002, 1995; Haroutune K. Armenian, 'Perceptions from epidemiologic research in an endemic war', *Social Science and Medicine*, vol. 28, no. 7, 1989; David Siegel, Robert Baron and Paul Epstein, 'The epidemiology of aggression: health consequences of war in Nicaragua', *Lancet*, vol. I, no. 8444, 1985; Michael J. Toole, Steven Galson and William Brady, 'Are war and public health compatible?' *Lancet*, vol. 341, no. 8854, 1993; M. Pavlovic *et al.*, 'Wartime migration and the incidence of tuberculosis in the Zagreb region, Croatia', *European Respiratory Journal*, vol. 12, no. 6, 1998.

15. Monographs of war epidemics by Prinzing (*Epidemics Resulting from Wars*) and Major (*War and Disease*) make no mention of TB, while paper-length reviews by Councell, 'War and infectious disease', Charles Ellenbogen, 'Infectious diseases of war', *Military Medicine*, vol. 147, no. 3, 1982, and Richard M. Garfield and Alfred I. Neugut, 'Epidemiologic analysis of warfare: a historical review', *Journal of the American Medical Association*, vol. 266, no. 5, 1991, are limited to a consideration of TB in twentieth-century conflicts. The sanitary dispatches can be found in US Marine Hospital Service, *Public Health Reports*, Washington, DC: Government Printing Office, 1895–1900. For a detailed description of the nature of the information included in the Public Health Reports, see: Andrew D. Cliff, Peter Haggett and Matthew Smallman-Raynor, *Deciphering Global Epidemics: Analytical Approaches to the Disease Records of World Cities, 1888–1912*, Cambridge: Cambridge University Press, 1998.

16. Smallman-Raynor and Cliff, 'The spatial dynamics of epidemic diseases'.

17. See: Philip S. Foner, *The Spanish-Cuban-American War and the Birth of American Imperialism*, New York: Monthly Review Press, 1972; John L. Offner, *An Unwanted War: The Diplomacy of United States and Spain over Cuba, 1895–1898*, London: University of North Carolina Press, 1992; Joseph Smith, *The Spanish-American War: Conflict in the Caribbean and the Pacific, 1895–1902*, London: Longman, 1994.

18. The population estimate is based on the post-war census of October 1899; see US War Department, *Census of Cuba Taken Under the Direction of the War Department, USA, Bulletin No. 1: Total Population by Province, Municipal Districts, Cities and Wards*, Washington, DC: Government Printing Office, 1900. Summarizing the sanitary condition of Havana at the beginning of the war, for example, one official of the US Marine Hospital Service observed that: 'More than two-thirds of the population live in densely crowded sections of the city, where the average house lot does not exceed 27 by 112 feet in dimensions and where all the local conditions are in the highest degree insanitary. Comparison of the statistics of other cities shows that three–fourths of the population of Habana live

in the most densely populated localities of the world. A tropical climate intensifies the enormous evil.' See: United States Marine Hospital Service, *Annual Report of the Supervising Surgeon-General of the Marine Hospital Service for the Fiscal Year 1895*, Washington, DC: Government Printing Office, 1896, p. 393.

19. See Foner, *The Spanish-Cuban-American War*; Smith, *The Spanish–American War*; David E. Trask, *The War with Spain in 1898*, New York: Macmillian, 1981.

20. USMHS Sanitary Inspector W. F. Brunner, sanitary report for Havana, dated 16 October 1897; reproduced in US Marine Hospital Service, *Public Health Reports*, 1897, pp. 1150–1.

21. USMHS Sanitary Inspector W. F. Brunner, sanitary report for Havana, dated 27 November 1897; ibid., p. 1330.

22. USMHS Sanitary Inspector W. F. Brunner, sanitary report for Havana, dated 4 October 1897; ibid., p. 1121.

23. USMHS Sanitary Inspector W. F. Brunner, sanitary report for Havana, dated 22 January 1898; reproduced in US Marine Hospital Service, *Public Health Reports*, 1898, p. 79. According to the same report, animals imported from the USA were taxed at thirty cents for a chicken and five dollars for a hog. USMHS Sanitary Inspector W. F. Brunner, sanitary report for Havana, dated 14 January 1898; ibid., p. 61.

24. USMHS Sanitary Inspector W. F. Brunner, sanitary report for Havana, dated 9 December 1898; ibid., p. 1528.

25. For details regarding the occurrence of TB in pre-war Havana, see: US Marine Hospital Service, *Public Health Reports*, 1900, pp. 1840–54.

26. Owing to the limitations of the available data, in Figure 4.2A the period 1890–94 refers to deaths from all forms of TB, while the period 1896–1902 refers exclusively to pulmonary TB. Writing in 1900, the newly instated Chief Quarantine Officer of Cuba, H. R. Carter, noted that 86 per cent of all TB deaths in the earlier period were attributable to pulmonary TB; ibid., p. 1853.

27. Anonymous, 'The success of sanitation in Havana', *Lancet*, vol. II, no. 3969, 1899.

28. Commenting on the early spread of yellow fever in the civilian population of Havana, for example, the Chief Quarantine Officer of Cuba could attribute the 'heavy mortality' of 1895 to 'the civil immigration . . . of the families of officers and of the civilian attaches who accompanied the [Spanish] army'. US Marine Hospital Service, *Public Health Reports*, 1900, p. 1849. On the later, minor outbreaks of diseases, see, for example, US Marine Hospital Service, *Public Health Reports*, 1898, p. 156.

29. US Marine Hospital Service, *Public Health Reports*, 1900, pp. 1853–4.

30. See, for example: James A. Doull, 'Tuberculosis mortality in England and certain other countries during the present war', *Medical Officer*, vol. 74, no. 19, 1945; Marc Daniels, 'Tuberculosis in Poland', *Lancet*, vol. II, no. 6424, 1946; Anon., 'Tuberculosis in Germany', *Lancet*, vol. II, no. 6465,

1947; Daniels, 'Tuberculosis in post-war Europe'; Esmond R. Long, 'Tuberculosis in Germany', *Proceedings of the National Academy of Sciences, USA*, vol. 34, no. 6, 1948; Daniels, 'Tuberculosis in Europe'; L. H. A. Hoefnagels, 'Tuberculosis in Holland', *Tubercle*, vol. 31, August 1950.

31. The selection of European countries in Table 4.3 has been dictated by the availability of TB data; information for several of the states most severely affected by the First World War and/or the Second World War (including Germany, Poland and Serbia) is either unavailable or too fragmentary to include in the analysis. The estimates for the change in tuberculosis mortality have been formed by expressing the mortality rate for the war period as a percentage deviation from the average of the rates in the periods immediately preceding and following the war.

32. See, for example, Heaf, 'Prevention of tuberculosis in war-time'; Daniels 'Tuberculosis in Europe'.

33. See, for example, Anon., 'Nutrition in enemy occupied Europe', *Journal of the American Medical Association*, vol. 124, no. 4, 1944.

34. See Daniels, 'Tuberculosis in post-war Europe'; Daniels, 'Tuberculosis in Europe'.

35. Medical Research Council, *Report of the Committee on Tuberculosis in War-Time*, London: HMSO, 1942, p. 34.

36. See, for example, Registrar-General of England and Wales, *Seventy-Ninth Annual Report of the Registrar-General of Births, Deaths and Marriages in England and Wales*, London: HMSO, 1918, p. lix.

37. Medical Research Committee, *An Inquiry into the Prevalence and Aetiology of Tuberculosis among Industrial Workers, with Special Reference to Female Munition Workers*, London: HMSO, 1919.

38. Ibid., p. 59.

39. As noted by the authors of the *Inquiry*, the formation of proportionate mortalities (rather than mortality rates) overcomes the difficulties associated with wartime population movements and related uncertainties regarding the size of the female population in a given borough.

40. Medical Research Committee, *An Inquiry into the Prevalence and Aetiology of Tuberculosis*, pp. 24, 15.

41. R. J. Reece, 'Report on cerebro-spinal fever and its epidemic prevalence among the civil population in England and Wales, with special reference to outbreaks in certain districts during the first six months of the year 1915', *Reports to the Local Government Board on Public Health and Medical Subjects, New Series*, no. 110, 1916.

42. See: Patrick Brogan, *World Conflicts*, 2nd edn., London: Bloomsbury, 1992; Guy Arnold, *Wars in the Third World since 1945*, 2nd edn., London: Cassell, 1995.

43. Arnold, *Wars in the Third World since 1945*.

44. See, for example, Levy and Sidel, *War and Public Health*.

45. Jerome H. Greenberg, 'Public health problems relating to the Vietnam

returnee', *Journal of the American Medical Association*, vol. 207, no. 4, 1969; Ray G. Cowley, 'Implications of the Vietnam War for tuberculosis in the United States', *Archives of Environmental Health*, vol. 21, no. 4, 1970.

46. Allukian and Atwood, 'Public health and the Vietnam War'.

47. G. Bahr, A. M. de L. Costello, Y. Alahdab and J. Stanford, 'Epidemic tuberculosis in north Lebanon', *Lancet*, vol. 337, no. 8747, 1991; R. G. Barr and R. Menzies, 'The effect of war on tuberculosis: results of a tuberculin survey among displaced persons in El Salvador and a review of the literature', *Tuberculosis and Lung Disease*, vol. 75, no. 4, 1994; L. N. Rybka and V. V. Punga, 'Tuberculosis in refugees from foreign countries', *Problemy Tuberkuleza*, no. 3, 1996 [in Russian] on Angola, Afghanistan and Somalia; Pavlovic *et al.*, 'Wartime migration and the incidence of tuberculosis' on Bosnia-Herzegovina; V. S. Odinets, L. A. Ioffe and O. K. Kikot, 'The impact of migratory processes on the epidemiology of tuberculosis in the Stavropol territory', *Problemy Tuberkuleza*, no. 1, 1997 [in Russian] on Chechnya.

48. M. E. Black and T. D. Healing, 'Communicable diseases in former Yugoslavia and in refugees arriving in the United Kingdom', *Communicable Disease Report, CDR Review*, vol. 3, no. 6, 1993; H. L. Rieder *et al.*, 'Tuberculosis control in Europe and international migration', *European Respiratory Journal*, vol. 7, no. 8, 1994; J. D. Fengler, 'Tuberkulose– Wiederkehr einer vergessenen Infektionskrankheit?' *Zeitschrift für Ärztliche Fortbildung und Qualitätssicherung*, vol. 89, no. 3, 1995; L. Loutan, D. Bierens de Haan and L. Subilia, 'La santé des demandeurs d'asile: du dépistage des maladies transmissibles à celui des séquelles post-traumatiques' (The health of asylum seekers: from screeing for communicable diseases to post-traumatic stress disorder), *Bulletin de la Société de Pathologie Exotique*, vol. 90, no. 4, 1997.

49. Black and Healing, 'Communicable diseases in former Yugoslavia'; Michael J. Toole, 'Displaced persons and war', in Levy and Sidel, *War and Public Health*, pp. 197–212.

50. Loutan *et al.*, 'La santé des demandeurs d'asile'; Rieder *et al.*, 'Tuberculosis control in Europe'. For one small cohort of sixty-eight Bosnian ex-detainees, evacuated on medical grounds from camps in Manjaca and Trnpolje and assigned to hospitals in London in 1992, the prevalence of confirmed and suspected TB exceeded 20 per cent. See Black and Healing, 'Communicable diseases in former Yugoslavia', p. R89.

51. Daniels, 'Tuberculosis in Europe', p. 1140.

5   The Present Global Burden of Tuberculosis

1. C. Dye *et al.*, 'Global burden of tuberculosis: estimated incidence, prevalence, and mortality by country', *Journal of the American Medical Association*, vol. 282, 1999, pp. 677–86.

2. World Health Organization, *World Health Report 2000. Health Systems: Improving Performance*, Geneva: World Health Organization, 2000 (http://www.who.int/whr/2000/en/report.htm).

3. D. Ahlburg, *The Economic Impact of Tuberculosis*. Stop TB Initiative 2000 series, Geneva: World Health Organization, 2000 (http://www.stoptb.org/conference/ahlburg.pdf).

4. World Health Organization, *Tuberculosis and Sustainable Development: The Stop TB initiative*, Geneva: World Health Organization, 2000.

5. M. C. Raviglione *et al.*, 'Tuberculosis and HIV: current status in Africa', *AIDS*, supplement 11, 1997, pp. S115–23.

6. World Health Organization, *Global Tuberculosis Control*, Geneva: World Health Organization, 2000.

7. Dye *et al.*, 'Global burden'.

8. World Health Organization, *Anti-tuberculosis Drug Resistance in the World*, World Health Organization Report no. 2, WHO/CDS/TB/2000.278. Geneva: WHO, 2000.

9. M. A. Espinal *et al.*, 'Standard short-course chemotherapy for drug-resistant tuberculosis, treatment outcomes in 6 countries', *Journal of the American Medical Association*, vol. 283, 2000, pp. 2537–45.

10. World Health Organization, *What is DOTS? A Guide to Understanding the WHO Recommended TB Control Strategy Known as DOTS*, Geneva: WHO, 1999.

11. C. Dye *et al.*, 'Prospect for worldwide tuberculosis control under the WHO DOTS strategy', *Lancet*, vol. 352, 1998, pp. 1886–91.

12. K. Styblo and A. Rouillon, 'Estimated global incidence of smear-positive pulmonary tuberculosis: unreliability of officially reported figures on tuberculosis', *Bulletin of the International Union Against Tuberculosis and Lung Disease*, vol. 56, 1981, pp. 118–26.

13. Dye *et al.*, 'Global burden'.

14. World Health Organization, *Global Tuberculosis Control*.

15. Ibid.

16. Ibid.

17. A. Bulla, 'Worldwide review of officially reported tuberculosis morbidity and mortality (1967–1971–1977)', *Bulletin of the International Union Against Tuberculosis and Lung Disease*, vol. 56, 1981, pp. 111–17.

18. Ibid.

19. World Health Organization, *Global Tuberculosis Control*.

20. P. Dolin, M. Raviglione and A. Kochi, *Global Tuberculosis Incidence and Mortality During 1990–2000*, World Health Organization Bulletin no. 72, 1994, pp. 213–20.

21. Dye *et al.*, 'Global burden'.

22. J. Narain, M. Raviglione and A. Kochi, 'HIV associated tuberculosis in developing countries: epidemiology and strategy for prevention', *International Journal of Tuberculosis and Lung Disease*, vol. 3, 1992, pp. 311–21; J. Jessurum, A. Angeles-Angeles and N. Gasman, 'Compara-

tive demographic and autopsy findings in acquired immunodeficiency syndrome in two Mexican populations', *Journal of Acquired Immune Deficiency Syndrome*, vol. 3, 1990, pp. 579–83; J. W. Pape *et al.*, 'The acquired immunodeficiency syndrome in Haiti', *Annals of Internal Medicine*, vol. 103, 1985, pp. 674–8.

23. Narain *et al.*, 'HIV associated tuberculosis in developing countries'.

24. H. Yanai *et al.*, 'Rapid increase in HIV-related tuberculosis, Chiang Rai, Thailand, 1990–1994', *AIDS*, vol. 10, 1996, pp. 527–31.

25. Narain *et al.*, 'HIV associated tuberculosis in developing countries'.

26. Kingdom of Cambodia, 'HIV seroprevalence survey among TB patients: tuberculosis report 1997 and 1999', Ministry of Health, National Tuberculosis Control Programme.

27. Dye *et al.*, 'Global burden'.

28. P. A. Selwyn *et al.*, 'A prospective study of the risk of tuberculosis among intravenous drug users with human immunodeficiency virus infection', *New England Journal of Medicine*, vol. 320, 1989, pp. 545–50; P. A. Selwyn *et al.*, 'High risk of active tuberculosis in HIV-infected drug users with cutaneous energy', *Journal of the American Medical Association*, vol. 268, 1992, pp. 504–9; S. Allen *et al.*, 'Two-year incidence of tuberculosis in cohort of HIV-infected and uninfected Rwandan women', *American Review of Respiratory Disease*, vol. 146, 1992, pp. 1439–44; A. Guelar *et al.*, 'A prospective study of the risk of tuberculosis among HIV-infected patients', *AIDS*, vol. 7, 1993, pp. 1345–9; G. Antonucci *et al.*, 'Risk factors for tuberculosis in HIV-infected persons', *Journal of the American Medical Association*, vol. 274, 1995, pp. 143–8.

29. A. D. Harries and D. Maher, *TB/HIV: A Clinical Manual*, Geneva: World Health Organization, 1996.

30. V. Payanandana *et al.*, Report of an internal evaluation of the National Tuberculosis Programme, Thailand, 1993. Bangkok, Tuberculosis Division, Department of Communicable Disease Control, Ministry of Public Health, 1993.

31. Espinal *et al.*, 'Standard short-course chemotherapy'.

32. World Health Organization, *Anti-tuberculosis Drug Resistance*.

33. Ibid.

34. M. C. Raviglione *et al.*, 'Secular trends of tuberculosis in Western Europe', *Bulletin of the World Health Organization*, vol. 71, 1993, pp. 297–306.

35. M. F. Cantwell *et al.*, 'Epidemiology of tuberculosis in the United States, 1985 through 1992', *Journal of the American Medical Association*, vol. 272, 1994, pp. 535–9.

36. Raviglione *et al.*, 'Secular trends of tuberculosis in Western Europe'; World Health Organization, *Global Tuberculosis Control*.

37. European Centre for the Epidemiological Monitoring of AIDS (CESES) and Royal Netherland Tuberculosis Association (KNCV), *Surveillance of Tuberculosis in Europe: Report on Tuberculosis Cases Notified in 1997*, The Hague: KNVC, 1998.

38. World Health Organization, *Western Pacific Regional Office: Epidemiological Review of Tuberculosis in the Western Pacific Region*, Geneva: WHO, 1995; World Health Organization, *Global Tuberculosis Control*.
39. M. Raviglione *et al.*, 'Tuberculosis trends in Eastern Europe and the former USSR', *Tubercle and Lung Disease*, vol. 75, 1994, pp. 400–16.
40. D. Maher and M. Raviglione, 'The global epidemic of tuberculosis: a World Health Organization perspective', in D. Schlossberg, ed., *Tuberculosis and Non tuberculosis Mycobacterial Infections*, 4th edn, W. B. Saunders, 1999, pp. 104–15.
41. World Health Organization, *Global Tuberculosis Control*.
42. C. J. L. Murray, K. Styblo and A. Rouillon, 'Tuberculosis', in D. T. Jamison, *et al.*, eds., *Disease Control Priorities in Developing Countries*, Oxford: Oxford University Press, 1993, pp. 233–59; C. J. L. Murray and A. Lopez, *The Global Burden of Disease*, Cambridge, MA: Harvard School of Public Health, 1996.
43. G. B. Migliori *et al.*, *Cost Effectiveness Analysis of Different Policies of Tuberculosis Control in Ivanovo Oblast*, Russian Federation, Working Paper of the Ministry of Health, n.d.
44. World Health Organization, *The Economic Impacts of Tuberculosis*, Geneva: World Health Organization, 2000.
45. P. Karnolratanalul *et al.*, 'Economic impact of tuberculosis at household level', *International Journal of Tuberculosis and Lung Disease*, vol. 3, 1999, pp. 1–7.
46. R. Rajeswari *et al.*, 'Socio-economic impact of tuberculosis on patients and family in India', *International Journal of Tuberculosis and Lung Disease*, vol. 3, 1999, pp. 869–77.
47. World Health Organization, *Tuberculosis and Sustainable Development*.
48. Liefooghe *et al.*, 'Perceptions, Social Consequences and Stages of Illness Behaviour: A Focus Group Study of Tuberculosis Patients in Salkot, Pakistan', Antwerp, Instituut voor Tropische Geneeskunde, Publication no. 21, n.d.
49. Rajeswari *et al.*; M. Uplekar and S. Rangan, 'Tackling TB: the search for solutions', Bombay: Foundation for Research in Community Health, 1996.
50. World Health Organization, *Tuberculosis and Sustainable Development*.
51. World Bank, *World Development Report 1993: Investing in Health*, Oxford: Oxford University Press, 1993; C. J. L. Murray, K. Styblo and A. Rouillon, 'Tuberculosis in developing countries: burden, intervention and cost', *Bulletin of the International Union Against Tuberculosis and Lung Disease*, vol. 65, 1990, pp. 6–24.
52. World Health Organization, *Status of Tuberculosis in the 22 High-Burden Countries*, Geneva: World Health Organization, 1999.
53. Ibid.; E. Netto, C. Dye and M. Raviglione, 'Progress in global tuberculosis control 1995–1996 with emphasis on 22 high-incidence countries', *Inter-*

national Journal of Tuberculosis and Lung Disease, vol. 3, 1999, pp. 310–20.

6   Tuberculosis and HIV Infection in Sub-Saharan Africa

1. Joint United Nations Programme on HIV/AIDS (UNAIDS), *AIDS Epidemic Update*, December 1999. UNAIDS/99.53E-WHO/CDS/CSR/EDC/99.9-WHO/FCH/HIS/99.6. UN AIDS, New York.
2. A.-G. Poulsen *et al.*, 'Nine-year HIV-2 associated mortality in an urban community in Bissau, West Africa', *Bulletin of the World Health Organization*, vol. 72, 1994, pp. 213–20.
3. F. J. Palella *et al.*, 'Declining morbidity and mortality among patients with advanced human immunodeficiency virus infection', *New England Journal of Medicine*, vol. 338, 1998, pp. 853–60; A. Mocroft *et al.*, 'Changing patterns of mortality across Europe in patients infected with HIV-1', *Lancet*, vol. 352, 1998, pp. 1725–30.
4. UNAIDS, *AIDS Epidemic Update*, December 1998. UN AIDS, New York.
5. A. D. Grant *et al.*, 'Spectrum of disease among HIV-infected adults hospitalised in a respiratory medicine unit in Abidjan, Côte d'Ivoire', *International Journal of Tuberculosis and Lung Disease*, vol. 2, 1998, pp. 926–34.
6. D. Morgan *et al.*, 'HIV-1 disease progression and AIDS-defining disorders in rural Uganda', *Lancet*, vol. 350, 1997, pp. 245–50.
7. M. C. Raviglione, D. E. Snider and A. Kochi, 'Global epidemiology of tuberculous morbidity and mortality of a worldwide epidemic', *Journal of the American Medical Association*, vol. 273, 1995, pp. 220–6.
8. C. Dye *et al.* for the WHO Global Surveillance and Monitoring Project, 'Global burden of tuberculosis: estimated incidence, prevalence and mortality by country', *Journal of the American Medical Association*, vol. 282, 1999, pp. 677–86.
9. P. J. Dolin, M. C. Raviglione and A. Kochi, 'Global tuberculosis incidence and mortality during 1990–2000,' *Bulletin of the World Health Organization*, vol. 72, 1994, pp. 213–20; P. A. Selwyn *et al.*, 'A prospective study of the risk of tuberculosis among intravenous drug users with human immunodeficiency virus infection', *New England Journal of Medicine*, vol. 320, 1989, pp. 545–50.
10. G. Di Perri *et al.*, 'Nosocomial epidemic of active tuberculosis among HIV-infected patients', *Lancet*, vol. 2, 1989, pp. 1502–4; C. L. Daley *et al.*, 'An outbreak of tuberculosis with accelerated progression among persons infected with the human immunodeficiency virus', *New England Journal of Medicine*, vol. 326, 1992, pp. 231–5.
11. P. Small *et al.*, 'The epidemiology of tuberculosis in San Francisco: a population-based study using conventional and molecular methods', *New England Journal of Medicine*, vol. 330, 1994, pp. 1703–9; D. Alland *et al.*, 'Transmission of tuberculosis in New York City: an analysis by DNA

fingerprinting and conventional epidemiologic methods', *New England Journal of Medicine*, vol. 330, 1994, pp. 1710–16.

12. D. Wilkinson *et al.*, 'Molecular epidemiology and transmission dynamics of Mycobacterium tuberculosis in rural Africa', *Tropical Medicine and International Health*, vol. 2, 1997, pp. 747–53; C. F. Gilks *et al.*, 'Recent transmission of tuberculosis in a cohort of HIV-1 infected female sex workers in Nairobi, Kenya', *AIDS*, vol. 11, 1997, pp. 911–18; A. van Rie *et al.*, 'Exogenous reinfection as a cause of recurrent tuberculosis after curative treatment', *New England Journal of Medicine*, vol. 341, 1999, pp. 1174–9.

13. D. S. Nyangulu *et al.*, 'Tuberculosis in a prison population in Malawi', *Lancet*, vol. 350, 1997, pp. 1284–7; J. Porter and C. Kessler, 'Tuberculosis in refugees: a neglected dimension of the "global epidemic of tuberculosis"', *Transactions of the Royal Society of Tropical Medicine and Hygiene*, vol. 89, 1995, pp. 241–2; A. D. Harries *et al.*, 'Tuberculosis in health care workers in Malawi', *Transactions of the Royal Society of Tropical Medicine and Hygiene*, vol. 93, 1999, pp. 32–5.

14. P. A. Reeve, 'HIV infection in patients admitted to a general hospital in Malawi', *British Medical Journal*, vol. 298, 1989, pp. 1567–8; D. Wadhawan and S. K. Hira, 'Tuberculosis and HIV-1 in medical wards', *Medical Journal of Zambia*, vol. 24, 1989, pp. 16–18; S. B. Lucas *et al.*, 'The mortality and pathology of HIV infection in a West African city', *AIDS*, vol. 7, 1993, pp. 1569–79.

15. A. D. Harries, 'The association between HIV and tuberculosis in the developing world', in P. D. O. Davies, ed., *Clinical Tuberculosis*, 2nd edn, London: Chapman and Hall Medical, 1998, pp. 315–45.

16. C. Chintu *et al.*, 'Seroprevalence of human immunodeficiency virus type 1 infection in Zambian children with tuberculosis', *Paediatric Infectious Diseases Journal*, vol. 12, 1993, pp. 499–504; M. Sassan-Morokro *et al.*, 'Tuberculosis and HIV infection in children in Abidjan, Côte d'Ivoire', *Transactions of the Royal Society of Tropical Medicine and Hygiene*, vol. 88, 1994, pp. 178–81.

17. World Health Organization, *Global Tuberculosis Control*, 1998, (WHO/TB/98.237.), Geneva: WHO, 1998.

18. D. Maher *et al.*, 'Tuberculosis care in community care organizations in sub-Saharan Africa: practice and potential', *International Journal of Tuberculosis and Lung Disease*, vol. 1, 1997, pp. 276–83.

19. D. Wilkinson, 'High-compliance tuberculosis treatment programme in a rural community', *Lancet*, vol. 343, 1994, pp. 647–8.

20. J. H. Perriens *et al.*, 'Increased mortality and tuberculosis treatment failure rate among human immunodeficiency virus (HIV) seropositive compared with HIV seronegative patients with pulmonary tuberculosis treated with "standard" chemotherapy in Kinshasa, Zaire', *American Review of Respiratory Disease*, vol. 144, 1991, pp. 750–5; A. Okwera *et al.*, 'Randomised trial of thiacetazone and rifampicin-containing regimens for

pulmonary tuberculosis in HIV-infected Ugandans', *Lancet*, vol. 344, 1994, pp. 1323–8.

21. P. Nunn *et al.*, 'The impact of HIV on resource utilization by patients with tuberculosis in a tertiary referral hospital, Nairobi, Kenya', *Tuberculosis and Lung Disease*, vol. 74, 1993, pp. 273–9.

22. P. Nunn *et al.*, 'Cutaneous hypersensitivity reactions due to thiacetazone in HIV-1 seropositive patients treated for tuberculosis', *Lancet*, vol. 337, 1991, pp. 627–30.

23. C. Chintu *et al.*, 'Cutaneous hypersensitivity reactions due to thiacetazone in the treatment of tuberculosis in Zambian children infected with HIV-1', *Archives of Diseases of Childhood*, vol. 68, 1993, pp. 665–8.

24. S. M. Graham *et al.*, 'Ethambutol usage in childhood tuberculosis – time to reconsider', *Archives of Diseases of Childhood*, vol. 79, 1998, pp. 274–8.

25. M. C. Raviglione *et al.*, 'Tuberculosis and HIV: current status in Africa', *AIDS*, vol. 11 (suppl. B), 1997, pp. S115–23.

26. C. J. L. Murray *et al.*, 'Cost effectiveness of chemotherapy for pulmonary tuberculosis in three sub-Saharan African countries', *Lancet*, vol. 338, 1991, pp. 1305–8.

27. A. D. Harries *et al.*, 'Treatment outcome of an unselected cohort of tuberculosis patients in relation to human immunodefiency virus serostatus in Zomba hospital, Malawi', *Transactions of the Royal Society of Tropical Medicine and Hygiene*, vol. 92, 1998, pp. 343–7.

28. P. Nunn *et al.*, 'Cohort study of human immunodeficiency virus infection in patients with tuberculosis in Nairobi, Kenya', *American Review of Respiratory Disease*, vol. 146, 1992, pp. 849–54; A. M. Elliott *et al.*, 'The impact of human immunodeficiency virus on mortality of patients treated for tuberculosis in a cohort study in Zambia', *Transactions of the Royal Society of Tropical Medicine and Hygiene*, vol. 89, 1995, pp. 78–82.

29. S. Z. Wiktor *et al.*, 'Efficacy of trimethoprim-sulphamethoxazole prophylaxis to decrease morbidity and mortality in HIV-1 infected patients with tuberculosis in Abidjan, Côte d'Ivoire: a randomised controlled trial', *Lancet*, vol. 353, 1999, pp. 1469–75.

30. S. D. Lawn, R. J. Shattock and G. E. Griffin, 'Delays in the diagnosis of tuberculosis: a great new cost', *International Journal of Tuberculosis and Lung Disease*, vol. 1, 1997, pp. 485–6.

31. Editorial, 'Impact of HIV on delivery of health care in sub-Saharan Africa: a tale of secrecy and inertia', *Lancet*, vol. 345, 1995, pp. 1315–17.

32. F. M. L. Salaniponi *et al.*, 'Loss of tuberculosis officers from a national tuberculosis programme: the Malawi experience, 1993–1997', *International Journal of Tuberculosis and Lung Disease*, vol. 3, 1999, pp. 174–5.

33. T. A. Kenyon *et al.*, 'Low levels of drug resistance amidst rapidly increasing tuberculosis and human immunodeficiency virus co-epidemics in Bot-

swana', *International Journal of Tuberculosis and Lung Disease*, vol. 3, 1999, pp. 4–11.

34. S. D. Lawn, B. Afful and J. W. Acheampong, 'Pulmonary tuberculosis: diagnostic delay in Ghanaian adults', *International Journal of Tuberculosis and Lung Disease*, vol. 2, 1998, pp. 636–40; B. R. Wandwalo and O. Morkve, 'Delay in tuberculosis case-finding and treatment in Mwanza, Tanzania', *International Journal of Tuberculosis and Lung Disease*, vol. 4, 2000, pp. 133–8; F. M. L. Salaniponi *et al.*, 'Care seeking behaviour and diagnostic practices in smear-positive pulmonary tuberculosis in Malawi', *International Journal of Tuberculosis and Lung Disease*, vol. 4, 2000, pp. 327–32.

35. D. Wilkinson, S. B. Squire and P. Garner, 'Effect of preventive treatment for tuberculosis in adults infected with HIV: systematic review of randomised placebo controlled trials', *British Medical Journal*, vol. 317, 1998, pp. 625–9.

36. T. Aisu *et al.*, 'Preventive chemotherapy for HIV-associated tuberculosis in Uganda: an operational assessment at a voluntary counselling and testing centre', *AIDS*, vol. 9, 1995, pp. 267–73.

37. T. R. Frieden *et al.*, 'The emergence of drug-resistant tuberculosis in New York city', *New England Journal of Medicine*, vol. 328, 1993, pp. 521–6; A. Pablos-Mendez *et al.*, 'Global surveillance for antituberculosis-drug resistance, 1994–1997', *New England Journal of Medicine*, vol. 338, 1998, pp. 1641–9.

38. UNAIDS/WHO, Joint United Nations Programme on HIV/AIDS (UNAIDS) and the World Health Organization, *Report on the Global HIV/AIDS Epidemic*, UNAIDS, New York, June 1998.

39. Poulson *et al.*, 'Nine-year HIV-2 associated mortality'; Grant *et al.*, 'Spectrum of disease among HIV-infected adults'.

40. M. C. J. Bosman, 'Health sector reform and tuberculosis control: the case of Zambia', *International Journal of Tuberculosis and Lung Disease*, vol. 4, 2000, pp. 606–14.

7   The Recent Tuberculosis Epidemic in New York City: Warning from the De-Developing World

This chapter is dedicated to the memory of our friend and great colleague Peter Gould whose work on AIDS and other scourges of humankind provides a model of humanism, creativity and solid methodology. Peter died on 22 January 2000 and is greatly missed as a scientist, educator, colleague and friend to many.

1. G. Youmans, *Tuberculosis*, Philadelphia: W. B. Saunders, 1979, p. 366.

2. Task Force on Tuberculosis in New York City, *A Plan to Control Tuberculosis in New York City*, New York: NYC Health Services Administration, 1968.

3. Letter to D. M. Wallace from the New York City Department of Health, 29 July 1979.
4. D. Wallace and R. Wallace, *A Plague on Your Houses: How New York Was Burned Down and National Public Health Crumbled*, New York: Verso, 1999, Chapter 4.
5. D. Wallace, 'The resurgence of tuberculosis in New York City: a mixed hierarchically and spatially diffused epidemic', *American Journal of Public Health*, vol. 84, 1994, pp. 1000–2.
6. On contagious processes, see Wallace and Wallace, *A Plague on Your Houses*, Chapter 3.
7. D. Wallace, 'Resurgence of tuberculosis'.
8. Ibid.
9. Wallace and Wallace, *A Plague on Your Houses*.
10. E. Drucker *et al.*, 'Childhood tuberculosis in the Bronx, New York', *Lancet*, vol. 343, 1995, pp. 1482–5.
11. D. Wallace, 'Resurgence of tuberculosis'.
12. N. T. J. Bailey, *The Mathematical Theory of Infectious Diseases and Its Applications*, 2nd edn, New York: Hafner Press, 1975.
13. A. Vennema, personal communication, 1983. Dr Vennema was the Director of TB Control, New York City.
14. K. Brudney and L. Dobkin, 'Resurgent tuberculosis in New York City: human immunodeficiency virus, homelessness, and the decline of tuberculosis control programs', *American Review of Respiratory Diseases*, vol. 144, 1991, pp. 745–9.
15. P. Bifani *et al.*, 'Origin and interstate spread of a New York City multidrug-resistant *Mycobacterium tuberculosis* clone family', *Journal of the American Medical Association*, vol. 272, 1996, pp. 452–7; P. Longuet *et al.*, 'A limited multidrug-resistant *Mycobacterium tuberculosis* (MDR-TB) outbreak: screening of contact hospitalized patients', in *Abstracts of the 35th Interscience Conference on Antimicrobial Agents and Chemotherapy, September 17–20, 1995, San Francisco*. Abstract J59.
16. T. Masciangelo and R. Awe, 'Cases of drug-resistant tuberculosis despite directly observed therapy', in *Abstracts, The Lancet Conference: The Global Challenge of Tuberculosis, Sept 14–15, 1995, Washington DC*. Abstract 113. W. Bradford, 'The changing epidemiology of acquired drug-resistant tuberculosis in San Francisco, USA', *Lancet*, vol. 348, 1996, pp. 928–31.
17. T. Frieden *et al.*, 'Tuberculosis in New York City – turning the tide', *New England Journal of Medicine*, vol. 333, 1995, pp. 229–33.
18. Youmans, *Tuberculosis*.
19. Wallace and Wallace, *Plague on Your Houses*.
20. Drucker *et al.*, 'Childhood tuberculosis in the Bronx'.
21. Department of Health of New York City 1970, 1980 and 1990 census data aggregated by health area. Received by RW on diskette from the Bureau of Biostatistics, New York. Data from 1980 is also held on the

online database infoshare organized by Leonard Rodberg of Queens College, New York.

22. This emigration was responsible for a decline in housing overcrowding and the steep decline in new TB cases in 1976–78. See R. Wallace, 'Homelessness, contagious destruction of housing, and municipal service cuts in New York City: 1. demographics of a housing deficit', *Environment and Planning A*, vol. 21, 1989, 1585–1603.

23. M. Stegman, *Housing in New York: Study of a City, 1984*, New York City: Department of Housing Preservation and Development, 1985.

24. Wallace and Wallace, *Plague on Your Houses*; R. Wallace, 'Contagion and incubation in New York City structural fires 1964–1976', *Human Ecology*, vol. 6, 1978, pp. 423–33.

25. M. Dear, 'Abandoned housing', in J. Adams, ed., *Urban Policy Making and Metropolitan Development*, Cambridge, MA: Ballanger, 1976.

26. R. Wallace and D. Wallace, 'Urban fire as an unstabilized parasite: the 1976–1978 outbreak in Bushwick, Brooklyn', *Environment and Planning A*, vol. 15, 1983, pp. 207–26.

27. D. Wallace and R. Wallace, *Report on Structural Fires to the Community Board and Neighborhood Office of HPD*, 1980. Available from the authors.

28. Wallace and Wallace, *Plague on Your Houses*; R. Wallace and D. Wallace, *Studies on the Collapse of Fire Service in New York City, 1972–1976: Impact of Pseudoscience on Public Policy*, Washington, DC: University Press of America, 1977.

29. For details of the misinterpretations, see Wallace and Wallace, *Plague on Your Houses*.

30. R. Starr, *Urban Choices: The City and its Critics*, Baltimore: Pelican Books, 1966–1969.

31. Wallace and Wallace, *Collapse of Fire Service*.

32. R. Wallace et al., 'The spatiotemporal dynamics of AIDS and TB in the New York metropolitan region from a sociogeographic perspective: understanding the linkages of central city and suburbs', *Environment and Planning A*, vol. 27, 1995, pp. 1085–1108.

33. R. Wallace et al., 'AIDS, tuberculosis, violent crime, and low birthweight in eight US metropolitan regions: public policy, stochastic resonance, and the regional diffusion of inner-city markers', *Environment and Planning A*, vol. 29, 1997, pp. 525–55.

34. R. Wallace et al., 'The hierarchical diffusion of AIDS and violent crime among US metropolitan regions: inner-city decay, stochastic resonance, and reversal of the mortality transition', *Social Science and Medicine*, vol. 44, 1997, pp. 935–47.

35. D. Wallace and R. Wallace, 'Scales of geography, time, and population: the study of violence as a public health problem', *American Journal of Public Health*, vol. 88, 1998, pp. 1853–8.

36. R. Wallace et al., 'Deindustrialization, inner-city decay, and the hierarchi-

cal diffusion of AIDS in the USA: how neoliberal and cold war policies magnified the ecological niche for emerging infections and created a national security crisis', *Environment and Planning A*, vol. 31, 1999, pp. 113–39.

37. R. Wallace and D. Wallace, 'The destruction of US minority urban communities and the resurgence of tuberculosis: ecosystem dynamics of the white plague in the dedeveloping world', *Environment and Planning A*, vol. 29, 1997, pp. 269–91.
38. Ibid.
39. Ibid.
40. Ibid.
41. China Tuberculosis Control Collaboration, 'Results of directly observed short-course chemotherapy in 112,842 Chinese patients with smear-positive tuberculosis', *Lancet*, vol. 347, 1996, pp. 358–62.
42. G. Condran, 'Changing patterns of epidemic disease in New York City', in D. Rosner, ed., *Hives of Sickness*, New Brunswick: Rutgers University Press, 1995, pp. 27–41.
43. Centers for Disease Control and Prevention, *Annual Summary of Notifiable Diseases, 1998*, Boston: Massachusetts Medical Society, 2000.
44. Bradford *et al.*, 'The changing epidemiology of acquired drug-resistant tuberculosis'; W. A. McCallion *et al.*, 'Helicobacter pylori infection in children: relation with current household living conditions', *Gut*, vol. 39, 1996, pp. 18–21.
45. Wallace and Wallace, 'Destruction of US minority urban communities'.
46. M. Smallman-Raynor, A. Cliff and P. Haggett, *Atlas of AIDS*, Oxford: Blackwell, 1993.

8   Private Wealth and Public Squalor: The Resurgence of Tuberculosis in London

1. ONS/CDSC Notification Data.
2. A. Hayward. *Tuberculosis Control in London: The Need for Change. A Report for the Thames Regional Directors of Public Health*, London: NHSE, 1998.
3. Colston, unpublished essay, London: Medical Research Council, n.d.
4. I. Smith, 'Tuberculosis in England and Wales: define high risk behaviours, not high risk groups', *British Medical Journal*, vol. 311, 1995, pp. 187–97.
5. P. Farmer, 'Social Scientists and the New Tuberculosis', *Social Science and Medicine*, vol. 44, 1997, pp. 347–58.
6. London NHS Executive website accessed 10/11/2000 (http://www.doh.gov.uk/london/income.htm).
7. Sir D. Acheson, *Acheson Report: Independent Inquiry into Inequalities in Health*, London: The Stationary Office, 1998; London Research Council, *The Capital Divided: Mapping Poverty and Social Exclusion in London*,

November 1996; G. Yamey, 'Study shows growing inequalities in health in Britain', *British Medical Journal*, vol. 319, December 1999, pp. 1453–8; M. Bardsley *et al.*, *The Health of Londoners: A Public Health Report for London*, London: Kings Fund, 1998.

8. M. T. Kearney *et al.*, 'Tuberculosis and poverty', *British Medical Journal*, vol. 307, 30 October 1993, p. 1143; D. P. Spence *et al.*, 'Tuberculosis and poverty', *British Medical Journal*, vol. 307, 1993, pp. 759–61.

9. N. Bhatti *et al.*, 'Increasing incidence of tuberculosis in England and Wales: a study of the likely causes', *British Medical Journal*, vol. 310, 1995, pp. 967–9.

10. M. Catchpole, 'Tuberculosis in England and Wales: incidence of tuberculosis in London is rising against general recent trend', *British Medical Journal*, vol. 311, 1995, p. 187; A. Pearson *et al.*, *The Surveillance, Prevention and Control of Tuberculosis in London*, London: Working Party on Tuberculosis of the London Group of Communicable Disease Control, 1995.

11. P. Cloke, P. Milbourne and A. Widdowfield, 'Change but no change: dealing with homelessness under the 1996 Housing Act', *Housing Studies*, vol. 15, 2000, pp. 739–56.

12. 'London Health Strategy: Outline Strategic Framework', London: NHS Executive, March 2000.

13. C. J. Martin, S. D. Platt and S. M. Hunt, 'Housing conditions and ill health', *British Medical Journal*, vol. 294, 2 May 1987, pp. 1125–7; P. Mangtani *et al.*, 'Socioeconomic deprivation and notification rates for tuberculosis in London during 1982–91', *British Medical Journal*, vol. 310, 15 April 1995, pp. 963–6; E. Drucker *et al.*, 'Childhood tuberculosis in the Bronx, New York', *Lancet*, vol. 343, 1994, pp. 1482–5; F. Elender, G. Bentham and I. Langford, 'Tuberculosis mortality in England and Wales during 1982–1992: its association with poverty, ethnicity and AIDS', *Society of Science and Medicine*, vol. 46, 1998, pp. 673–81.

14. Association of London Government, 1997.

15. M. Wilson, 'Travel and the emergence of infectious diseases', *Emerging Infectious Diseases*, vol. 1, April–June 1995; F. G. Cobelens *et al.*, 'Risk of infection with Mycobacterium tuberculosis in travellers to areas of high tuberculosis endemicity', *Lancet*, vol. 356, 2000, pp. 461–5.

16. O. R. McCarty, 'Asian immigrant tuberculosis – the effect of visiting Asia', *British Journal of Diseases of the Chest*, vol. 78, 1984, pp. 248–53.

17. S. Hargreaves, 'System to detect tuberculosis in new arrivals to UK must be improved', *British Medical Journal*, vol. 320, 2000, pp. 870–3.

18. G. Daly, 'Migrants and gate keepers: the links between immigration and homelessness in Western Europe', *Cities*, vol. 13, 1996, pp. 11–23.

19. Red Cross, *World Disasters Report 1998*, New York: Oxford University Press, 1999.

20. London Health Strategy. See also A. McMichael and R. Beaglehole, 'The

changing global context of public health', *Lancet*, vol. 356, 2000, pp. 495–9; Audit Commission, *Another Country*, London: Audit Commission, 2000.

21. M. Bardsley and M. Storkey, 'Estimating the numbers of refugees in London', *Journal of Public Health Medicine*, vol. 22, 2000, pp. 406–12. On the social exclusion and deprivation of refugees, see 'London Health Strategy'.

22. R. M. Hardie and J. M. Watson, 'Screening migrants at risk of tuberculosis', *British Medical Journal*, vol. 307, 1993, pp. 1539–40.

23. S. Hargreaves, A. Holmes and J. S. Friedland, 'Health-care provision for asylum seekers and refugees in the UK', *Lancet*, vol. 353, May 1999, pp. 1497–8; J. Aldous, *Refugee Health in London: Key Issues for Public Health*, London: NHS Executive North Thames Regional Office, 1999.

24. C. Van den Bosch and J. Roberts, 'Tuberculosis screening of new entrants: how can it be made more effective?' *Journal of Public Health Medicine*, vol. 22, 2000, pp. 220–3.

25. S. Bakhshi, 'Screening immigrants at risk of tuberculosis', *British Medical Journal*, vol. 308, 1994, p. 416.

26. G. H. Bothamley *et al.*, 'Detecting tuberculosis in new arrivals to the UK: failure to register with a general practice compounds the problem', *British Medical Journal*, vol. 321, 2000, p. 570.

27. D. Jones and P. S. Gill, 'Refugees and primary care: tackling the inequalities', *British Medical Journal*, vol. 317, 1998, pp. 1444–6.

28. Hargreaves, Holmes and Friedland, 'Health care provision for asylum seekers'.

29. Jones and Gill, 'Refugees and primary care'.

30. Van den Bosch and Roberts, 'Tuberculosis screening'.

31. J. Connelly and M. Schweiger, 'The health risks of the UK's new asylum act', *British Medical Journal*, vol. 321, 2000, pp. 5–6.

32. UK Home Office, *Fairer, Faster and Firmer: A Modern Approach to Immigration and Asylum*, Cm 4018, London: HMSO, 1998.

33. H. Hogan, 'Meeting health needs of asylum seekers: white paper will make access to health care more difficult', *British Medical Journal*, vol. 318, 1999, p. 671.

34. United Nations Office for Drug Control and Crime Prevention, *Global Programme against Trafficking in Human Beings: An Outline for Action*, New York: United Nations Interregional Crime and Justice Research Institute, February 1999.

35. D. Bamber, 'Most prostitutes are illegal immigrants', *Sunday Telegraph* (London), 28 November 1999.

36. R. Horton, 'Health and the UK Human Rights Act 1998', *Lancet*, vol. 356, 2000, pp. 1186–8.

37. G. Daly, *Homeless: Policies, Strategies and Lives on the Street*, London: Routledge, 1996.

38. K. Chahal, *Minority Ethnic Homelessness in London: Findings from a Rapid Review*, London: NHS Executive, 1999.
39. Ibid. C. Small and T. Hinton, *Reaching Out: A Study of Black and Minority Ethnic Single Homelessness and Access to Primary Health Care*, London: Health Action for Homeless People, 1997.
40. J. Smith, 'Youth homelessness in the UK: a European perspective', *Habitat International*, vol. 23, 1999, pp. 63–77.
41. Crisis Annual Review 1999, London: Crisis, 1999.
42. Smith, 'Youth homelessness'.
43. Crisis Annual Review.
44. P. Grenier, *Still Dying for a Home*, London: Crisis, 1996.
45. M. Bardley, *Housing and Health in London*, London: Health of Londoners Project, London, 1998.
46. N. Pleace and D. Quilgers, *Health and Homelessness in London: A Review*, London: Kings Fund, 1996. Definitions of homelessness range from the specific to the all-encompassing. See Bardley, *Housing and Health in London*.
47. Shelter, *Health and Housing: How Homelessness and Bad Housing Impact on Physical Health*, London: Shelter, 2000.
48. UK Social Exclusion Unit, *Rough Sleeping: Report by the Social Exclusion Unit*, London: HMSO, 1998.
49. Shelter, *Go Home and Rest? The Use of an Accident and Emergency Department by Homeless People*, London: Shelter, 1996.
50. A. Pablos-Mendez *et al.*, 'Nonadherence in tuberculosis treatment: predictors and consequences in New York City', *American Journal of Medicine*, vol. 102, 1997, pp. 164–70; N. Schluger *et al.*, 'Comprehensive tuberculosis control for patients at high risk for noncompliance', *American Journal of Respiratory and Critical Care Medicine*, vol. 151, 1995, pp. 1486–90.
51. A. Southern *et al.*, 'Tuberculosis among homeless people in London: an effective model of screening and treatment', *International Journal of Tuberculosis and Lung Disease*, vol. 3, 1999, pp. 1001–8; K. M. Citron, *Coming out of the Shadow: A National Survey of Provision for Detecting and Treating Tuberculosis amongst Single Homeless People*, London: Crisis 1997.
52. D. Banerjee *et al.*, 'Molecular epidemiology of tuberculosis in London: genetic fingerprinting of isolates of *Mycobacterium tuberculosis*: results of a multi-centre pan-London collaborative study', 1998. Available from the authors.
53. J. M. Watson, personal communication with the authors; P. F. Barnes, 'Tuberculosis among inner city poor', *International Journal of Tuberculosis and Lung Disease*, vol. 2, 1998, pp. S41–5.
54. M. Hickman *et al.*, 'A sexual health ready reckoner: summary indicators of sexual behaviour and HIV in London and South East England', London: The Health of Londoners Project, 1997.

55. D. Churchill *et al.*, 'HIV associated culture proved tuberculosis has increased in north central London from 1990 to 1996', *Sexually Transmitted Infections*, vol. 76, 2000, pp. 43–5.

56. A. Ferguson, D. Bennet and S. Conning, 'Notification of tuberculosis in patients with AIDS', *Journal of Public Health Medicine*, vol. 20, 1998, pp. 218–20; M. A. Balogun, P. G. Wall and A. Noone, 'Undernotification of tuberculosis in patients with AIDS', *International Journal of STD and AIDS*, vol. 7, 1996, pp. 58–60; B. G. Marshall *et al.*, 'HIV and tuberculosis co-infection in an inner London hospital – a prospective anonymised seroprevalence study', *Journal of Infection*, vol. 38, 1999, pp. 162–6.

57. Joint Tuberculosis Committee of the British Thoracic Society, 'Control and prevention of tuberculosis in the United Kingdom: code of practice', *Thorax*, vol. 55, 2000, pp. 887–901.

58. M. H. Levy and G. Alperstein, 'Patients with tuberculosis can be managed effectively in the community', *British Medical Journal*, vol. 319, 1999, p. 455.

59. T. R. Frieden *et al.*, 'Tuberculosis in New York City – turning the tide', *New England Journal of Medicine*, vol. 333, 1995, pp. 229–33; M. R. Gasner *et al.*, 'The use of legal action in New York City to ensure treatment of tuberculosis', *New England Journal of Medicine*, vol. 340, February 1999, pp. 359–66.

60. R. Cocker, 'Public health, civil liberties, and tuberculosis', *British Medical Journal*, vol. 318, May 1999, pp. 1434–5.

61. *Results of Pan London Multidisciplinary Workshops on Tuberculosis Control*, Report to the Director of Public Health for London, 1999.

62. Frieden *et al.*, R. Cocker, 'Tuberculosis, non-compliance and detention for the public health', *Journal of Medical Ethics*, vol. 26, 2000, pp. 157–9.

63. S. Rangan, *Tuberculosis Control in India: A State of the Art Review*, Dehli: Department for International Development (DFID), 1997.

64. J. Ogden, 'The resurgence of tuberculosis in the tropics: improving tuberculosis control – social science inputs', *Transactions of the Royal Society of Tropical Medicine and Hygiene*, vol. 94, March–April 2000, pp. 135–40.

65. M. Hadley and D. Maher, 'Community involvement in tuberculosis control: lessons from other health care programmes', *International Journal of Tuberculosis and Lung Disease*, vol. 4, May 2000, pp. 401–8; W. el-Sadr, F. Medard and M. Dickerson, 'The Harlem family model: a unique approach to the treatment of tuberculosis', *Journal of Public Health Management and Practice*, vol. 1, Fall 1995, pp. 48–51.

66. L. Gelberg, R. M. Andersen and B. D. Leake, 'The behavioral model for vulnerable populations: application to medical care use and outcomes for homeless people', *Health Service Research*, vol. 34, February 2000, pp. 1273–302; E. Diez *et al.*, 'Evaluation of a social health intervention among homeless tuberculosis patients', *Tuberculosis and Lung Disease*, vol. 77, October 1996, pp. 420–4.

67. A. C. Hayward and R. J. Cocker, 'Could a tuberculosis epidemic occur in London as it did in New York?' *Emerging Infectious Diseases*, vol. 6, January–February 2000, pp. 12–26.
68. Results from Pan London Disciplinary Workshops.
69. Hickman *et al.*, 'A sexual health ready reckoner'.

9   The Social Impact of Multi-drug-resistant Tuberculosis: Haiti and Peru

1. G. P. Youmans, E. H. Williston and W. H. Feldman, 'Increase in resistance of tubercle bacilli to streptomycin; a preliminary report', *Mayo Clinic Proceedings*, vol. 21, 1946, pp. 126–7; E. Wolinsky, A. Reginster and W. Steenken Jr, 'Drug-resistant tubercle bacilli in patients under treatment with streptomycin', *American Review of Tuberculosis*, vol. 58, 1948, pp. 335–43; S. Bernstein, N. D. D'Esopo and W. Steenken, 'Streptomycin resistant tubercle bacilli', *American Review of Tuberculosis*, vol. 58, 1948, pp. 344–52; D. A. Mitchison, 'Development of streptomycin resistant strains of tubercle bacilli in pulmonary tuberculosis', *Thorax*, vol. 5, 1950, pp. 144–61.
2. C. Canetti, 'Present aspects of bacterial resistance in tuberculosis', The J. Burns Amberson Lecture, *American Review of Respiratory Diseases*, vol. 92, 1965, pp. 687–703; M. Zierski, 'Treatment of patients with cultures resistant to the primary antituberculosis drugs', *Tubercle*, vol. 45, 1964, pp. 96–100; Anon., 'Drug resistance in patients with pulmonary tuberculosis presenting at chest clinics in Hong Kong: A Hong Kong Government Tuberculosis Service/British Medical Research Council co-operative investigation', *Tubercle*, vol. 45, 1964, pp. 77–95.
3. M. Goble, M. D. Iseman and L. A. Madsen, 'Treatment of 171 patients with pulmonary tuberculosis resistant to isoniazid and rifampin', *New England Journal of Medicine*, vol. 328, 1993, pp. 527–32.
4. C. M. Beck-Sague *et al.*, 'Hospital outbreak of multidrug-resistant *Mycobacterium tuberculosis* infections: factors in transmission to staff and HIV-infected patients', *Journal of the American Medical Association*, vol. 268, 1992, pp. 1280–6; V.G. Coronado *et al.*, 'Transmission of multidrug-resistant *Mycobacterium tuberculosis* among persons with human immunodeficiency virus infection in an urban hospital: epidemiologic and restriction fragment length polymorphism analysis', *Journal of Infectious Diseases*, vol. 168, 1993, pp. 1052–5; S. E. Valway *et al.*, 'Outbreak of multidrug-resistant tuberculosis in a New York State prison, 1991', *American Journal of Epidemiology*, vol. 140, 1994, pp. 113–22; E. A. Nardell *et al.*, 'Exogenous reinfection with tuberculosis in a shelter for the homeless', *New England Journal of Medicine*, vol. 315, 1986, pp. 1570–5.
5. D. L. Cohn, F. Bustreo and M. C. Raviglione, 'Drug-resistant tuberculosis: review of the worldwide situation and the WHO/IUATLD Global Surveillance Project', *Clinical Infectious Diseases*, vol. 24, 1997, pp. S121–130;

World Health Organization, *Anti-tuberculosis Drug Resistance in the World: The WHO/IUATLD Global Project on Anti-tuberculosis Drug Resistance Surveillance 1994-1997*, WHO/TB/97.229. Geneva: World Health Organization, 1997.

6. M. C. Becerra, P. E. Farmer and J. Y. Kim, 'The problem of drug-resistant tuberculosis: an overview', in Program in Infectious Disease and Social Change, *The Global Impact of Drug-Resistant Tuberculosis*, Boston: Harvard Medical School, 1999.

7. W. A. Githui *et al.*, 'Antituberculosis drug resistance surveillance in Kenya, 1995', *International Journal of Tuberculosis and Lung Disease*, vol. 2, 1998, pp. 499-505.

8. In a 1998 publication, WHO estimated global case detection rates to be between 39 and 51 per cent. See World Health Organization Global Tuberculosis Programme, *Global Tuberculosis Control: World Health Organization Report 1998*, WHO/TB/98-237. Geneva: World Health Organization, 1998.

9. See World Health Organization, *WHO Tuberculosis Programme: Framework for Effective Tuberculosis Control*, WHO/TB/94.175. Geneva: World Health Organization, 1994; A. Kochi, 'Tuberculosis control – is DOTS the health breakthrough of the 1990s?' *World Health Forum*, vol. 18, 1997, pp. 225-32.

10. The World Bank has committed over $350 million to TB control since 1989, making it the leading source of external funding for TB control in resource-poor countries. See the Bank's website, www.worldbank.org, particularly the 'Issue Briefs' section on TB, accessible at http://www.worldbank.org/html/extdr/pb/tbpb.htm

11. World Health Organization, *Global Tuberculosis Control: WHO Report 1999*, Geneva: World Health Organization, 1999.

12. In particular, critics have argued that the cost of treating MDR TB is prohibitive, detracting resources from pan-susceptible disease treatment. See, for example, A. D. Harries and D. Maher, *TB/HIV: A Clinical Manual*, WHO/TB/96.200. Geneva: World Health Organization, 1996.

13. M. A. Espinal *et al.*, 'Standard short-course chemotherapy for drug-resistant tuberculosis', *Journal of the American Medical Association*, vol. 283, 2000, pp. 2537-45.

14. Centers for Disease Control and Prevention, 'Primary multidrug-resistant tuberculosis – Ivanovo Oblast, Russia, 1999', *Morbidity and Mortality Weekly Report*, vol. 48, 1999, pp. 661-3.

15. P. E. Farmer *et al.*, 'The dilemma of MDRTB in the global era', *International Journal of Tuberculosis and Lung Disease*, vol. 2, 1998, pp. 869-76.

16. A. Pablos-Mendez *et al.*, 'Nonadherence in tuberculosis treatment: predictors and consequences in New York City', *American Journal of Medicine*, vol. 102, 1997, pp. 164-70.

17. Compare, for example, the following assessments: M. C. Becerra *et al.*,

'Using treatment failure under effective directly observed short-course chemotherapy programs to identify patients with multidrug-resistant tuberculosis', *International Journal of Tuberculosis and Lung Disease*, vol. 4, 2000, pp. 108–14; M. C. Becerra *et al.*, 'Redefining MDR-TB transmission "hot spots"', *International Journal of Tuberculosis and Lung Disease*, vol. 4, 2000, pp. 387–94; Program in Infectious Disease and Social Change, *Global Impact*; C. Dye, 'A rational basis for the control of drug-resistant tuberculosis', *International Journal of Tuberculosis and Lung Disease*, vol. 3, 1999, p. S8; World Health Organization, *Anti-tuberculosis Drug Resistance in the World. Report No. 2: The WHO/IUATLD Global Project on Anti-tuberculosis Drug Resistance Surveillance 2000*, Geneva: World Health Organization, 2000.

18. F. Manalo *et al.*, 'Community-based short-course treatment of pulmonary tuberculosis in a developing nation: initial report of an eight-month, largely intermittent regimen in a population with a high prevalence of drug resistance', *American Review of Respiratory Diseases*, vol. 142, 1990, pp. 1301–5; T. Shimao, 'Drug resistance in tuberculosis control', *Tubercle*, vol. 68, 1987, pp. 5–18.

19. 'TB carriers see clash of liberty and health', *New York Times*, 14 October, 1992, p. A1.

20. J. Y. Kim, 'Making DOTS-Plus work: the challenge of rational drug procurement', 30th ASTER Challenge Lecture Madrid, 16 September 1999.

21. World Health Organization, *TB: a Crossroads, WHO Report on the Tuberculosis Epidemic*, WHO/TB/98.247. Geneva: World Health Organization, 1998; New York City Department of Health, '1993 Annual summary–tuberculosis', *City Health Inform*, November/December 1994, p. 14.

22. P. E. Farmer, 'Managerial successes, clinical failures', *International Journal of Tuberculosis and Lung* Disease, vol. 3, 1999, pp. 365–7; P. E. Farmer *et al.*, 'Recrudescent tuberculosis in the Russian Federation, Program in Infectious Disease and Social Change', in *The Global Impact of Drug-resistant Tuberculosis*, Boston, MA: Harvard Medical School and the Open Society Institute, 1999, pp. 39–84.

23. This has long been the case. Although the debate is brisk, we often fail to refer to surveys from the pre-antibiotic era. See, for example, E. R. Long and H. W. Hetherington, 'A tuberculosis survey in the Papago Indian area of southern Arizona', *American Review of Tuberculosis*, vol. 33, 1936, pp. 407–33. Among contacts of MDR-TB patients, see the important study by A. L. Kritski *et al.*, 'Transmission of tuberculosis to close contacts of patients with multidrug-resistant tuberculosis', *American Journal of Respiratory Critical Care Medicine*, vol. 153, 1996, pp. 331–5.

24. P. E. Farmer, 'Pathologies of power: rethinking health and human rights', *American Journal of Public Health*, vol. 89, 1999, pp. 1486–96.

25. M. Iseman, personal communication with the authors.

26. P. E. Farmer *et al.*, 'Responding to outbreaks of multidrug-resistant tuberculosis: introducing DOTS-Plus', in L. B. Reichman and E. S. Hershfield, eds., *Tuberculosis: A Comprehensive International* Approach, 2nd edn, New York: Marcel Dekker, 2000; P. E. Farmer *et al.*, 'Making DOTS-Plus work', in I. Bastian and F. Portaels, eds., *Multidrug-resistant Tuberculosis*, Dordrecht: Kluwer, 2000.

27. M. C. Becerra *et al.*, 'Redefining MDR-TB transmission "hot spots" '; World Health Organization, *Anti-tuberculosis Drug Resistance in the World: The WHO/IUATLD Global Project on Anti-tuberculosis Drug Resistance Surveillance 1994–1997*, Geneva: World Health Organization, 1997; World Health Organization, *Anti-tuberculosis Drug Resistance in the World. Report no. 2.*

28. K. Weyer *et al.*, 'A noxious synergy: tuberculosis and HIV in South Africa', in Program in Infectious Disease and Social Change, ed., *Global Impact*.

10   *The House of the Dead* Revisited: Prisons, Tuberculosis and Public Health in the Former Soviet Bloc

I would like to thank Vivien Francis and Anton Shelupanov, researchers at the International Centre for Prison Studies, Kings College, University of London, for their assistance in writing this chapter.

1. S. McConville, *A History of English Prison Administration, Vol. 1, 1750–1877*, London: Routledge and Kegan Paul, 1981, p. 50.

2. C. Harding *et al.*, *Imprisonment in England and Wales: A Concise History*, London: Croom Helm, 1985, pp. 9–95.

3. McConville, *A History of English Prison Administration*, p. 51.

4. Harding *et al.*, *Imprisonment in England and Wales* p. 115

5. Ibid., p. 117.

6. J. Howard, *Prisons and Lazarettos: Volume One, the State of the Prisons in England and Wales, and Volume Two, An Account of the Principal Lazarettos in Europe*, London: 1777.

7. McConville, *A History of English Prison Administration*, p. 85.

8. It was after attending to a prisoner with typhus at Kherson in the Ukraine that Howard became ill. He died on 20 January, 1790 at the age of 64. He was buried in Russia. http://www.acjnet.org/jhsa/

9. Vivien Stern, *A Sin Against the Future: Imprisonment in the World*, Harmondsworth: Penguin, 1998, Part Two, pp. 105ff.

10. *Puerto Rico Daily News*, 16 May 2000.

11. A. Bone *et al.*, *Tuberculosis Control in Prisons: A Manual for Programme Managers*, Geneva: World Health Organization, 2000, p. 22 (text version).

12. Program in Infectious Disease and Social Change, *The Global Impact of Drug-resistant Tuberculosis*, Boston: Harvard Medical School, 1999, p. 43.

13. M. Raviglione et al., 'Tuberculosis trends in Eastern Europe and the Former USSR', in Vivien Stern, ed., Sentenced to Die? The Problem of TB in Prisons in Eastern Europe and Central Asia, London: Centre for Prison Studies, 1999, p. 237.

14. World Health Organization, Global Tuberculosis Control: WHO Report 2000, Geneva: WHO, 2001 p. 121.

15. J. Y. Kim et al., 'The Russian health crisis', in J. Y. Kim et al., eds., Dying for Growth, Maine: Common Courage Press, 2000, p. 161.

16. D. Peter and O. Davies, 'Multi-drug resistant tuberculosis', p. 1. Available online at http://www.priory.co.uk/cmol/TBMultid.htm

17. Nicholas Banatvala and Gennady Georgievich Peremitin, 'Tuberculosis, Russia and the Holy Grail', Lancet, vol. 353, 1999.

18. Stern, ed., Sentenced to Die? p. 22.

19. Banatvala and Peremitin, 'Tuberculosis, Russia and the Holy Grail'.

20. Stern, A Sin Against the Future, Part One, pp. 64ff.

21. Ibid.

22. Official statistics of the penal system, Ministry of Interior/Ministry of Justice of the Russian Federation, 1989–1999.

23. Personal communication from Roy Walmsley, author of Research Findings No. 116: World Prison Population List, Home Office Research, Development and Statistics Directorate.

24. The latest figures show imprisonment rates, per 100,000, of 363 in Latvia, 577 in Belarus, 275 in Moldova, 323 in Azerbaijan. Source: World Prison Brief Online, available at http://www.prisonstudies.org/

25. Roy Walmsley, Research Findings No. 116: World Prison Population List Home Office Research, Development and Statistics Directorate.

26. Personal communication from Dr Andrew Coyle.

27. Radio Free Europe, Radio Liberty, Moscow, 26 April 2000.

28. Hans Kluge, 'Implementing a TB treatment programme in Colony 33, Marinsk, Siberia', in Stern, ed., Sentenced to Die? pp. 97–103.

29. Kees van der Loo and Andrew Coyle, 'Penal reform and the control of tuberculosis in Pawlodar', in Stern, ed., Sentenced to Die? pp. 107–16.

30. Newsletter of the Penal Reform Project in Eastern Europe and Central Asia, no. 3, 1998, p. 2, Penal Reform International.

31. Bone et al., Tuberculosis Control in Prisons, p. 13.

32. Ibid.

33. Research carried out in the prisons of Barcelona in Spain between 1994 and 1996 suggests that half of the 247 culture-positive cases there became infected whilst in prison.

34. Public Health Research Institute, Russian Criminal Correction System Overview, May 2000.

35. Bone, Tuberculosis Control in Prisons, p. 57.

36. Ibid., p. 19.

37. Ibid., p. 32.

38. Stern, ed., Sentenced to Die? p. 110.

39. Information Pack 1: Measures to Reduce Overcrowding in Prisons – Kazakhstan Penal Reform International Central and Eastern Europe and Central Asia Programme, 1999. Penal Reform International, Washington, DC.

40. S. Bryans et al., 'Report of a delegation to the corrections department of Mongolia, 16–23 September 1997'.

41. Program in Infectious Disease and Social Change, Global Impact, p. 55.

42. Boston Globe, 21 March 2000, 3rd edn.

43. Banatvala and Peremitin, 'Tuberculosis, Russia and the Holy Grail'.

44. Program in Infectious Disease and Social Change, Global Impact, p. 54.

45. F. Portaels, L. Rigouts and I. Bastian, 'Addressing multi-drug resistant tuberculosis in penitentiary hospitals and in the general population in the former Soviet Union', International Journal of Tuberculosis and Lung Disease, vol. 3, 1999, pp. 583–8.

46. World Health Organization, Global Tuberculosis Control: WHO Report 2000, Annex 3 (European Region).

47. John Porter and John Grange, Tuberculosis: An Interdisciplinary Perspective, London: Imperial College Press, 1999, p. 14.

48. Personal communication from the Moscow office of MSF.

49. Bone et al., Tuberculosis Control in Prisons, p. 21 (text version).

50. Ibid. p. 20. The 1999 figure is given in Russian Criminal Correction System Overview, May 2000, PHRI.

51. See the chapters by Kluge and Van der Loo and Coyle in Stern, ed., Sentenced to Die?

52. Rudi Coninx, 'Tuberculosis in prisons: the work of the International Committee of the Red Cross – case study: Baku, Azerbaijan', in Stern, ed., Sentenced to Die? pp. 89–96.

53. Newsletter of the Penal Reform Project in Eastern Europe and Central Asia, Penal Reform International, Autumn 2000.

54. A. I. Zubkov, Punitive Policy in Russia, Moscow: Penal Reform International, 2000.

55. Alternatives to Imprisonment in the Republic of Kazakstan, Penal Reform International, 1999.

56. Newsletter of the Penal Reform Project in Eastern Europe and Central Asia, Penal Reform International, Autumn 2000.

11   Rethinking the Social Context of Illness: Interdisciplinary Approaches to Tuberculosis Control

The authors wish to thank John Porter who helped to develop many of the ideas discussed in this chapter. They also wish to thank the Department for International Development, UK, who fund the Tuberculosis Knowledge Programme at the London School of Hygiene and Tropical Medicine, and contribute to the joint funding of the West African TB Initiative Project that is mentioned in this chapter, in association with the Direction Générale de la

Coopération et du Développement International, France. Lastly, the authors are grateful to the partners of the West African TB Initiative who participated fully in the development of the project. Despite all this support, the opinions expressed and any errors made are the authors' alone.

1. E. H. Kass, 'Infectious diseases and social change', *Journal of Infectious Disease*, vol. 123, 1971, pp. 110–14; L. C. Rodrigues, 'Tuberculosis in developing countries and methods for its control', *Transactions of the Royal Society of Tropical Medicine and Hygiene*, vol. 84, 1990, pp. 739–44; C. J. L. Murray, K. Styblo and A. Rouillon, 'Tuberculosis in developing countries: burden, intervention and cost', *Bulletin of the International Union against Tuberculosis and Lung Diseases*, vol. 65, 1990, pp. 6–24; J. Porter, J. A. Ogden and P. Pronyk, 'Infectious disease policy: towards the production of health', *Health Policy and Planning*, vol. 14, 1999; J. A. Ogden *et al.*, 'Shifting the paradigm in tuberculosis control: illustrations from India', *International Journal of Tuberculosis and Lung Diseases*, vol. 3, 1999, pp. 1–7.
2. Tuberculosis Chemotherapy Centre, 'A concurrent comparison of home and sanatorium treatment of pulmonary tuberculosis in India', *Bulletin of the World Health Organization*, vol. 29, 1959; M. S. Westaway, P. W. Condrie and L. Remmers, 'Supervised outpatient treatment of TB: evaluation of a South African rural programme', *Tubercle*, vol. 72, 1991, pp. 140–4; D. Wilkinson, 'High-compliance tuberculosis treatment programme in a rural community', *Lancet*, vol. 343, 1994, pp. 647–8; D. Wilkinson and D. Moore, 'Tuberculosis treatment programmes in low-income countries', *Lancet*, vol. 344, 1994, pp. 259–60.
3. J. A. Ogden, 'Improving tuberculosis control: social science inputs', *Transactions of the Royal Society of Tropical Medicine and Hygiene*, vol. 94, 2000, pp. 1–6. On this theme, see the work done on leprosy, which shares many social determinants with TB: J. A. Ogden and J. Porter, 'Leprosy: applying qualitative techniques to research and intervention', *Leprosy Review*, vol. 70, 1999, pp. 129–35.
4. World Health Organization Tuberculosis Programme, *Framework for Effective Tuberculosis Control* (WHO/TB/94.179.), Geneva: WHO, 1994.
5. For an extensive review of methods of TB control, see L. C. Rodrigues, 'Tuberculosis in developing countries and methods for its control', *Transactions of the Royal Society of Tropical Medicine and Hygiene*, vol. 84, 1990, pp. 739–44; J. F. Broekmanns, 'Control strategies and programme management', in K. McAdam and J. Porter, eds., *Tuberculosis: Back to the Future*, London: John Wiley and Sons, 1994, pp. 171–88; K. Jochem and J. Walley, 'Tuberculosis in high prevalence countries: current control strategies and their technical and operational limitations', in J. Porter and J. Grange, eds., *Tuberculosis: An Interdisciplinary Perspective*, London: Imperial College Press, 1999.
6. On concepts and structures of TB control programmes, see the following

works. World Health Organization, *Tuberculosis Control: Report of a joint WHO/IUAT Study Group*, Technical Report Series No. 571, Geneva: WHO 1982. World Health Organization, *Treatment of Tuberculosis: Guidelines for National Programmes* (WHO/TB/97.220.), WHO: Geneva, 1997. D. A. Enarson and A. Rouillon, 'The epidemiological basis of tuberculosis control', in P. D. O. Davies, ed., *Clinical Tuberculosis*, London: Chapman and Hall, 1994; D. A. Enarson *et al.*, *Tuberculosis Guide for Low Income Countries*, Frankfurt: PMI, 1996. On passive and active case finding, see: H. Rieder, 'Case finding', in L. B. Reichman and E. S. Hershfield, eds., *Tuberculosis: a Comprehensive International Approach*, New York: Marcel Dekker, 1993, pp. 167–82.

7. P. I. Fujiwara, 'Tide pools: what will be left after the tide has turned?' *International Journal of Tuberculosis and Lung Diseases*, vol. 4, 2000, pp. S111–16.

8. For information on the various reported delays, see the following works. N. Beyers *et al.*, 'Delay in the diagnosis, notification and initiation of treatment and compliance in children with tuberculosis', *Tubercle*, vol. 74, 1994, pp. 260–5 (South Africa). P. Mathur *et al.*, 'Delayed diagnosis of pulmonary tuberculosis in city hospitals', *Archives of Internal Medicine*, vol. 54, 1994, pp. 306–10. T. W. Steen and G. N. Mazonde, 'Pulmonary tuberculosis in Kweneng District, Botswana: delays in diagnosis in 212 smear-positive patients', *International Journal of Tuberculosis and Lung Diseases*, vol. 2, 1998, pp. 627–34 (Botswana). S. D. Lawn, B. Afful and J. W. Acheampong, 'Pulmonary tuberculosis: diagnostic delay in Ghanaian adults', *International Journal of Tuberculosis and Lung Diseases*, vol. 2, 1998, pp. 635–40 (Ghana). J. F. Pirkis *et al.*, 'Time to initiation of anti-tuberculosis treatment', *Tubercle Lung Diseases*, vol. 77, 1996, pp. 401–6 (Australia).

9. For further information on risk factors for delay, see the following articles. K. Brudney and J. Dobkin, 'Resurgent tuberculosis in New York City: human immuno-deficiency virus, homelessness and the decline of tuberculosis control programme', *American Review of Respiratory Diseases*, vol. 144, 1991, pp. 745–9. P. Hudelson, 'Gender differentials in tuberculosis: the role of socio-economic and cultural factors', *Tuberculosis and Lung Diseases*, vol. 77, 1996, pp. 391–400. R. Liefooghe *et al.*, 'From their own perspective: a Kenyan community's perception of tuberculosis', *Tropical Medicine and International Health*, vol. 2, 1997, pp. 809–11; D. M. Needham, P. Godfrey-Faussett and S. D. Foster, 'Barriers to tuberculosis control in urban Zambia: the economic impact and burden on patients prior to diagnosis', *International Journal of Tuberculosis and Lung Diseases*, vol. 2, 1998, pp. 811–17. C. Lienhardt *et al.*, 'Factors affecting time delay to treatment in a Tuberculosis Control Programme in a Sub-Saharan country: the experience of The Gambia', *International Journal of Tuberculosis and Lung Disease*, vol. 5, 2001, pp. 1–7.

10. Liefooghe *et al.*, 'From their own perspective'; P. E. Farmer, 'Social

scientists and the new tuberculosis', *Social Science and Medicine*, vol. 43, 1997, pp. 347–58.

11. E. Sumartojo, 'When tuberculosis treatment fails: a social behavioural account of patient adherence', *American Review of Respiratory Diseases*, vol. 147, 1993, pp. 1311–20.

12. Farmer, 'Social scientists and the new tuberculosis'.

13. Fujiwara, 'Tide pools'.

14. A series of abstracts was produced from India on this subject: V. Singh *et al.*, 'Tuberculosis Programme, India', *International Journal of Tuberculosis and Lung Diseases*, vol. 2, 1998, p. S367 (Abstract no. 691-PC); V. Singh *et al.*, 'Social vulnerability and the treatment of tuberculosis in Delhi: can DOTS fill the gap?' *International Journal of Tuberculosis and Lung Diseases*, vol. 2, 1998, p. S364 (Abstract no. 368-PC); V. Singh *et al.*, 'Patient experiences with the Revised National Tuberculosis Programme, India', *International Journal of Tuberculosis and Lung Diseases*, vol. 2, 1998, p. S354. (Abstract no. 367-PC); R. Sarin *et al.*, 'Obstacles to TB treatment for women in Delhi', *International Journal of Tuberculosis and Lung Diseases*, vol. 2, 1998, p. S350. (Abstract no. 598-PC).

15. M. A. Seetha *et al.*, 'Influence of motivation of patients and their family members on the drug collection by patients', *Indian Journal of Tuberculosis*, vol. 28, 1981, p. 182; A. J. Rubel and L. A. Garro, 'Social and cultural factors in the successful control of tuberculosis', *Public Health Report*, vol. 107, 1992, p. 626; F. Barnhoorn and H. Adriaanse, 'In search of factors responsible for non-compliance among tuberculosis patients in Wardha district, India', *Social Science and Medicine*, vol. 34, 1992, p. 291; M. Uplekar and S. Rangan, 'Alternative approaches to improve treatment adherence in tuberculosis control programme', *Indian Journal of Tuberculosis*, vol. 42, 1995, pp. 67–74; R. Liefooghe *et al.*, 'Perception and social consequences of tuberculosis: a focus group study of tuberculosis patients in Sialkot, Pakistan', *Social Science and Medicine*, vol. 41, 1995, pp. 1685–92. This has been noted in the case of other illnesses as well: see for example, M. H. Becker and L. W. Green, 'A family approach to compliance with medical regimens: a selective review of the literature', *International Journal Health Education*, vol. 18, 1975, pp. 173–82.

16. D. A. Enarson, 'Principles of IUATLD collaborative TB programmes', *Bulletin of the International Union Against Tuberculosis*, vol. 66, 1991, pp. 195–200; A. Kochi, 'The global tuberculosis situation and the new control strategy at the World Health Organisation', *Tubercle*, vol. 72, 1991, pp. 1–6. See also K. Styblo, 'Epidemiology of tuberculosis', in *Selected Papers of the KNCV*, vol. 24, The Hague: KNCV. Netherlands, 1991.

17. A. Kochi, B. Vareldzis and K. Styblo, 'Multidrug resistant tuberculosis and methods for its control', *Research in Microbiology*, vol. 144, 1993, pp. 104–10.

18. WHO 1994; WHO 1997. When initially launched, DOTS was promoted as standing for Directly Observed Therapy, Shortcourse. In mid-2001, however, WHO took the decision to drop the full name and market DOTS as a 'brandname' in order to reduce confusion between DOTS – the comprehensive strategy – and DOT, which is only one element of the strategy. WHO Strategic and Technical Advisory Group for Tuberculosis, *DOTS: Do We Need to Change the Name?* Working Paper 4, Geneva: WHO, 2001.

19. M. C. Raviglione *et al.*, 'Assessment of world-wide tuberculosis control', *Lancet*, vol. 350, 1997, pp. 624–9; World Health Organization, *Global Tuberculosis Control: World Report 2000* (WHO/CDS/TB/ 2000.275.), Geneva: WHO, 2000; C. Dye *et al.*, 'Prospects for world-wide tuberculosis control under the WHO DOTS strategy', *Lancet*, vol. 352, 1998, pp. 1886–91.

20. A series of papers has been published, originating from the work of the Cochrane collaboration on the systematic review of clinical trials of DOT regimens in TB. See: J. Volminck and P. Garner, 'Systematic review of randomised trials of strategies to promote adherence to TB treatment', *British Medical Journal*, vol. 315, 1997, pp. 1403–6; J. Volminck, P. Matchaba and P. Garner, 'Directly Observed Therapy and treatment adherence', *Lancet*, vol. 355, 2000, pp. 1345–50.

21. For the South African trial, see M. Zwarenstein *et al.*, 'Randomised controlled trial of self-supervised and directly observed treatment of tuberculosis', *Lancet*, vol. 352, 1998, pp. 1340–3. For the Thai trial, see P. Kamolratanakul *et al.*, 'Randomized controlled trial of DOT for patients with pulmonary TB in Thailand', *Transactions of the Royal Society of Tropical Medicine and Hygiene*, vol. 93, 1999, pp. 552–7. For the trial in Pakistan, see J. D. Walley *et al.*, 'Effectiveness of the direct observation component of DOTS for tuberculosis: a randomised controlled trial in Pakistan', *Lancet*, vol. 357, 2001, pp. 664–9.

22. Volminck and Garner, 'Systematic review'; Volminck, Matchaba and Garner, 'Directly Observed Therapy'.

23. K. Jochem and J. Walley, 'Tuberculosis in high prevalence countries: current control strategies and their technical and operational limitations', in J. Porter and J. Grange, eds., *Tuberculosis: An Interdisciplinary Perspective*, London: Imperial College Press, 1999, p. 146; J. Walley, J. Newell and A. Khan, 'Directly Observed Therapy and treatment adherence (letter)', *Lancet*, vol. 356, 2000, pp. 1031–2.

24. Jochem and Walley, 'Tuberculosis in high prevalence countries'.

25. A. J. Rubel and L. A. Garro, 'Social and cultural factors in the successful control of tuberculosis', *Public Health Report* vol. 107, 1992, p. 626; F. Barnhoorn and H. Adriaanse, 'In search of factors responsible for non-compliance among tuberculosis patients in Wardha district, India', *Social Science and Medicine*, vol. 34, 1992, p. 291; M. Uplekar and S. Rangan, 'Alternative approaches to improve treatment adherence in tuberculosis

control programme', *Indian Journal of Tuberculosis*, vol. 42, 1995, pp. 67–74; R. Liefooghe *et al.*, 'Perception and social consequences of tuberculosis: a focus group study of tuberculosis patients in Sialkot, Pakistan', *Social Science and Medicine*, vol. 41, 1995, pp. 1685–92. See also, for the debate on the ethics of the approach, J. Porter, J. A. Ogden and P. Pronyk, 'Infectious disease policy: towards the production of health', *Health Policy and Planning*, vol. 14, 1999.

26. World Health Organization, *Global Tuberculosis Control: World Report 2000*.

27. A. B. Block, E. Sumartojo and K. Castro, 'Directly observed therapy for tuberculosis in New York City' (reply to Klein *et al.* 1994), *Journal of the American Medical Association*, vol. 272, 1994, pp. 435–6 (emphasis in the text added).

28. Volminck, Matchaba and Garner, 'Directly observed therapy'.

29. World Health Organization Strategic and Technical Advisory Group for Tuberculosis, *DOTS: Do We Need to Change the Name?*

30. The concept and structure of a qualitative approach to infectious diseases is proposed in J. Green and N. Britten, 'Qualitative research and evidence based medicine', *British Medical Journal*, vol. 316, 1998, pp. 1230–2; J. A. Ogden and J. D. H. Porter, 'Leprosy: applying qualitative techniques to research and intervention', *Leprosy Review*, vol. 70, 1999, pp. 129–35.

31. *Pace* R. Firth, 'Degrees of intelligibility', in J. Overing, ed., *Reason and Morality*, ASA Monograph no. 24, London: Tavistock, pp. 29–46.

32. J. A. Ogden, 'Improving tuberculosis control: social science inputs', *Transactions of the Royal Society of Tropical Medicine and Hygiene*, vol. 94, 2000, pp. 1–6; J. A. Ogden and J. Porter, 'Leprosy: applying qualitative techniques to research and intervention', *Leprosy Review*, vol. 70, 1999, pp. 129–35.

33. C. Lienhardt, 'From exposure to disease: the role of environmental factors in susceptibility to TB', *Epidemiology Review*, vol. 23, 2001.

34. A. S. Pym and S. T. Cole, 'Post DOTS, post genomics: the next century of tuberculosis control', *Lancet*, vol. 353, 1999, pp. 1004–5; J. Porter, J. A. Ogden and P. Pronyk, 'Infectious disease policy: towards the production of health', *Health Policy and Planning*, vol. 14, 1999; C. Lienhardt, J. Rowley and K. Manneh, 'Directly Observed Treatment for Tuberculosis', *Lancet*, vol. 353, 1999, pp. 145–6.

12 Reflections on the Role of Science in Tuberculosis Control

The authors would like to acknowledge with gratitude the Marie Curie Individual Fellowship (MCFI-1999–01114) received by Martin Munk.

1. G. A. Rook and J. L. Stanford, 'The Koch phenomenon and the immunopathology of tuberculosis', *Current Topical Microbiology*, vol. 215, 1996, pp. 239–62.

2. Attenuation is the process of growing a disease-causing organism outside its normal host for many generations. Most pathogens are highly adapted to life inside their hosts and as they adapt to life in a laboratory flask, they become less capable of growing (and causing disease) in their original host. Many of the first vaccines were attenuated pathogens.

3. J. M. Grange et al., 'What is BCG?' Tubercle, vol. 64, 1983, pp. 129–39.

4. Ibid.

5. Anon., 'The role of BCG vaccine in the prevention and control of tuberculosis in the United States: a joint statement by the Advisory Council for the Elimination of Tuberculosis and the Advisory Committee on Immunization Practices', Morbility and Mortality Weekly Report, vol. 45, pp. 1–18.

6. Ibid.

7. M. A. Behr et al., 'Comparative genomics of BCG vaccines by whole-genome DNA microarray', Science, vol. 284, 1999, pp. 1520–3; S. V. Gordon et al., 'Identification of variable regions in the genomes of tubercle bacilli using bacterial artificial chromosome arrays', Molecular Microbiology, vol. 32, 1999, pp. 643–55; T. Oettinger et al., 'Development of the Mycobacterium bovis BCG vaccine: review of the historical and biochemical evidence for a genealogical tree', Tubercle Lung Disease, vol. 79, 1999, pp. 243–50.

8. L. C. Rodrigues and P. G. Smith, 'Tuberculosis in developing countries and methods for its control', Transactions of the Royal Society of Tropical Medicine and Hygiene, vol. 84, 1990, pp. 739–44; G. A. Colditz et al., 'Efficacy of BCG vaccine in the prevention of tuberculosis: meta-analysis of the published literature', Journal of the American Medical Association, vol. 271, 1994, pp. 698–702.

9. P. D. Hart. 'Efficacy and applicability of mass BCG vaccination in tuberculosis control', British Medical Journal, vol. 1, 1967, pp. 587–92.

10. A. van Rie et al., 'Exogenous reinfection as a cause of recurrent tuberculosis after curative treatment', New England Journal of Medicine, vol. 341, 1999, pp. 1174–9.

11. J. B. Milstien and J. J. Gibson, 'Quality control of BCG vaccine by WHO: a review of factors that may influence vaccine effectiveness and safety', Bulletin of the World Health Organisation, vol. 68, 1990, pp. 93–108; T. W. Osborn, 'Changes in BCG strains', Tubercle, vol. 64, 1983, pp. 277–81. A discussion of vaccination necessarily involves a large number of technical terms. Definitions for the most commonly used are given here. Proteins are one of the basic building blocks of all cells – whether bacterial or human. Many of these are closely related, but most organisms contain proteins which are unique to their species. An antigen is a protein that is recognized by the host's immune system. These can be the same thing – to most people, the proteins in milk are simply proteins. However, to someone with a milk allergy, some of these proteins are antigens – his or her body makes an immune response to them. Some proteins stimulate

strong immune responses in most individuals. These are said to be *immunogenic*. These are the basic tools for vaccine construction, since the goal of vaccination is to induce an immune response against an antigen which is present in the disease-causing organism, but not the recipient of the vaccine. If successful, the vaccinated person's immune system can then identify and destroy the organism, if the person is later infected.

12. I. M. Orme, 'Characteristics and specificity of acquired immunologic memory to Mycobacterium tuberculosis infection', *Journal of Immunology*, vol. 140, 1988, pp. 3589–93.

13. D. N. McMurray, 'Cell-mediated immunity in nutritional deficiency', *Progress of Food and Nutrition Science*, vol. 8, 1984, pp. 193–228.

14. D. N. McMurray et al., 'Mycobacterium bovis BCG vaccine fails to protect protein-deficient guinea pigs against respiratory challenge with virulent Mycobacterium tuberculosis', *Infection and Immunity*, vol. 50, 1985, pp. 555–9; D. N. McMurray, R. A. Bartow and C. L. Mintzer, 'Protein malnutrition alters the distribution of FcyR+ (Ty) and FcuR+ (Tu) T lymphocytes in experimental pulmonary tuberculosis', *Infection and Immunity*, vol. 58, 1990, pp. 563–5.

15. S. M. Vidal et al., 'Natural resistance to infection with intracellular parasites: isolation of a candidate for BCG', *Cell*, vol. 73, 1993, pp. 469–85.

16. I. Kramnik, P. Demant and B. B. Bloom, 'Susceptibility to tuberculosis as a complex genetic trait: analysis using recombinant congenic strains of mice', *Novartis Foundation Symposium*, vol. 217, 1998, pp. 120–31; R. Bellamy, 'Identifying genetic susceptibility factors for tuberculosis in Africans: a combined approach using a candidate gene study and a genome-wide screen', *Clinical Science (Colch)*, vol. 98, 2000, pp. 245–50.

17. W. W. Stead et al., 'Racial differences in susceptibility to infection with M. tuberculosis', *New England Journal of Medicine*, vol. 322, 1990, pp. 422–7; G. W. Comstock, 'Tuberculosis in twins: a re-analysis of the Prophit survey', *American Review of Respiratory Disease*, vol. 117, 1978, pp. 621–4; P. E. M. Fine, 'Immunogenetics of susceptibility to leprosy, tuberculosis and leishmaniasis: an epidemiological perspective', *International Journal of Leprosy*, vol. 49, 1981, pp. 337–454.

18. J. A. Hank et al., 'Influence of the virulence of Mycobacterium tuberculosis on protection induced by Bacille Calmette-Guerin in guinea pigs', *Journal of Infectious Diseases*, vol. 143, 1981, pp. 734–8.

19. The balance between Type 1 and Type 2 immunity is maintained by soluble factors called cytokines which are produced by immune cells. Cytokines regulate immune functions, including their own production – augmenting or decreasing immune responses – in an attempt to kill invading organisms as effectively as possible while at the same time reducing the damage caused to host tissues in the process. Type 1 cells produce many cytokines, such as interferons or tumour necrosis factor, which are essential for the killing of M. *tuberculosis*. Unfortunately, in

high doses, they are also lethal for human cells – and the symptoms of TB (and many other diseases) are an unavoidable side effect of the body's attempt to deal with infection.

20. E. Pearlman et al., 'Modulation of murine cytokine responses to mycobacterial antigens by helminth-induced T helper 2 cell responses', Journal of Immunology, vol. 151, 1993, pp. 4857–64; G. R. Stewart et al., 'Onchocerciasis modulates the immune response to mycobacterial antigens', Clinical Experimental Immunology, vol. 117, 1999, pp. 517–23.

21. On this correlation, see P. E. M. Fine, 'Leprosy and tuberculosis – an epidemiological comparison', Tubercle, vol. 65, 1984, pp. 137–53.

22. E. Lozes et al., 'Cross-reactive immune responses against Mycobacterium bovis BCG in mice infected with non-tuberculous mycobacteria belonging to the MAIS-Group', Scandinavian Journal of Immunology, vol. 46, 1997, pp. 16–26.

23. Advisory Council for the Elimination of Tuberculosis (ACET), 'Tuberculosis elimination revisited: obstacles, opportunities, and a renewed commitment', Morbidity and Mortality Weekly Report, 1999.

24. J. S. Bergmann and G. L. Woods, 'Clinical evaluation of the Roche AMPLICOR PCR Mycobacterium tuberculosis test for detection of M. tuberculosis in respiratory specimens', Journal of Clinical Microbiology, vol. 34, 1996, pp. 1083–5; E. Carpentier et al., 'Diagnosis of tuberculosis by Amplicor Mycobacterium tuberculosis test: a multicenter study', Journal of Clinical Microbiology, vol. 33, 1995, pp. 3106–10.

25. N. Manjunath et al., 'Evaluation of a polymerase chain reaction for the diagnosis of tuberculosis', Tubercle, vol. 72, 1991, pp. 21–7.

26. A. B. Andersen et al., 'Interspecies reactivity of five monoclonal antibodies to Mycobacterium tuberculosis as examined by immunoblotting and enzyme-linked immunosorbant assay', Journal of Clinical Microbiology, vol. 23, 1986, pp. 446–51; A. R. Coates et al., 'Antigenic diversity of Mycobacterium tuberculosis and Mycobacterium bovis detected by means of monoclonal antibodies', Lancet, vol. 2, 1981, pp. 167–9.

27. R. Turcotte, 'The participation of common and species-"specific" antigens of mycobacteria in the tuberculin skin reaction', Canadian. Journal of Microbiology, vol. 21, 1975, pp. 774–83.

28. S. T. Cole et al., 'Deciphering the biology of Mycobacterium tuberculosis from the complete genome sequence', Nature, vol. 393, 1998, pp. 537–44.

29. G. G. Mahairas et al., 'Molecular analysis of genetic differences between Mycobacterium bovis BCG and virulent M. bovis', Journal of Bacteriology, vol. 178, 1996, pp. 1274–82.

30. Behr et al., 'Comparative genomics'; Gordon et al., 'Identification of variable regions'; R. Brosch et al., 'Use of Mycobacterium tuberculosis H37Rv bacterial artificial chromosome library for genome mapping, sequencing, and comparative genomics', Infection and Immunity, vol. 66, 1998, pp. 2221–9.

31. P. Andersen et al., 'Recall of long-lived immunity to Mycobacterium

tuberculosis infection in mice', *Journal of Immunology*, vol. 154, 1995, pp. 3359–72; F. X. Berthet *et al.*, 'A mycobacterium tuberculosis operon encoding ESAT-6 and a novel low-molecular-mass culture filtrate protein (CFP-10)', *Microbiology*, vol. 144, 1998, pp. 3195–203; L. A. H. van Pinxteren *et al.*, 'Diagnosis of tuberculosis based on the two specific antigens ESAT-6 and CFP10', *Clinical Diagnosis and Laboratory Immunology*, vol. 7, 2000, pp. 155–60; R. L. Skjot *et al.*, 'Comparative evaluation of low-molecular-mass proteins from Mycobacterium tuberculosis identifies members of the ESAT-6 family as immunodominant T-cell antigens', *Infection and Immunity*, vol. 68, 2000, pp. 214–20; M. Harboe *et al.*, 'Evidence for occurrence of the ESAT-6 protein in Mycobacterium tuberculosis and virulent Mycobacterium bovis and for its absence in Mycobacterium bovis BCG', *Infection and Immunity*, vol. 64, 1996, pp. 16–22.

32. Van Pinxteren *et al.*, 'Diagnosis of tuberculosis'; J. M. Pollock and P. Andersen, 'The potential of the ESAT-6 antigen secreted by virulent mycobacteria for specific diagnosis of tuberculosis', *Journal of Infectious Diseases*, vol. 175, 1997, pp. 1251–4; B. M. Buddle *et al.*, 'Differentiation between mycobacterium bovis BCG-vaccinated and M. bovis-infected cattle by using recombinant mycobacterial antigens', *Clinical Diagnosis and Laboratory Immunology*, vol. 6, 1999, pp. 1–5.

33. T. Ulrichs *et al.*, 'Differential T cell responses to Mycobacterium tuberculosis ESAT-6 in tuberculosis patients and healthy donors', *European Journal of Immunology*, vol. 28, 1998, pp. 3949–58; A. S. Mustafa *et al.*, 'Comparison of antigen-specific T-cell responses of tuberculosis patients using complex or single antigens of Mycobacterium tuberculosis', *Scandinavian Journal of Immunology*, vol. 48, 1998, pp. 535–43; A. D. Lein *et al.*, 'Cellular immune responses to ESAT-6 discriminate between patients with pulmonary disease due to Mycobacterium avium complex and those with pulmonary disease due to Mycobacterium tuberculosis', *Clinical Diagnosis and Laboratory Immunology*, vol. 6, 1999, pp. 606–9; P. Ravn *et al.*, 'Human T cell responses to the ESAT-6 antigen from Mycobacterium tuberculosis', *Journal of Infectious Diseases*, vol. 179, 1999, pp. 637–45.

34. J. M. Ponnighaus *et al.*, 'Efficacy of BCG vaccine against leprosy and tuberculosis in northern Malawi', *Lancet*, vol. 339, 1992, pp. 636–9; C. Lanckriet *et al.*, 'Efficacy of BCG vaccination of the newborn: evaluation by a follow-up study of contacts in Bangui', *International Journal of Epidemiology*, vol. 24, 1995, pp. 1042–9; S. P. Zodpey *et al.*, 'Effectiveness of Bacillus Calmette Guerin (BCG) vaccination in the prevention of childhood pulmonary tuberculosis: a case control study in Nagpur, India', *Southeast Asian Journal of Tropical Medicine and Public Health*, vol. 29, 1998, pp. 285–8.

35. J. L. Flynn *et al.*, 'An essential role for interferon gamma in resistance to Mycobacterium tuberculosis infection', *Journal of Experimental Medicine*,

vol. 178, 1993, pp. 2249–54; T. H. Ottenhoff, D. Kumararatne and J. L. Casanova, 'Novel human immunodeficiencies reveal the essential role of type-I cytokines in immunity to intracellular bacteria', *Immunology Today*, vol. 19, 1998, pp. 491–4; A. K. Abbas, K. M. Murphy and A. Sher, 'Functional diversity of helper T lymphocytes', *Nature*, vol. 383, 1996, pp. 787–93.

36. C. H. Ladel, S. Daugelat and S. H. Kaufmann, 'Immune response to Mycobacterium bovis bacille Calmette Guerin infection in major histo-compatibility complex class I- and II-deficient knock-out mice: contribution of CD4 and CD8 T cells to acquired resistance', *European Journal of Immunology*, vol. 25, 1995, pp. 377–84; S. Stenger *et al.*, 'Differential effects of cytolytic T cell subsets on intracellular infection', *Science*, vol. 276, 1997, pp. 1684–7; J. P. Rosat *et al.*, 'CD1-restricted microbial lipid antigen-specific recognition found in the CD8+ alpha beta T cell pool', *Journal of Immunology*, vol. 162, 1999, pp. 366–71; D. Jullien *et al.*, 'CD1 presentation of microbial nonpeptide antigens to T cells', *Journal of Clinical Investigations*, vol. 99, 1997, pp. 2071–4.

37. M. A. Behr and P. M. Small, 'Has BCG attenuated to impotence?' *Nature*, vol. 389, 1997, pp. 133–4.

38. L. Slobbe *et al.*, 'An in vivo comparison of bacillus Calmette-Guerin (BCG) and cytokine-secreting BCG vaccines', *Immunology*, vol. 96, 1999, pp. 517–23.

39. R. A. McAdam *et al.*, 'In vivo growth characteristics of leucine and methionine auxotrophic mutants of Mycobacterium bovis BCG generated by transposon mutagenesis', *Infection and Immunity*, vol. 63, 1995, pp. 1004–12; I. Guleria *et al.*, 'Auxotrophic vaccines for tuberculosis', *Nature Medicine*, vol. 2, 1996, pp. 334–7; M. Jackson *et al.*, 'Persistence and protective efficacy of a Mycobacterium tuberculosis auxotroph vaccine', *Infection and Immunity*, vol. 67, 1999, pp. 2867–73.

40. Guleria *et al.*, 'Auxotrophic vaccines'.

41. A. Kochi, 'Tuberculosis: distribution, risk factors, mortality', *Immunobiology*, vol. 191, 1994, pp. 325–36.

42. Ponnighaus *et al.*, 'Efficacy of BCG vaccine'.

43. F. M. Collins, 'Immunogenicity of various mycobacteria and the corresponding levels of cross-protection developed between species', *Infection and Immunity*, vol. 4, 1971, pp. 688–96.

44. For results, so far, see Durban Immunotherapy Trial Group, 'Immunotherapy with Mycobacterium vaccae in patients with newly diagnosed pulmonary tuberculosis: a randomised controlled trial', *Lancet*, vol. 354, 1999, pp. 116–19.

45. X. Zhu *et al.*, 'Vaccination with recombinant vaccinia viruses protects mice against Mycobacterium tuberculosis infection', *Immunology*, vol. 92, 1997, pp. 6–9; J. Hess and S. H. Kaufmann, 'Live antigen carriers as tools for improved anti-tuberculosis vaccines', *FEMS: Immunology and Medical Microbiology*, vol. 23, 1999, pp. 165–73.

46. R. L. Anacker *et al.*, 'Effectiveness of cell walls of Mycobacterium bovis strain BCG administered by various routes and in different adjuvants in protecting mice against airborne infection with Mycobacterium tuberculosis strain H37Rv', *American Review of Respiratory Disease*, vol. 99, 1969, pp. 242–8. Adjuvants are chemical mixtures which augment the immunogenicity of vaccine antigens. They generally do this by stimulating specific types of immune response, so the choice of the appropriate adjuvant for vaccination is crucial.

47. Rook and Stanford, 'The Koch phenomenon'; K. N. Masihi *et al.*, 'Immunobiological activities of nontoxic lipid A: enhancement of nonspecific resistance in combination with trehalose dimycolate against viral infection and adjuvant effects', *International Journal of Immunopharmacology*, vol. 8, 1986, pp. 339–45.

48. P. Andersen, 'Effective vaccination of mice against Mycobacterium tuberculosis infection with a soluble mixture of secreted mycobacterial proteins', *Infection and Immunity*, vol. 62, 1994, pp. 2536–44.

49. Ibid. See also M. A. Horwitz *et al.*, 'Protective immunity against tuberculosis induced by vaccination with major extracellular proteins of Mycobacterium tuberculosis', *Proceedings of the National Academy of Science*, vol. 92, 1995, pp. 1530–4; J. Hess *et al.*, 'Superior efficacy of secreted over somatic antigen display in recombinant Salmonella vaccine induced protection against listeriosis', *Proceedings of the National Academy of Science*, vol. 93, 1996, pp. 1458–63.

50. E. B. Lindblad *et al.*, 'Adjuvant modulation of immune response to tuberculosis sub-unit vaccines', *Infection and Immunity*, vol. 65, 1997, pp. 623–9; A. K. Sharma *et al.*, 'Adjuvant modulation of T-cell reactivity to 30-kDa secretory protein of Mycobacterium tuberculosis H37Rv and its protective efficacy against experimental tuberculosis', *Journal of Medical Microbiology*, vol. 48, 1999, pp. 757–63.

51. Lindblad *et al.*, 'Adjuvant modulation'.

52. L. Brandt *et al.*, 'ESAT-6 subunit vaccination against Mycobacterium tuberculosis', *Infection and Immunity*, vol. 68, 2000.

53. J. B. Ulmer *et al.*, 'DNA vaccines against tuberculosis', *Novartis Foundation Symposium*, vol. 217, 1998, pp. 239–46; R. E. Tascon *et al.*, 'Vaccination against tuberculosis by DNA injection', *Nature Medicine*, vol. 2, 1996, pp. 888–92; K. Huygen, 'DNA vaccines: application to tuberculosis', *International Journal of Tuberculosis and Lung Disease*, vol. 2, 1998, pp. 971–8.

54. O. Denis *et al.*, 'Vaccination with plasmid DNA encoding mycobacterial antigen 85A stimulates a CD4+ and CD8+ T-cell epitopic repertoire broader than that stimulated by Mycobacterium tuberculosis H37Rv infection', *Infection and Immunology*, vol. 66, 1998, pp. 1527–33; C. L. Silva, V. L. Bonato and V. M. Lima, 'DNA encoding individual mycobacterial antigens protects mice against tuberculosis', *Brazilian Journal of Medical and Biological Research*, vol. 32, 1999, pp. 231–4.

55. D. B. Lowrie *et al.*, 'Therapy of tuberculosis in mice by DNA vaccination', *Nature*, vol. 400, 1999, pp. 269–71.

56. P. R. Hernandez *et al.*, 'Pathogenesis of tuberculosis in mice exposed to low and high doses of an environmental mycobacterial saprophyte before infection', *Infection and Immunity*, vol. 65, 1997, pp. 3317–27; A. D. Howard and B. S. Zwilling, 'Reactivation of tuberculosis is associated with a shift from Type 1 to Type 2 cytokines', *Clinical Experimental Immunology*, vol. 115, 1999, pp. 428–34; T. Mustafa *et al.*, 'A mouse model for slowly progressive primary tuberculosis', *Scandinavian Journal of Immunology*, vol. 50, 1999, pp. 127–36; C. A. Scanga *et al.*, 'Reactivation of latent tuberculosis: variations on the Cornell murine model', *Infection and Immunity*, vol. 67, 1999, pp. 4531–8.

57. S. L. Baldwin *et al.*, 'Evaluation of new vaccines in the mouse and guinea pig model of tuberculosis', *Infection and Immunity*, vol. 66, 1998, pp. 2951–9.

13   Global Poverty and Tuberculosis: Implications for Ethics and Human Rights

1. S. R. Benatar, 'Prospects for global health: lessons from tuberculosis', *Thorax*, vol. 50, 1995, pp. 487–9.

2. D. L. Cohn, F. Bustreo and M. Raviglione, 'Drug-resistant tuberculosis: review of the worldwide situation and the WHO/IUATLD global surveillance project', *Clinical Infectious Diseases*, vol. 24, 1997, pp. S121–30.

3. M. A. Espinal, ed., *Report: Multidrug resistant tuberculosis*, (WHO/TB/ 99.26.), Geneva: World Health Organization, 1999.

4. C. Holden, 'Stalking a killer in Russia's prisons', *Science*, vol. 286, 1999, p. 1670.

5. P. Alcock, *Understanding Poverty*, 2nd edn, London: Macmillan, 1993.

6. S. R. Benatar, 'Global disparities in health and human rights', *American Journal of Public Health*, vol 88, 1998, pp. 285–300; R. L. Sivard, *World Military and Social Expenditure*, 16th edn, Washington, DC: World Priorities, 1996; I. Heath *et al.*, 'Poverty and health – an open invitation to health professionals', *South African Medical Journal*, vol. 90, 2000 pp. 126–7.

7. D. Logie and S. R. Benatar, 'Realistic priorities for AIDS control', *Lancet*, vol. 356, 2000, pp. 1535–6.

8. S. George and F. Sabelli, *Faith and Credit: the World Bank's Secular Empire*, London: Penguin, 1994; A. Pettifor, *Debt, the Most Potent Form of Slavery: A Discussion of the Role of Western Lending Policies in Supporting the Economies of Poor Countries*, London: Christian Aid, 1996.

9. A. J. McMichael, *Planetary Overload: Global Environmental Change and the Health of the Human Species*, Cambridge: Cambridge University Press, 1993.

10. S. Huntington, 'The clash of civilisations', *Foreign Affairs*, vol. 72, 1993, pp. 22–49; B. R. Barber, *Jihad versus McWorld: How Globalism and Tribalism are Reshaping the World*, New York: Ballantine Books, 1995.

11. 'The health of nations', *Economist*, 24 June 2000, p. 118; R. G. Wilkinson, *Unhealthy Societies: The Afflictions of Inequality*, London: Routledge, 1996.

12. Wilkinson, *Unhealthy Societies*.

13. *Final Report of Meeting on Policy-oriented Monitoring of Equity in Health and Health Care* (WHO/ARA/98.2.), Geneva: World Health Organization, 1998.

14. Ibid.

15. G. Gunatilleke, *Poverty and Health in Developing Countries*, (WHO/CO/MESD.16.), Geneva: World Health Organization, 1995.

16. Ibid.

17. World Health Organization, *World Health Report 1998: Life in the 21st Century – a Vision for All*, Geneva: World Health Organization, 1999.

18. World Health Organization, *World Health Report 1996: Fighting Disease, Fostering Development*, Geneva: World Health Organization, 1997.

19. B. R. Bloom *et al.*, 'Investing in the World Health Organisation', *Science*, vol. 284, 1999, p. 911.

20. B. Loff and S. Gruskin, 'Getting serious about the right to health', *Lancet*, vol. 356, 2000, p. 1435.

21. M. Ignatieff, 'Human Rights: the Midlife Crisis', *New York Review of Books*, 20 May 1999, pp. 58–62.

22. A. R. Chapman and L. S. Rubenstein, eds., *Human Rights and Health*, Washington, DC: American Association for the Advancement of Science, 1998; Amnesty International, *United States of America: Rights for All*, London: Amnesty International, 1998.

23. E. Hobsbawm, *The Age of Extremes: The Short Twentieth Century, 1914–1991*, London: Pantheon Books, 1994; J. Grey, *False Dawn: the Delusions of Global Capitalism*, London: Granta Books, 1998; World Health Organization, *Health and Environment in Sustainable Development: Five Years After the Summit*, Geneva: World Health Organization, 1997; I. Hauchler and P. M. Kennedy, eds., *Global Trends: The World Almanac of Development and Peace*, New York: Continuum, 1994. See also note 6 above, and McMichael, *Planetary Overload*.

24. A. Richmond, *Global Apartheid*, Oxford: Oxford University Press, 1994; T. Alexander, *Unravelling Global Apartheid: An Overview of World Politics*, Cambridge: Polity Press, 1996.

25. J. Geiger, 'The political context of health care: some warnings from the US', in M. A. Seedat, ed., *Health Care Team: Unity in Action*, Westville: University of Durban, 1995, pp. 2–19.

26. N. Gardels, 'The post-Atlantic capitalist order', *New Perspectives Quarterly*, vol. 2/3, 1993, pp. 2–3.

27. R. Heilbroner, 'The rest of the world off the track: growth and the lumpen planet', *New Perspectives Quarterly*, vol. 2/3, 1993, pp. 48–53.

28. R. Howard, 'Monitoring human rights: problems of consistency', *Ethics and International Affairs*, vol. 4, 1990, pp. 33–51.

29. R. Howard, 'Human rights and the search for community', *Journal of Peace Research*, vol. 32, 1995, pp. 1–8.

30. J. Grange and A. Zumla, 'Tuberculosis – an epidemic of injustice', *Journal of the Royal College of Physicians of London*, vol 31, 1997, pp. 637–9.

31. R. Sennett, *The Corrosion of Character: The Personal Consequences of Work in the New Capitalism*, New York: W. W. Norton and Co., 1998.

32. A. R. Jonsen, *The Birth of Bioethics*, Oxford: Oxford University Press, 1998.

33. McMichael, *Planetary Overload*.

34. H. R. Friman and P. Andreas, eds., *The Illicit Global Economy and State Power*, New York: Rowman and Littlefield, 1999.

35. McMichael, *Planetary Overload*.

36. S. R. Benatar, 'The importance of medical ethics as an international endeavour', *World Medical Journal*, vol. 41, 1995, pp. 20–5.

37. S. R. Benatar and J. Coovadia, Preface to H. M. Coovadia and S. R. Benatar, eds., *A Century of Tuberculosis: South African Perspectives*, Oxford: Oxford University Press, 1991.

Epilogue: Politics, Science and the 'New' Tuberculosis

1. For optimistic views on the role of science in the eradication of disease see: N. Letvin, B. Bloom and S. L. Hoffman, 'Prospects for vaccines to protect against AIDS, tuberculosis and malaria', *Journal of the American Medical Association*, vol. 285, pp. 606–11; I. M. Orme, 'The search for new vaccines against tuberculosis', *Journal of Leucocyte Biology*, vol. 70, 2001, pp. 1–10.

2. See, for example, T. R. Frieden, B. H. Lerner and B. R. Rutherford, 'Lessons from the 1800s: tuberculosis control in the new millenium', *Lancet*, vol. 355, 2000, pp. 1088–92; M. Gandy, 'Science, society, and disease: emerging perspectives', *Current Opinion in Pulmonary Medicine*, vol. 7, 2001, pp. 170–2; A. Zumla and J. Grange, 'Science, medicine and the future: the future of tuberculosis', *British Medical Journal* vol. 316, 1998, pp. 1962–4; A. Zumla and J. Grange, 'Tuberculosis and the poverty–disease cycle', *Journal of the Royal Society of Medicine*, vol. 92, 1999, pp. 105–7; D. N. Wallace, 'Discriminatory public policies and the New York City tuberculosis epidemic, 1975–1993', *Microbes Infect*, vol. 3, 2001, pp. 515–24.

3. F. Williams, 'WHO programme under fire', *Financial Times*, 5 October 2000.

4. C. Ainsworth and D. MacKenzie, 'Coming home', *New Scientist*, vol. 171, 7 July 2001, pp. 28–33; C. Cookson, 'Resistant strains of TB continue to spread', *Financial Times*, 24 March 2000.

5. V. Griffith, 'New alliance to fight TB threat', *Financial Times*, 10 October 2000.
6. D. Piling, 'A shot in the arm for the drugs industry: scientific advances and a change in public attitudes are fuelling the revival of the vaccine', *Financial Times*, 23 February 2000.
7. Editorial comment, 'Cheaper medicine exposes Africa's woes: pharmaceutical companies may have cut drug prices but poor countries still face many other obstacles', *Financial Times*, 19 May 2000.
8. R. Brugha and G. Watt, 'A global health fund: a leap of faith', *British Medical Journal*, vol. 323, 2001, pp. 152–9.
9. G. Tett, 'The G8 summit: G8 leaders sign up to anti-disease targets', *Financial Times*, 24 July 2000.

About the Contributors

Peter Andersen is head of the Department of Infectious Disease Immunology at the Statens Serum Institute in Copenhagen. He is a World Health Organization adviser on the development of a vaccine against tuberculosis, a member of the European Union expert panel on vaccines against TB and Chairman of the WHO task force for the evaluation of experimental tuberculosis vaccines.

Solomon R. Benatar is Professor of Medicine at the University of Cape Town Medical School and the Director of the University of Cape Town Bioethics Centre. He is President of the International Association of Bioethics and his current research is focused on international research ethics and international health.

Léopold Blanc is based in the Communicable Disease Cluster of the WHO, Geneva with responsibility for developing strategies for tuberculosis control. He has worked for the Institut Marchoux (Mali) and was for six years the WHO Regional Adviser for tuberculosis control and leprosy elimination in the Western Pacific Region.

Ken Citron was formerly a consultant physician at the Royal Brompton Hospital, London. He is a trustee of TB Alert and has written influential reports on the relationship between tuberculosis and homelessness.

Andrew D. Cliff is Professor of Geography at the University of Cambridge. He has co-authored (with Matthew Smallman-Raynor) several books at the interface of geography and epidemiology, including: *International Atlas of AIDS* (Blackwell, 1992), *Measles: An Historical Geography from Global Expansion to Local Retreat* (Blackwell, 1993), *Deciphering Global Epidemics* (Cambridge University Press, 1998) and *Island Epidemics* (Oxford University Press, 2000).

Vinod K. Diwan is Professor in the Nordic School of Public Health, Gothenburg, and the Division of International Health Care Research, Karolinska Institute, Stockholm, Sweden. He is the co-author of *Gender and Tuberculosis* (Nordic School of Public Health, 1998). His current research interests include gender and tuberculosis, access to health care, and the impact of migration on disease epidemiology. His research includes studies in China, India, Sweden, Vietnam and Zambia.

T. Mark Doherty is a senior scientist in the Department of Infectious Disease Immunology at the Serum Statens Institut, Copenhagen, Denmark. He has worked on the immunology of intracellular infections (particularly the mycobacteria), cytokine biology and the intersection of these fields for the past twelve years, leading to many publications in leading journals such as *Science*. He has also been involved in the initiation of clinical trials of immunotherapy of mycobacterial infections in the United States, and has been a WHO distinguished visiting professor in Brazil and adviser for the WHO, the Centers for Disease Control and Prevention, and the EU. He currently co-ordinates the department's clinical research programme in Africa.

Paul Farmer is an infectious disease physician and anthropologist. He is a professor in the Harvard Medical School and divides his clinical time between Boston, Haiti and Peru. He is author of *AIDS and Accusation: Haiti and the Geography of Blame* (University of California Press, 1992) and *Infections and Inequalities: The Modern Plagues* (University of California Press, 2001) and is co-author of *The Uses of Haiti* (Common Courage Press, 1994) and *Women, Poverty and AIDS: Sex, Drugs and Structural Violence* (Common Courage Press, 1996).

Matthew Gandy is Reader in Geography at University College London. He has published widely on urban, environmental and cultural themes. His most recent book is *Concrete and Clay: Reworking Nature in New*

York City (MIT Press, 2002). His current research interests are focused on cultural histories of water, sanitation and urban infrastructure with research in Germany, India, Nigeria and the USA.

Nicola J. Hargreaves is Lecturer in Tropical Medicine at the Liverpool School of Tropical Medicine. She is also co-ordinator of the PROTEST Project, National Tuberculosis Control Programme, Lilongwe, Malawi.

Anthony D. Harries is Foundation Professor of Medicine, Malawi, and Technical Adviser to the National Tuberculosis Control Programme, Malawi. He is also an honorary professor at the Liverpool School of Tropical Medicine and the London School of Hygiene and Tropical Medicine. He is co-author of *TB/HIV: A Clinical Manual* (World Health Organization, 1996) and *Clinical Problems in Tropical Medicine* (W. B. Saunders, 1998).

Nicholas B. King is the J. Alfred Royer Postdoctoral Fellow in the Department of Anthropology, History and Social Medicine at the University of California, San Francisco. He is currently writing a book on emerging diseases, globalization, and biological terrorism.

Richard Levins is the John Rock Professor of Population Sciences in the Department of Population and International Health, Harvard University. Richard Levins is a former tropical farmer turned ecologist, biomathematician and philosopher of science. He is author of many influential publications including (with Richard Lewontin) *The Dialectical Biologist* (Harvard University Press, 1985). He is a pioneer of the ecology movement in Puerto Rico.

Richard Lewontin is the Alexander Agassiz Research Professor in the Museum of Comparative Zoology at Harvard University, and an evolutionary geneticist, philosopher of science and social critic. His books include (with Richard Levins) *The Dialectical Biologist* (Harvard University Press, 1985), *Biology as Ideology: The Doctrine of DNA* (Harper Collins, 1991) and *The Triple Helix: Gene, Organism and Environment* (Harvard University Press, 2000).

Christian Lienhardt is a clinical epidemiologist and coordinator of the TB Research Programme at the Institut de Recherche pour le Développement (IRD) in Dakar, Senegal. He has worked for many years in the field of leprosy and tuberculosis research and is currently the coordinator of a multicentre project in West Africa to explore problems of access to health care and develop long-term strategies for tuberculosis control.

Martin E. Munk is originally from Brazil and has worked in Germany and Denmark for more than fifteen years, most recently at the Max Planck Institute for Infection Biology in Berlin and the Statens Serum Institute in Copenhagen, where he was a Marie Curie Fellow. His work has focused on human responses to infection with *M. tuberculosis*, and diagnosis of latent infection. He currently works as a senior scientist at Genemab, Copenhagen.

Jessica Ogden is Senior Lecturer in Social Anthropology at the London School of Hygiene and Tropical Medicine. Her doctoral research focused on the relationship between gender, reproductive identity and HIV/AIDS in Kampala, Uganda. Since joining the London School in 1995 she has conducted research on tuberculosis in India and West Africa and health policy research in South Africa and Mozambique. Her current research is concerned with the interface between biomedicine and the social sciences in the development of effective and sustainable infectious disease interventions.

Matthew Smallman-Raynor is Reader in Geography at the University of Nottingham. He has co-authored (with Andrew Cliff) several books at the interface of geography and epidemiology, including: *International Atlas of AIDS* (Blackwell, 1992), *Measles: An Historical Geography from Global Expansion to Local Retreat* (Blackwell, 1993), *Deciphering Global Epidemics* (Cambridge University Press, 1998) and *Island Epidemics* (Oxford University Press, 2000).

Oumou Younoussa Sow is a Medical Doctor and specialist in Pneumology and International Health. Professor Sow is the Head of the Pneumology Unit at the Ignace Deen Teaching Hospital in Conakry (Guinée). She initiated and headed the National Tuberculosis Control Programme in Guinée until 2001. Her current research is focused on TB in Africa and she has organized several courses on the management of TB in resource-poor countries.

Vivien Stern is Director of the International Centre for Prison Studies at King's College, University of London, and Honorary Secretary-General of Penal Reform International. She is author of *A Sin Against the Future: Imprisonment in the World* (Northeastern University Press, 1998) and editor of *Sentenced to Die? The Problem of TB in Prisons in Eastern Europe and Central Asia* (Centre for Prison Studies, 1999).

Alistair Storey is a trained TB nurse with extensive experience of community-based and outpatient nursing. He is currently based in the Tuberculosis Division of the Public Health Laboratory Service, London, and is a member of the London TB Link Project.

Anna Thorson is based in the Division of International Health Care Research in the Nordic School of Public Health, Gothenburg, Sweden. She is co-author of *Gender and Tuberculosis* (Nordic School of Public Health, 1998).

Mukund Uplekar works for the WHO in Geneva and is a Takemi Fellow in International Health of the Harvard School of Public Health. He has had a long association with the Foundation for Research in Community Health based in Mumbai and Pune, India. His current research is focused on access to health care and gender issues related to tuberculosis control.

Deborah N. Wallace is President of Public Interest Scientific Consulting Service Inc. Her current research involves the application of ecosystem ecology to the understanding of the spatiotemporal dynamics of AIDS, tuberculosis and health care inequalities. Her many publications include (with Rodrick M. Wallace) *A Plague on Your Houses: How New York Was Burned Down and Public Health Crumbled* (Verso, 1998).

Rodrick M. Wallace is research scientist in the Epidemiology of Mental Disorders Research Department at the New York State Psychiatric Institute. He has carried out extensive research into the socioeconomic factors behind the incidence of AIDS, tuberculosis, violence and low-weight births. He is author (with Deborah N. Wallace) of *A Plague on*

Your Houses: How New York Was Burned Down and Public Health Crumbled (Verso, 1998).

David Walton is a research fellow in the Harvard Medical School Programme in Infectious Disease and Social Change and also works at the Clinique Bon Saveur in Haiti's Central Plateau. His research is focused on the management of tuberculosis, HIV and sexually transmitted diseases.

Alimuddin Zumla is Professor of Infectious Diseases and International Health at the Royal Free and University College Medical School and Director of the Centre for Infectious Diseases and International Health, Windeyer Institute of Medical Sciences, University College London. He has published extensively on the clinical, scientific, operational and medical aspects of a variety of infectious diseases and is co-editor of several books including *AIDS and Respiratory Medicine* (Chapman and Hall, 1997), *Granulomatous Disorders* (Cambridge University Press, 1999) and *Manson's Tropical Diseases* (Saunders, 2002).

Resource List

American Lung Association
http://www.lungusa.org/

British Lung Foundation
http://www.lunguk.org/research/

Centers for Disease Control and Prevention
National Center for HIV, STD and TB Prevention
http://www.cdc.gov/nchstp/tb/

Columbia University Information Website
http://www.cpmc.columbia.edu/tbcpp/index.html

Global list of Tuberculosis websites
http://www.cpmc.columbia.edu/tbcpp/extres.html

IUATLD
International Union Against Tuberculosis and Lung Disease
68 boulevard Saint Michel
75006 Paris
France
union@iuatld.org
http://www.iuatld.org

Johns Hopkins Center for Tuberculosis Research
http://www.hopkins-tb.org/

National Institutes of Health, Division of Microbiology and Infectious Diseases
http://www.niaid.nih.gov/dmid/tuberculosis/

New Jersey Medical School National Tuberculosis Center
http://www.umdnj.edu/ntbcweb/tbsplash.html

New York City Department of Health Chest Clinics
http://www.cpmc.columbia.edu/tbcpp/tbclinic.html

Public Health Research Institute Tuberculosis Center
International Center for Public Health
225 Warren Street
Newark, NJ 07103–3535
USA
http://www.phri.org/tb.htm

Stop TB
http://www.stoptb.org/

Stop TB / Haltez à la Tuberculose Canada
http://www.stoptb.ca/

TB Alert
22 Tiverton Rd
London NW10 3HL
UK
tbalert@somhealy.demon.co.uk
http://www.tbalert.org

Tuberculosis: Annotated Internet Resources
http://www.comeunity.com/adoption/health/tuberculosis/resources.html

Tuberculosis.net
http://tuberculosis.net/

Tuberculosis Control – India
Central TB Division
Directorate General of Health Services
Nirman Bhavan
New Delhi – 110 001
India
postmaster@tbcindia.org
http://www.tbindia.org

Tuberculosis Research Unit
Case Western Reserve University
http://www.cwru.edu/affil/tbru

Tuberculosis Resources
http://www.cpmc.columbia.edu/resources/tbcpp/

USAID Tuberculosis Web Resources
http://www.usaid.gov/pop_health/id/tuberculosis/resources/

WHO
Communicable Diseases
World Health Organization
20 Avenue Appia
CH-1211 Geneva 27
Switzerland
http://www.who.int/gtb/
http://www.who.int/gtb/publications/index.html

Acknowledgements

The first stages of this project were completed with a small grant from University College London that facilitated a unique collaboration between the UCL Department of Geography and the Windeyer Institute in the UCL Medical School. Special thanks must go to Martin Harradine who participated in this project and helped to track down many key bibliographic sources for the collection. Our editor at Verso, Jane Hindle, has played a pivotal role in bringing this complex project to fruition. Other critical inputs from Verso include Tim Clark, Peter Hinton and Stuart Smith. We would also like to thank our copy editor Pat Harper for her invaluable contribution to the final outcome. Thanks also to Jamie Quinn in the UCL Cartographic Laboratory for his assistance in the preparation of maps and figures. We are grateful for permission from Guilford Press to reproduce the essay by Richard Lewontin and Richard Levins which originally appeared in *Capitalism, Nature, Socialism*, vol. 7, June 1996, pp. 103–7. The painting by Alice Neel is reproduced with permission from the National Museum of Women in the Arts, Washington, DC.

Index

Page numbers in italics denote references to figures/tables.

access to health care
  anti-essentialism 43
  as cornerstone of TB control
    programmes 197
  equitable 232
  fees for provision 106
  gender differences 64
  HIV infection 11
  homeless people 156
  immigrants 48, 153–4, 155
  influence on DOTS strategy 201
  interdisciplinary approach 196
  multi-drug-resistant TB 164, 175–6
  qualitative approach to TB control 205
  racial disparities 51, 52
  rural/urban differences 198
  social vulnerability 199
  stigmatization 57
  transnational geographies of difference
    53
  unequal 32
  urban poor 31
  World Medical Association proposed
    code 236
active case finding 58, 61, 64, 121, 197
adjuvants 218–19
adverse skin reactions to drugs 119
Advocacy Forum for Massive Effort
    Against Diseases of Poverty 238
Afghanistan
  estimated number of cases 109
  refugees 91

Africa
  cholera pandemic 1
  deterioration in healthcare delivery
    systems 224
  European colonial explanations for
    disease 42
  health-seeking behaviour differences
    197–8
  HIV/AIDS 8, 35–6, 42, 95, 100–2, 101,
    105, 112–24, 239
  male/female prevalence ratios 60, 64
  malnutrition 210
  notified cases 97, 98, 98, 99, 102, 105
  racial arguments 29
  rural urban differences in 198
  West African TB Research Initiative 205
African-Americans 28–9, 42, 51, 129,
    135, 136
agriculture schools 5
AIDS see HIV/AIDS
Alaska, female progression from infection
    to disease 61
Algeria, effective TB case management
    strategies 104
American Region
  HIV attributable cases 101
  notified cases 98, 99
  see also North America; South America
'amplifier effect' 35, 165
Amsterdam Declaration 110, 239
Angola, refugees 91
animal diseases 3
anti-essentialism 43–4
anti-urbanism 18, 19, 20
antibiotics 2, 8, 18, 119, 120

antibiotics (*cont.*)
    advances in treatment 32, 33
    decline of TB in the United Kingdom
        148
    resistance to 134, 145–6, 177
    see also drugs; isoniazid; streptomycin
antiretroviral drugs 114–15, 120, 122–3,
    159, 240
apartheid 32, 229, 230, 235
Argentina, drug-resistant TB 103
Argentine haemorrhagic fever 1
Armenia, conflicts 180
Asia
    developing economies 105
    fees for health care provision 106
    HIV infections 100, *101*, 102, 239
    notified cases 100
    see also South Asia; Southeast Asia
asylum seekers 91, 152, 153–4, 155
    see also refugees
Australia
    delay in diagnosis 197
    immigrants 44, *45*
    notified cases 104
    wartime TB mortality 84, *85*
Austria, wartime TB mortality 84, *85*
Austro-Prussian War 71, 74
Azerbaijan, prison infections 184, 186,
    187, 188, 190

Bacille Calmette-Guérin vaccine *see* BCG
    vaccination
bacteria 3, 4, 9, 10, 208–9, 218
bacteriology 15, 17, 22, 27, 28
Bailey, Norman 130
Bangladesh
    costs of TB 106–7
    DOTS-Plus projects 176
    estimated number of cases *109*
    GNP 226
    multi-drug-resistant TB 176
    women 65
Barnes, David 26
BCG (Bacille Calmette-Guérin) vaccination
    122, 206, 208–12, 213, 220, 241
    beneficial effects 216, 221
    development of 31–2
    former Soviet bloc 180, 181
    gender differences in scar size 60
    genes 215, 216–17
    immigrants to London 153
    response of patients to PPD 214
Beach, William 16–17
Becerra, Mercedes 179
Belgium

decline of TB 27
    wartime TB mortality 84, *85*
'Benign Neglect' 139, 141
Benin, notified cases 105
biological terrorism 7
Black Death 3
Blackmore, Richard 16
bloodstream infections 115, 120
Bolivia, female fatality rate 67
Bolivian haemorrhagic fever 1
Bosnia-Herzegovina, refugees 91
Botswana
    delay in diagnosis 197
    HIV infections 114
bovine tuberculosis 17, 24, 208
Brazil
    estimated number of cases *109*
    prison infections 179, 185
Brehmer, Herman 20
bronchitis 16
Brontë sisters 10
Brunner, W. F. 77–8
Bryce, Peter 30
Buenos Aires, HIV infections 102
Bulgaria, wartime TB mortality 84, *85*
Burundi, HIV infections 117
Bushnell, George 29–30

Cahill, Kevin 126
Calmette, Albert 31, 208
Cambodia
    estimated number of cases *109*
    HIV infections 100, 102
    war 76, 91
Canada
    BCG vaccine 31
    immigrants 39, *45*
    TB as social disease 30
    wartime TB mortality 84, *85*
capitalism 5–6, 230
Carter, H. R. 82
Castiglioni, Arturo 15
catastrophes 144–5, 146
cerebrospinal meningitis 71, 90
CFP-10 protein 215
Chechnya, refugees 91
Chekhov, Anton 10
chemotherapy 104, 108, 213–14, 220
    DOTS strategy 200
    multi-drug-resistant TB 163, 165, 216
    short-course (SCC) 165, 168, 173, 174,
        175, 176
children
    effect of parental death on 107
    India 95, 107

New York City epidemic 129–30, 135
Trieste Declaration of Human Duties
234
tuberculin test 60
Chile, effective TB case management
strategies 104
China
DOTS strategy 108
drug costs 174
estimated number of cases *109*
female fatality rate 67
GNP 226
HIV infections 100
multi-drug-resistant TB 103, 239
notified cases 97
war 91
Chinese community, New York City
epidemic 126, 136
cholera
nineteenth-century epidemics 140, 237
pandemics 1
recent resurgence 8
scientific conception of 4–5
wartime epidemics 71
Chopin, Frédéric 10
chronic fatigue syndrome 1
cities *see* urban areas
civic citizenship 232
Clark, James 16
class 12, 18, 28
gender relationship 56
stigmatization 31
United States 29, 30
see also middle class; socioeconomic
status; working class
climate 19, 20
Cold War 4, 224
Colombia, leishmaniasis 58
communism
challenges to World Bank/IMF approach
4
end of 180, 182, 183
community
community-based care 161
destruction of New York communities
140, 143
qualitative approach to TB control 204,
205
support 154, 199
compliance
antibiotic revolution 32
gender issues 59, 66–8, 69
social context 198, 199
see also non-compliance
compulsory notification 16, 28

Congo, Democratic Republic of
Ebola virus 42
estimated number of cases *109*
conservatism 30, 230
contact tracing 36, 213
contagion 10, 17
institutional segregation 22
New York City epidemic 130
stigmatized groups 31
'contagionists' 22, 24, 27
Convention on the Rights of the Child
228
cost-effectiveness
assessment of 202
developed world 213
DOTS programmes 111, 164
lowering standards of care 175
multi-drug-resistant TB treatment
176
passive case-finding 197
Costa Rica, infant mortality 226
costs
development of new drugs 213
of doing nothing 175
DOTS programmes 201
drugs 103, 106, 123, 171–2, 173–4,
213–14, 240
HIV-positive patient care 119, 120
multi-drug-resistant TB 35, 107, 173–4,
186, 213–14, 222
for patients 106–7, 197, 198, 201
World Bank promotion of cost-recovery
224
Côte d'Ivoire, HIV infections 117, 120
cotrimoxazole 120
Crimean-Congo haemorrhagic fever 1
cryptosporidiosis 1, 8
Cuba
effective TB case management strategies
104
Havana case study 71, 76–82, 91
infant mortality 226
Cummins, Lyle 28–9
Czechoslovakia, wartime TB mortality *85*

Daniels, Marc 71, 92
Davies, Peter 181
De Carle Woodcock, H. 22
De Schweinitz, G. E. 31
de-development, United States 37, 145,
146
debt 224–5, 241
see also structural adjustment
programmes
debt relief 225, 241

decentralization
 Africa 118–19, 122, 123
 United Kingdom 161
deforestation 3
Demeulenare, Tine 185
Denmark
 gender and notification rates 63
 immigrant cases *45*
 notified cases 104
 wartime TB mortality 84, *85*
detection 65, 69, 96, 97
 active case finding 58, 61, 64, 121, 197
 DOTS strategy 108, 200
 passive case finding 58, 62, 64, 121,
   197, 200
 UK medical approach 159
detention of patients 159–60
developed countries
 decline in TB 103, 104
 diagnosis 216
 drug therapy effect on 181
 income differentials 226
 TB control 213
developing countries
 antiretroviral drugs 240
 BCG vaccination 209
 deaths from TB *95*, 227
 DOTS programmes 108, 200–1
 drug availability 239
 failure of national TB control
   programmes 104
 helminthic infections 212
 high prevalence of TB 33, 36
 HIV infections 105, 111, 115
 passive case finding 197
 poor diagnosis 107
 poverty 223, 224
 pressures to reduce social expenditure
   241
 resources 4, 145
 women 57
 see also resource-poor countries
development 4
DFID *see under* United Kingdom,
   Department for International
   Development
diagnosis 164, 214, 241
 delay before 65, 107, 121, 197–8
 developed countries 216
 developing countries 107
 DOTS strategy 108
 gender issues *59*, 63–6
 HIV/AIDS *114*, 115, 122
 immunodiagnosis 214–15
diarrhoea 115, 119, 120

Dickens, Charles 10
difference, geographies of 52–4
Dinkins, David N. 126
diphtheria 2, 36
directly observed therapy, short-course
   programme *see* DOTS programme
discrimination
 exclusion 223
 gender 56
 HIV/AIDS pandemic 40
 racial 51–2, 229, 234
 screening of immigrants to the UK 152
 social 107
 Trieste Declaration of Human Duties
   234
 see also stigmatization
DNA vaccines 219
doctors
 compliance 67
 medical ethics 231–2
 see also general practitioners; health care
   professionals
Dostoevsky, Fyodor 10, 179, 182
DOTS (directly observed therapy, short-
   course) programme 11, 96, 106,
   108–11, 170–1, 200–3
 case notifications 97
 compliance 66–7
 costs of 174
 former Soviet bloc 181, 184
 gender issues 66–7
 high-HIV-prevalent countries 118, 121,
   122
 homeless people 157
 multi-drug-resistant TB 164, 165, 168,
   176
 New York City epidemic 130, 132–4,
   143
 number of new cases *109*
 projected expansion rate *110*
 self-supervised treatment comparison
   201, 206
DOTS-Plus projects 176
drug resistance 4, 8, 12, 35, 53, 163–77
 decline due to DOTS strategy 108, 110
 immigrants 44
 increase in 33, *95*–6, 238, 239
 London 147, 157
 monitoring difficulties 200
 New York City epidemic 132, 133–4
 United States 145–6
 see also multi-drug-resistant TB
drug users 43, 140, 156, 161, 198–9
drugs 2, 12
 access to 239

adverse skin reactions 119
antiretroviral 114–15, 120, 122–3, 159, 240
  costs of 103, 106, 123, 171–2, 173–4, 213–14, 240
  first-line 157, 164, 167–8, 170, 173, 174
  Global Alliance for TB Drug Development 239
  Global TB Drug Facility 239
  HIV-positive patient care 119, 120
  New York City epidemic 131–2, 133
  reduction of need for hospitalization 181
  regular supply of 108, 200
  second-line 103, 167, 170, 173–4, 176
  side effects 132, 157, 159, 198
  Soviet prison infections 187
  third-line 171
  see also antibiotics; isoniazid; rifampicin; streptomycin
Dubos, Jean 7
Dubos, René 7
dysentery 71

Eastern Europe
  economic dislocation 106
  end of communism 182
  HIV attributable cases 101
  notified cases 98, 100, 105
  prison infections 191
Eastern Mediterranean
  developing economies 105
  notified cases 97, 98, 99
Ebola virus 1, 8, 42
economic burden on patients 197, 198
economic conditions 27, 33, 36–7, 38
  costs for patients 106–7
  former Soviet bloc 182, 183
  human rights abuses 230
  ignored by biomedical focus 160
  unemployment in United States 143, 144, 146
  see also poverty; structural factors
economic growth 225, 227
El Salvador, war 91
Emerson, Ralph Waldo 10
employment
  TB mortality during wartime 87–90
  transnational geographies of difference 53
Engels, Friedrich 3, 7
England
  gender and notification rates 63
  imprisonment rate 183

  wartime TB mortality 74, 74, 84–90, 85, 86, 88, 89
  see also Great Britain; United Kingdom
Enlightenment 19
enteric fever 76, 79, 80, 81, 91
environmental issues
  ethical challenges 233
  spread of infectious diseases 3, 7
  Trieste Declaration of Human Duties 234
epidemiological transition 1, 2, 23–8
epidemiology 195–6
  changing dynamics of 12
  development hampered by false dichotomies 5
  pre-bacteriological 19
  reductionism 42
equity
  ethical issues 232
  global health 176–7
  prisoners 189
  see also inequalities
ESAT-6 protein 215
essentialism 41–4, 50, 53, 55
Estonia, multi-drug-resistant TB 103, 239
ethical issues 231–6
  individual versus society 159
  prison reform 179, 191
Ethiopia, estimated number of cases 109
ethnic violence 226
ethnicity
  anti-essentialism 43–4
  gender relationship 56
  health disparities 49–52
  homelessness amongst minority ethnic groups 155
  see also race
eugenicism 42, 52
Europe
  anti-immigrant sentiments 46, 47
  decline of TB 2, 23–7, 31, 104
  immigrants 44, 46, 47
  imprisonment rate 183
  multi-drug-resistant TB 103, 164, 223
  nineteenth-century cities 15, 18, 38
  notified cases 97, 98, 98, 99
  sanatoria 20, 22
  social stigma 63
  wartime TB mortality 82–4, 92
  see also Eastern Europe
evolutionary theory
  disease organism evolution 4
  immunological transition 30
exclusion, social 11, 156, 157, 223

extra-pulmonary tuberculosis 63, 118, 122

family structure 57, 68
famine 3
Farmer, Paul 179, 198–9
feminism 55, 56
filariasis 57
Finland, wartime TB mortality 85
fire damage to New York City housing 137–40, *138*
First World War
  impact on TB 71, 73, 75, 82–90, *83*, *85*, *86*
  Russian deaths from TB 179
Ford, Henry 5
Fracastoro, Gerolamo 17
France
  BCG vaccine 31
  decline of TB 27
  high mortality rate for TB 24–6
  notified cases 104
  syphilis 41
  wartime TB mortality 84, *85*
Franco-Prussian War 71, 74
free trade 225
fungal meningitis 115

G8 Summit 240, 241
gastrointestinal abnormalities 146
Geiger, Jack 230
gender blindness 65
gender issues 12, 55–69
  deaths from TB 55
  diagnosis 63–6, 197
  inability of patients to complete treatment 198–9
  isolation 68–9
  progression from infection to disease 61–2
  symptoms recognition 62–3
  treatment compliance 66–8
  see also women
general practitioners (GPs) 153, 156
  see also doctors
genetics
  DNA vaccines 219
  immune responses 211, 216–17
  racial differences 50
  Trieste Declaration of Human Duties 234
  understanding of bacteria 195
Georgia
  conflicts 180
  prison infections 186, 187

rates for TB 180
'germ theories' 17–18, 30
Germany
  decline of TB 26, 27
  HIV/AIDS blamed on the United States 42
  Nazism and tuberculosis 31
  sanatoria 20
Ghana, delay in diagnosis 197
ghettoes 136, 139–40, 141
'gibbus' 16
GLA see Greater London Authority
glandular tuberculosis (scrofula) 11, 16, 22
Glasgow 27
Global Alliance for TB Drug Development 239
Global Alliance on Vaccines and Immunization 240
Global Health Fund 240, 241
Global TB Drug Facility 239
globalization 37, 225–6
GNP see gross national product
Goethe, Johann Wolfgang von 10
GPs see general practitioners
Great Britain
  decline of TB 24, 26, 27
  housing disparities 27
  workhouses 24
  see also England; United Kingdom; Wales
Greater London Authority (GLA) 161
Greece, mortality records lost during war 76
gross national product (GNP) 226–7, 227
Guérin, Camille 31, 208

haemoptysis 167, 168, 170, 171
Haiti
  HIV infections 41, 42, 102
  multi-drug-resistant TB 166–9, 175
hanta virus 1
Harvard Medical School 164, 185, 186
Harvard School of Public Health 1
Havana 71, 76–82, 91
health care centres 118
health care professionals 2–3, 12
  advocacy role 158
  DOTS programmes 66
  expertise of 197
  former Soviet bloc 181
  HIV/AIDS in Africa 118, 121, 122, 123
  London 154
  South Africa 229

World Medical Association proposed
  code 236
see also doctors
health education
  condom use 102
  high-HIV-prevalent countries 122
health sector reform 123
health-seeking behaviour
  rural/urban differences in Africa 197–8
  women 57, 59, 61, 62–3, 69
heart attacks 65
Heine, Heinrich 10
helminthic infections 212
Helsinki Declaration 233–5
hepatitis C 179
hereditarian views of TB 16, 17, 18, 19,
  28, 31
Hinsdale, Guy 31
Hippocrates 15, 19
HIV/AIDS 1, 8, 11, 223, 235, 238
  Africa 8, 35–6, 42, 95, 100–2, 101,
    105, 112–24, 239
  co-infection 36, 95, 100–2, 116, 147,
    158
  costs of TB 107
  developing countries 105, 111, 115
  discrimination 40
  DOTS programme 110
  drug resistance 133, 163
  effect on immune system 8, 9
  essentialist attitudes 43
  funding 37
  gastrointestinal abnormalities 146
  Haiti 41, 42
  impact of 12, 100–2
  London 147, 158–9
  multi-drug-resistant TB 163
  New York City 134–5
  population stress 144
  prison populations 179, 187, 188
  regionalization 141–3
  spread of 7, 239
  TB notification rates 105
  United States 33, 36, 104
  user charges 224
  vaccine development 217
  Vietnam 91
  Western fears about 240
Holm, John 33
homelessness
  anti-essentialism 43
  inability of patients to complete
    treatment 198–9
  London 147, 150, 155–8
  New York City 33, 132

racial minorities 51, 52
United Kingdom 147, 149, 150, 155–8
United States 33, 51, 132
Hong Kong, short-course chemotherapy
  165
hospitals
  facilities 27
  London 148, 160, 161
  military disruption 75
  overcrowding 118
housing 18, 36, 146
  apartheid South Africa 32
  decline of TB in the United Kingdom
    148
  design 27, 28
  French cities 26
  immigrants 48, 152
  improvements in 24, 27
  London 149–50, 152, 161
  New York City epidemic 135–7, 136
  transnational geographies of difference
    53
  see also overcrowding
Howard, John 178–9, 185, 191
Howard, Rhoda 230
Hulliger, Pierre 20–2
human immuno-deficiency virus see HIV/
  AIDS
human rights 225, 228–30, 233
  prisoners 179, 189, 190, 191
  Trieste Declaration of Human Duties
    233, 234
  World Medical Association proposed
    code 236
Human Rights Act (UK 1998) 154–5
Hungary, wartime TB mortality 85
hygiene 28, 29
  see also sanitation

ICHD see International Council of
  Human Duties
illegal immigrants 46–7, 154–5
illicit global economy 226
IMF see International Monetary Fund
immigrants 39–40, 44–6, 45
  epidemiological knowledge 48–9
  essentialism 41–2
  London 150–5
  New York City 126, 145
  politics of blame 46–7
  screening of 46, 133, 151–3
  see also asylum seekers; refugees
immunity
  differential 29, 30
  genes 211, 216–17

immunity (*cont.*)
  HIV infection 35–6, 116, 121
  innoculation experiments 31
  malnutrition effect on 210
  new adjuvants 218–19
  protein vaccines 218
  racial arguments 29
  stress effect on 144
  Type 1/Type 2 distinction 211–12,
    216, 219
immunization *see* vaccination
immunodiagnosis 214–15
India
  children 95, 107
  compliance 199
  costs of TB 107
  estimated number of cases 109
  female fatality rate 67
  female progression from infection to
    disease 61
  HIV infections 100
  infant mortality 226
  leprosy 58
  male prevalence of TB 60
  notified cases 97
  racial arguments 29
  stigma against women 107
  syphilis 41
  TB rate compared to London 8
Indonesia
  cholera pandemic 1
  estimated number of cases 109
Industrial Revolution 3
inequalities
  antibiotic revolution 32, 177
  apartheid South Africa 32
  food allocation 68
  gender 56, 57, 58, 69
  inability of patients to complete
    treatment 198–9
  London 147, 149–50
  'new' TB 8
  profit-driven health care 37
  racial arguments of difference 28
  racial discrimination 51
  World Medical Association proposed
    code 236
  see also equity; wealth disparities
infant mortality 143, 223, 226, 227
infectious diseases 1, 7
  claimed decline of 2, 3, 8
  most common cause of death 57
  poverty relationship 7, 36, 57
  qualitative approach 203
  war effect on 70–1, 83, 91

inflammation 207, 212, 216, 218
influenza 71
innoculation 31
Institute of Tropical Medicine 186
institutionalization
  anti-essentialism 43
  immigrants 48
  nineteenth-century 20
  racial disparities 51
  see also sanatoria; segregation
interdisciplinary approaches to TB control
  195–206
International Committee of the Red Cross
  184, 188
International Council of Human Duties
  (ICHD) 233
International Covenant on Civil and
  Political Rights 191
International Covenant on Social,
  Economic and Cultural Rights 228
International Monetary Fund (IMF) 4
International Union against Tuberculosis
  and Lung Diseases (IUATLD) 33,
  103, 108, 163–4, 200, 223
Iran, multi-drug-resistant TB 239
Ireland
  decline of TB 27
  wartime TB mortality 84, 85
isoniazid 18, 32, 119, 121–2, 157
  multi-drug-resistant TB 35, 163, 166–7,
    171, 173, 175, 239
  short-course chemotherapy 165
Israel, immigrant cases 45
Italy
  eighteenth-century 17
  great plague 3
  immigrants 39, 45
  syphilis 41
  wartime TB mortality 84, 85
IUATLD *see* International Union against
  Tuberculosis and Lung Diseases

Japan
  HIV/AIDS blamed on the United States
    42
  notified cases 104
  syphilis 41
  tuberculin test 60
Jews 31, 42
Jochem, Klaus 201
Joint United Nations Programme on HIV/
  AIDS (UNAIDS) 112, 187, 238
Jordan, effective TB case management
  strategies 104

justice 232, *236*
    see also social justice

Kalinin, Yuri Ivanovitch 182
Kant, Immanuel 10
Kaposi's sarcoma 115
Kazakhstan
    prisons 182, 184, 186, 190
    rates for TB 180
Keats, John 10, 20
Kenya, estimated number of cases *109*
Kim, Jim Yong 179
King, Nicholas B. 39–54
Kluge, Hans 184
Koch phenomenon 207
Koch, Robert 17, 26–7, 31, 207–8, 214, 218, 222
Korea, Republic of
    effective TB case management strategies 104
    male prevalence of TB 60
Kuwait, tuberculin test 60
Kyrgystan, rates for TB 180

Lassa fever 1
latent infections 48
Latin America
    HIV infections 8, 100, *101*
    multi-drug-resistant TB 103, 223
    notified cases 98–100
    see also South America
Latinos, New York City epidemic 129, 135, 136
Latvia
    multi-drug-resistant TB 103, 239
    prison infections 188
    rates for TB 180
Lawrence, D. H. 10
Lebanon, war 76, 91
Legionnaire's disease 1, 3
Leicester outbreak 8
leishmaniasis 58
leprosy 37, 57, 216, 217
life expectancy
    HIV infection in Africa 115
    homeless people 156
    poverty 223, 226, *227*
liver failure 132, 133
London 12, 15, 147–62
    ad hoc committee on 1998 epidemic 108
    cholera epidemic 140
    Engels' description of 7
    higher TB incidence than India 8

'lupus' 16
Lyme disease 1

McKeown thesis 18, 23–7
McKeown, Thomas 23–4
macrophages 9
'magic bullet' approaches to disease control 4, 6, 32–3, 240
malaria 1, 2, 7, 240
    funding for control 37
    recent resurgence 8
    Thailand 58
Malawi
    HIV infections 102, 117
    notified cases *105*, *117*
Mallon, Mary 41–2
malnutrition 11, 106, 190
    immune system 210–11
    poverty 223, 224
    wartime 75
    see also nutrition
Manchester 3
mandatory screening 36
Mansfield, Katherine 10
marginalized groups 28, 30, 238
    compliance 199
    stigmatization 40, 43, 51, 63
    transnational factors for high incidence of disease 49
    United Kingdom 148–9, *159*
    see also social exclusion
market economy 49, 180, 184
Marr, John 126
marriage 57, 58, 63, 68
mass screening 16
MDR-TB *see* multi-drug-resistant TB
Médecins Sans Frontières (MSF) 184, 185, 187, 238–9
medical ethics 231–2
Medical Research Council 148
medical schools 5
meningitis
    cerebrospinal 71, 90
    fungal 115
    tubercular 11
mental illness 149, 161, 191
Merlin 186
Mexico, HIV infections 102
mice 3
middle class
    New York City epidemic 127, 135, 136, 140, 143, *145*
    US attitudes 29
middle-income countries 103–4

migration
  globalization 226
  London 147
  New York City epidemic 136, 141, 142, 143, 144
  reactivation of dormant infection 9, 48
  social/economic changes 36
  Trieste Declaration of Human Duties 234
  see also immigrants
Mitchell, Allan 26
modernism 20
Mongolia, prison infections 186
monitoring
  DOTS strategy 108, 200
  health sector reform 123
moral arguments 30
morality 28
mortality
  anti-essentialism 43, 44
  decline due to antibiotics 32
  development of treatments 31
  DOTS strategy 108
  Great Britain 27
  Havana 78–81, 79, 80, 82
  HIV-related 115, 119–20, 122–3, 158
  immigrants 40
  McKeown thesis 24, 26
  prison infections 185, 186
  racial differences 28, 29, 41, 49–50
  Russia 106, 179, 185
  social deprivation in the United States 197
  wartime 72–4, 78–81, 79–80, 82–90, 83, 85–6, 88–9, 91
  women 55, 58, 67–8
Moynihan, Daniel Patrick 139
Mozambique, GNP 226
MSF see Médecins Sans Frontières
multi-drug-resistant TB (MDR-TB) 35, 52, 102–3, 163–77, 223
  costs of 35, 107, 173–4, 186, 213–14, 222
  Haiti 166–9, 175
  HIV co-infection 36
  increase in 52, 96, 216, 235, 239
  London 157
  New York City epidemic 8, 35, 132, 133–4
  Peru 169–73, 174, 175
  Russian prisons 185, 186–7, 188
  social-structural factors 199
  United States 122, 146, 163, 223
  Vietnam War 91

Western fears about 240
  see also drug resistance
multinational corporations 225
Munk, Martin E. 207–21
Myanmar
  estimated number of cases 109
  HIV infections 100
mycobacteria 65, 68, 208, 212, 214–15, 217–18, 219

Namibia
  HIV infections 114
  notified cases 105
National Health Service (NHS) 153, 161
nationality 44, 50
native Americans 3
nativism 41, 42, 43, 46
neocolonialism 145
neoliberalism 225
Nepal, active/passive case finding 64
Netherlands
  immigrants 44, 45
  notified cases 104
  wartime TB mortality 84, 85
New York City 12, 33, 125–46, 237
  decline in drug resistance 108
  detention of patients 159–60
  DOTS programme 108, 202
  drug costs 174
  multi-drug-resistant TB 8, 35, 132, 133–4
  nineteenth-century public health policies 27–8
  notifications 148
  poorest areas 199
New York City-Rand Institute 138, 139, 140
  see also Rand Corporation
New Zealand
  immigrant cases 45
  notified cases 104
NGOs see non-governmental organizations
NHS see National Health Service
Nicaragua
  GNP 226–7
  war 76
Nigeria
  estimated number of cases 109
  GNP 226
non-compliance 32, 159, 168
'non-economic' poverty 223, 231
non-governmental organizations (NGOs) 111, 184

North America
  decline of TB 2, 23, 24, 31
  European conquest of 3
  multi-drug-resistant TB 164
  nineteenth-century cities 15, 18, 38
  sanatoria 20, 22
  see also Canada; United States
Norway
  decline of TB 27
  gender and notification rates 63
  inadequate hospital provision 27
notification 96–100, *98, 99,* 102
  African countries with high rates of HIV
    infection *105*
  compulsory 16, 28
  developed countries 104
  Eastern Europe trends *100*
  gender relationship 63–4, 66
  London 147, *148,* 149
  Malawi *117*
  New York *148*
  United States 36
  Zambia *117*
Novalis (Friedrich von Hardenburg) 20
Nuffield Institute for International Health
    201
nutrition
  anti-essentialism 43
  decline of TB in the United Kingdom
    148
  height relationship *56*
  immigrants 48
  primary prevention measures 146
  prison infections 185
  TB relationship 67–8
  see also malnutrition
'nutritionists' 24, 27

Open Society Institute 185, 186
origin narratives 41, 42
Orwell, George 10
overcrowding 36, 106, 146, 190
  anti-essentialism 43
  during wartime 70, 74–5, 77, 78
  hospitals 118
  immigrants 48
  London 150, 157
  New York City epidemic 135–7, *136*
  Soviet prisons 35, 183, 185, 189
  see also housing

Pakistan
  costs of treatment 201
  estimated number of cases *109*
  self-supervised treatment 201

  women 65
pan-susceptible tuberculosis 174
Paris 15, 26
passive case finding 58, 62, 64, 121, 197,
    200
Pasteur, Louis 207–8
PCR *see* polymerase chain reaction
Penal Reform International 184, 190
Peru
  DOTS strategy 108
  DOTS-Plus programmes 176
  estimated number of cases *109*
  multi-drug-resistant TB 169–73, 174,
    175, 176
  short-course chemotherapy 165
pesticide analogy 145
pharmaceutical industry 6, 239, 240
Philippines, estimated number of cases
    109
plague
  Black Death 3
  wartime epidemics 71
plant diseases 3–4
pneumonia 115
Poland, mortality records lost during war
    75
policy
  global health equity 176–7
  London public health 161
  treatment of prisoners 188, 190
  see also social policy
polio 2
political economy 49
political issues 11, 38, 238
  political commitment to TB control
    108, 196, 200
  poor leadership 241
  reductionism 43
  South Africa's transformation 235
polymerase chain reaction (PCR) testing
    214
population reconcentrations 71, 77
population stress 144
Portugal, syphilis 41
post-structuralism 55
'Pott's disease' 16
poverty 4, 11, 95, 96, 106, 241
  African-Americans 29–30
  anti-essentialism 43
  apartheid South Africa 32
  former Soviet bloc 180, 182
  gender relationship 57
  global 33–8, 222–36
  inability of patients to complete
    treatment 198–9

poverty (*cont.*)
  infectious disease relationship 7, 36, 57
  international initiatives 238–9
  London 149, 154
  multi-drug-resistant TB 177
  New York City epidemic 126, 134, 141
  nineteenth-century conceptions of TB
    22
  'non-economic' 223, 231
  obscured by biomedical approach 18
  racial disparities 51
  refugees 154
  shifting patterns of 8
  strategies for TB control 195
  TB as cause of 220
  transnational geographies of difference
    53
  United States 33, 104
  see also social deprivation
power relations 55, 56
PPD *see* Purified Protein Derivative
pregnancy 61–2
prevention
  focus on pulmonary TB 63
  HIV/AIDS 121–2, 159
  interdisciplinary approach 206
  New York City epidemic 134
  primary 134, 145, 146
  secondary 145
prisons
  former Soviet bloc 35, 179, 181–91,
    223
  Howard arguments for improvement
    178–9
  New York City 8
  overcrowding 35, 183, 185, 189
profit-driven health care 37
prostitution 154
proteins 214–15, 217, 218
Public Health Act (UK) 159
public health campaigns 37
public health care
  reduction in expenditure 35, 36, 180,
    224
  structural adjustment impact on 5,
    105–6, 224, 241
public health movement 24, 28
Puerto Rico
  female progression from infection to
    disease 61
  prison infections 179
pulmonary tuberculosis 10, 15
  BCG vaccination 209
  climate discourse 19
  diagnosis 122, 164

DOTS treatment 110
First World War 73, 87–90
gender issues 63, 65
global incidence of 97
HIV-positive patients 120
smear positive/smear negative distinction
  118
transmission 197
Purified Protein Derivative (PPD) 214

qualitative approach 203–5, 206
quarantine 36
  see also segregation

race 12, 18, 28–31
  essentialism 41, 42, 43–4
  health disparities 40, 49–52
  New York neighbourhoods of colour
    126, 136, 139–40, 143
  social construction of 50
  see also apartheid; ethnicity; immigrants;
    racism
racial discrimination 51–2, 229, 234
racism
  essentialism 53
  health disparities 51
  immigrants 46
  inability of patients to complete
    treatment 198–9
  London 149
  medical research 52
  reductionism 43
  United States 230
Rand Corporation 144
  see also New York City-Rand Institute
reactivation of dormant infection
  BCG efficacy studies 209
  DNA vaccines 219
  HIV as risk factor 116
  migration 9, 48
  New York City epidemic 126, 143
recombinant vaccinia viruses 217–18
reconcentrations of populations 71, 77
reductionism 42–3, 57
refugees 91, 152, 153–4, 155, 214, 229
  see also asylum seekers; immigrants
Rehberg, Dennis 43
reinfection 209
reporting systems 96–7, 108
reproductive health 57, 61–2
research
  racial biases 52
  vaccinations 195, 216, 220–1
resource-poor countries 118, 164, 165,
  168

respiratory tract infections 71
rifampicin 120, 157, 200
  multi-drug-resistant TB 35, 163, 166–7, 171, 173, 239
  short-course chemotherapy 165
Robbins, Jessica 30
rodent-borne diseases 3
Romania, rates for TB 180
Romanticism 18, 19–20, 22
Rousseau, Jean-Jacques 10
Royal Netherlands TB Association 184, 190
Rubin, Gayle 55
rural areas
  health-seeking behaviour 198
  Trieste Declaration of Human Duties 234
Ruskin, John 10
Russia
  HIV/AIDS 187
  market economy transition 49
  multi-drug-resistant TB 35, 174, 175, 239
  prison infections 179, 185–6, 187, 188, 190, 223
  resurgence of TB 174
  short-course chemotherapy 165, 174
  syphilis 41
  Tsarist 179, 182
  see also Soviet Union, former
Russian Federation
  drug-resistant TB 103
  estimated number of cases 109
  mortality rate 106
  notified cases 105
  prisons 179, 183, 187
  rates for TB 180
  see also Soviet Union, former
Russo-Japanese War 71
Rwanda, prison infections 185

sanatoria 18, 20–2, 21, 104
  closing of 148
  drug therapy effect on 181
  former Soviet bloc 180
  military disruption 75
sanitation
  Havana during insurrection 77
  poverty 106, 223, 224, 227
  social/economic changes 36
  urban areas 28
  see also hygiene
SCC see short-course chemotherapy
Schengen Agreement 39
schistosomiasis 57

Schulze, Ernst 20
science 4–5, 15, 207–21
screening
  former Soviet bloc 180
  immigrants 46, 133, 151–3
  immunodiagnosis 214
  mandatory 36
  mass 16
  multi-drug-resistant TB 216
  New York City epidemic 143
scrofula (glandular tuberculosis) 11, 16, 22
Second World War 71, 75–6, 82–4, 83, 85, 86, 87, 92
secondary cases 48–9
segregation 22, 24, 27, 39
  see also institutionalization; quarantine
self-supervised treatment 66, 201, 206
service delivery 123, 160, 161, 196
sex-gender distinction 55
sexually transmitted infections 71
shared care 158–9
short-course chemotherapy (SCC) 165, 168, 173, 174, 175, 176
  see also DOTS programme
Siberia
  DOTS-Plus projects 176
  prisons 182, 184
  syphilis 41
  TB institutions 181
Sierra Leone, GNP 226
skin test 60, 207, 214
sleeping sickness 36
smallpox
  eradication of 2, 8
  European conquests 3
  wartime epidemics 71, 76, 79, 80, 81, 82, 91
Smith, I. 55
Snider, Gordon L. 7
social class see class
social conditions 30, 33, 36–8, 53
  African-Americans 29
  anti-essentialism 43–4
  human rights abuses 230
  ignored by biomedical focus 160
  McKeown thesis 23–7
  prisons 190
  UK homelessness 155
  see also structural factors
social contacts 60
social deprivation
  delay in diagnosis 197
  London 147, 149–50, 152
  United States 197

social exclusion 11, 156, 157, 223
  see also marginalized groups
social factors
  influence on biology 56
  interdisciplinary approaches to TB
    control 195–206
social isolation of women 68–9
social justice 44, 160, 195
  health relationship 37
  transnational geographies of difference
    53
social networks 53, 145
social policy
  attitudes towards BCG vaccine 32
  essentialist understandings of difference
    53
  health disparities 40, 43
social sciences 195, 196, 205
social services
  illegal immigrants 47
  racial discrimination 52
  support from 202, 205
social vulnerability 199
socioeconomic status 51
  see also class
Socios En Salud 172, 173
soil exposure 212
Somalia, refugees 91
Sontag, Susan 19
South Africa
  AIDS summit 240
  apartheid 32, 229, 235
  decentralized TB treatment 119
  DOTS-Plus projects 176
  estimated number of cases *109*
  healthcare professionals 229
  multi-drug-resistant TB 176
  new case incidence 129
  political transformation 235
  self-supervised treatment 66, 201
South America
  cholera pandemic 1
  European conquest of 3
  see also Latin America
South Asia
  European colonial explanations for
    disease 42
  HIV/AIDS 8, 239
  immigrants from 49
  see also Southeast Asia
South Korea
  effective TB case management strategies
    104
  male prevalence of TB 60
Southeast Asia

HIV infections 100, *101*, 102
  male/female prevalence ratios 64
  malnutrition 210
  notified cases 97, *98*, 99
  see also South Asia
Soviet Union, former 178–91
  economic dislocation 106
  HIV/AIDS blamed on the United States
    42
  multi-drug-resistant TB 35, 214
  poverty 37
  prisons 35, 179, 181–91
  resurgence of TB 174
  transition to market economy 49, 180,
    184
  see also Russia; Russian Federation
Spain
  BCG vaccine 31
  wartime TB mortality 84, *85*
spatial diffusion 127, 129, 130, 141, 143
sputum testing 65–6, 168, 171, 200, 214
Sri Lanka
  effective TB case management strategies
    104
  GNP 227
staff *see* health care professionals
state intervention 20, 31
statistics 40, 75–6
Stevenson, Robert Louis 10
stigmatization 31, 40, 43, 106, 107
  contact with health care services 66
  essentialism 53
  ethnic minorities 51
  HIV/AIDS 36, 158
  immigrants 47
  nineteenth-century stigma of poverty 22
  as obstacle to treatment 201–2
  women 57–8, 62–3, 68, 107
  see also social exclusion
Stop TB initiative 96, 239
streptomycin 18, 32, 119
  multi-drug-resistant TB 35, 163, 166,
    168
  short-course chemotherapy 165
stress
  effect on immune system 9, 144
  prison infections 185
  reactivation of latent infections 48
  wartime 75
structural adjustment programmes 5, 105,
    224, 241
  see also debt
structural factors 11, 30
  attention shifted from 18, 240
  gender 56

nineteenth-century public health policies 27, 28
  transmission of TB 49
  treatment failures 199
  see also economic conditions; social conditions
Sumartojo, Esther 198
support
  community 154, 199
  family 199
  social services 202, 205
  structures of 204
  women 68
susceptible individuals 29, 30, 143, 144, 145
Sweden
  immigrant cases *45*
  notified cases 104
Switzerland
  immigrant cases *45*
  wartime TB mortality *85*
symptom recognition *59* 62–3, 69
syphilis 41, 64
systemic lupus erythomatosus 64

Tahiti, syphilis 41
Tajikistan, conflicts 180
Tanzania
  estimated number of cases *109*
  HIV infections 102
  notified cases *105*
targeted interventions 53
TB *see* tuberculosis
technology
  globalization 225
  impact on infectious diseases 2
terrorism, biological 7
testing
  HIV 158
  improvement in laboratory tests 2
  polymerase chain reaction (PCR) 214
  skin test 60, 207, 214
  sputum testing 65–6, 168, 171, 200, 214
tetanus 2
Thailand
  delay before diagnosis 107
  estimated number of cases *109*
  HIV infections 100, 102
  immigrants 39–40
  malaria clinics 58
  self-supervised treatment 201
thiacetazone 119
Third World debt 224–5, 241
threshold of epidemics 130, 144
tick-borne diseases 3

Tolstoy, Leo 182
Torchia, Marion 30
toxic shock syndrome 1
trade 4, 5, 241
transmission
  conventional TB control 197
  DOTS strategy 121, 200
  epidemiology 196
  immigrants blamed for 48, 49
  latent infections 48
  London 157
  New York City 129–30
  wartime 70, 74–5
  see also spatial diffusion
transnational social networks 53
travel
  intensification of 42
  recommended as cure 16–17, 19
treatment 222, 237–8
  completion of 196, 198, 203
  decentralization of 118–19
  DOTS strategy 108, 200
  failure to complete 132, 157, 173
  gender analysis *59*, 66–8
  HIV/AIDS *114*
  homeless people 132, 157
  interdisciplinary approach 196, 206
  long duration of 106, 157, 198
  medical approach 159, 160–1, 202, 205
  multi-drug-resistant TB 164–5, 166–73
  New York City epidemic 131–4, 143
  prisoners 184, 186, 188, 189
  self-supervised 66, 201, 206
  see also chemotherapy; compliance; drugs
Trieste Declaration of Human Duties 233, *234*
Trudeau, Edward Livingston 31
Tsarist Russia 179, 182
TST *see* tuberculin skin test
tubercular meningitis 11
'tubercularization' thesis 28–9
tuberculin 60, 207, 214
tuberculin skin test (TST) 60, 207
Tuberculosis Research Unit, University of Liverpool 181
tuberculosis (TB)
  annual cases 8
  biological description of 9–11
  biomedical approach 18, 159, 160, 202, 206, 238
  decline of 2, 18, 23–7, *23*, 31, 103, 104
  economic considerations 7
  European conquests 3
  former Soviet bloc 178–91

tuberculosis (*cont.*)
  gender perspective 55–69
  geographies of difference 52–4
  global incidence of *34*
  global poverty 222–36
  historical context 15–38
  immigrants 39–42, 44–9, 126, 133,
    145, 150–5
  interdisciplinary approaches to control
    195–206
  as leading cause of death 1
  London case study 147–62
  New York City case study 125–46
  political responsibility for action 241
  present global burden of 95–111
  in prisons 8, 35, 178–9, 181–91, 223
  racial disparities 40, 49–52
  resurgence 8, 18
  role of science in tuberculosis control
    207–21
  Sub-Saharan Africa 112–24
  symptoms 10–11, *59*, 62–3, 65
  war 70–92
  see also multi-drug-resistant TB;
    pulmonary tuberculosis
Turkmenistan, rates for TB 180
Tuskeegee Syphilis Study 52
typhoid
  TB confusion with 16
  wartime epidemics 71
Typhoid Mary 41–2
typhus 71

UDHR *see* Universal Declaration of
  Human Rights
Uganda
  costs of TB 106
  estimated number of cases *109*
  HIV/AIDS infections 102, 115, 117,
    123
Ukraine, prison infections 188
UN *see* United Nations
UNAIDS *see* Joint United Nations
  Programme on HIV/AIDS
unemployment
  developing countries 36
  former Soviet bloc 180
  immigrants 152
  United Kingdom 155
  United States 143, 144, 146
United Kingdom
  Department for International
    Development (DFID) 161–2
  ethnic groups 50
  immigrants 49, 150–5

notified cases 104
poverty 149
see also England; Great Britain; London;
  Wales United Nations Relief and
  Rehabilitation Administration
  (UNRRA) 75–6 United Nations (UN)
  Committee on Economic, Social, and
    Cultural Rights 228
  proposed 'Universal Declaration of
    Human Duties' 233
United States
  aid budget cuts 224
  anti-immigrant sentiments 46–7
  class issues 29, 30
  de-development 37, 145, 146
  decline in TB 104
  Environmental Protection Agency 132
  failure to pay World Health
    Organization 228
  HIV infection 158
  immigrants 41–2, 44, *45*, 46–7, 48–9,
    145
  imprisonment rate 183, 191
  increase of TB in urban areas 33
  Legionnaire's disease 1
  Lyme disease 1
  minority groups 49–50, 51
  multi-drug-resistant TB 122, 146, 163,
    223
  non-ratification of human rights treaties
    228
  notifiable diseases 146
  poverty 230
  punitive public health strategies 36
  racial arguments 29–30, 42
  racism 230
  rejection of BCG vaccine 31
  social deprivation 197
  wartime TB mortality 84, *85*
  wealth 226
  see also New York City
'Universal Declaration of Human Duties'
  proposal 233
Universal Declaration of Human Rights
  (UDHR) 228–9
UNRRA *see* United Nations Relief and
  Rehabilitation Administration
urban areas 18–19, 22, 28
  health-seeking behaviour 198
  population reconcentrations during
    wartime 77
  racial disparities 51
  transnational social networks 53
  Trieste Declaration of Human Duties
    234

United States 33
  see also London; New York City
US Maritime Hospital Service (USMHS)
  76, 77–8, 82

vaccination 2, 12, 207–21, 237, 239–40
  development of new vaccines 206
  DNA vaccines 219
  genetic engineering 216–18, 219
  live/whole cell 216–18
  new adjuvants 218–19
  protein vaccines 214–15, 218
  research on 195, 216, 220–1
  see also BCG vaccination
Venezuela haemorrhagic fever 1
ventilation
  hostels 157
  prisons 185, 189
Vietnam
  compliance of women 67
  diagnosis of women 65
  estimated number of cases *109*
  female symptom recognition 62
  HIV infections 100
  scaling down of public health care 36
  stigma attached to women 63, 68
  war 76, 90–1
Villemin, Jean-Antoine 17
violent crime 140, 141–3, 144
Virchov, Rudolf 17
viruses
  Ebola 1, 8, 42
  recombinant vaccinia 217–18
Volmink, J. 202
vulnerability 199

Waksman, Selman 32
Wales
  gender and notification rates 63
  imprisonment rate 183
  wartime TB mortality 74, *74*, 84–90,
    85, 86, 88, 89
  see also Great Britain; United Kingdom
Walley, John 201
war 12, 70–92
  former Soviet bloc 180
  inability of patients to complete
    treatment 199
  mass movements of people 36
  reactivation of dormant infection 9
  Trieste Declaration of Human Duties
    234
  US diversion of resources for 144
water
  access to safe 223, 224, *227*

untreated 212
wealth disparities
  global 223–4, 226
  London 149–50
  see also inequalities
West African TB Research Initiative 205
Western Pacific region
  HIV attributable cases *101*
  male/female prevalence ratios 64
  notified cases 97, *98, 99*
whooping cough 2
Wilson, Leonard 24
women 55–69, 95
  deaths from TB 55
  diagnosis 63–6
  First World War TB incidence 73, 87,
    88, 89
  isolation 68–9
  progression from infection to disease
    61–2
  stigma against 107
  symptoms recognition 62–3
  treatment compliance 66–8
  Trieste Declaration of Human Duties
    234
  see also gender issues
workhouses 24
working class
  nineteenth-century sanatoria 20
  United States 30
  urban 28
working conditions 18–19, 26, 28
  apartheid South Africa 32
  immigrants 48
  women during First World war 87
World Bank 4, 5
  DOTS strategy 108, 164
  Global Alliance on Vaccines and
    Immunization 240
  poverty study 180
  structural adjustment programmes 224
World Health Organization (WHO) 12
  Advocacy Forum for Massive Effort
    Against Diseases of Poverty 238
  cases reported to 97
  classical public health paradigms 196
  DFID funding 162
  diagnosis 65
  DOTS programme 11, 96, 108–111,
    132, 200–3
    compliance 66–7
    costs of 174
    former Soviet bloc 181
    gender issues 66–7
    high-HIV-prevalent countries 122

World Health Organization (*cont.*)
  number of new cases *109*
  projected expansion rate *110*
  DOTS-Plus projects 176
  former Soviet bloc rates of TB 180
  Global Alliance on Vaccines and
    Immunization 240
  global ethics 232
  health definition 37
  HIV infection 102, 122
  multi-drug-resistant TB 163–4, 223
  prison infections 185, 187, 188
  projected number of deaths averted *111*
  short-course chemotherapy 165
  Stop TB initiative 96, 239
  TB declared as global emergency 40,
    96, 237, 241
  TB prevalence surveys 64
  US failure to pay 228
World Medical Association 235, *236*

xenophobia 152, 153

yellow fever, wartime epidemics 71, 76,
    79, *80*, 81, 82, 91
Youmans, Guy P. 134
Yugoslavia, former, war 76, 91

Zaire
  Ebola virus 42
  see also Congo, Democratic Republic of
Zambia
  economic burden on patients 198
  health sector reform 123
  HIV infections 102, 117, 224
  notified cases *105*, 117
Zimbabwe
  estimated number of cases *109*
  GNP 227
  HIV infections 102, 114
  notified cases 105, *105*